# MEDICAL BREAKTHROUGHS 2004

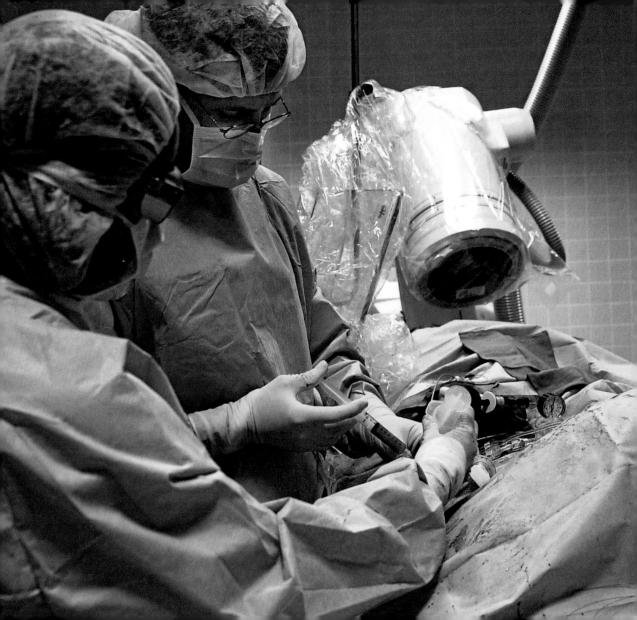

# Reader's Digest
## MEDICAL BREAKTHROUGHS
## 2004

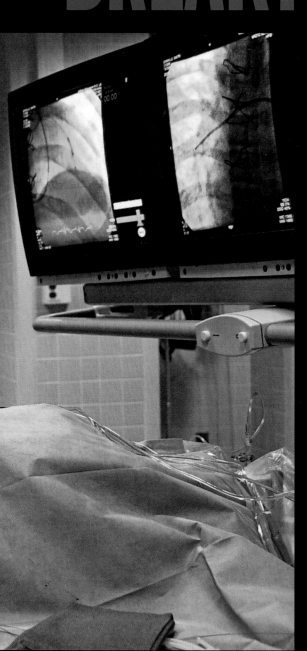

The year's most
important health
developments

Published by
The Reader's Digest Association Limited
London • New York • Sydney • Montreal

## MEDICAL BREAKTHROUGHS 2004

### READER'S DIGEST PROJECT STAFF

**Consultant**
Vince Forte

**Project editor**
Rachel Warren Chadd

**Art editor**
Kate Harris

**Assistant editors**
Caroline Boucher
Celia Coyne
Henrietta Heald
Jill Steed

**Proofreader**
Ken Vickery

**Indexer**
Marie Lorimer

### READER'S DIGEST GENERAL BOOKS

**Editorial director**
Cortina Butler

**Art director**
Nick Clark

**Executive editor**
Julian Browne

**Managing editor**
Alastair Holmes

**Picture resource manager**
Martin Smith

**Pre-press account manager**
Penelope Grose

**Origination**
Colour Systems Limited, London
**Printing and binding**
Mateu Cromo, Spain

**Medical Breakthroughs 2004** was originated by the editorial team of The Reader's Digest Association, Inc., USA

This edition was adapted and published by The Reader's Digest Association Limited, London

First edition copyright © 2004
The Reader's Digest Association Limited,
11 Westferry Circus, Canary Wharf,
London E14 4HE

We are committed to both the quality of our products and the service we provide to our customers. We value your comments, so please feel free to contact us on **08705 113366** or via our web site at: **www.readersdigest.co.uk**
If you have any comments or suggestions about the content of our books, email us at: gbeditorial@readersdigest.co.uk

Any references in this book to any products or services do not constitute or imply an endorsement or recommendation.

Concept code  IE 0088A/IC
Book code  440-104-01
ISBN  0 276 42863 3
Oracle code  250007951H.00.24

# READER'S DIGEST USA

## PROJECT STAFF

**Senior Editor**
Marianne Wait

**Senior Design Director**
Elizabeth Tunnicliffe

**Production**
Katherine S. Frattarola

**Production Technology Manager**
Douglas A. Croll

**Manufacturing Manager**
John L. Cassidy

**Special thanks to**
Chandni Jhunjhunwala and
Jennifer Samuels

## CONTRIBUTORS

**Editor**
Jeff Bredenberg

**Writers**
Alisa Bauman, Susan Freinkel,
Kelly Garrett, Debra Gordon,
Eric Metcalf, Rob Waters

**Designers**
Susan Bacchetti
Andrew Ploski

**Copy Editor**
Jane Sherman

**Indexer**
Ann Cassar

**Picture Research**
Carousel Research, Inc.
Laurie Platt Winfrey, Van Bucher,
Mary Teresa Giancoli,
Cristian Pena, Fay Torres-yap

## MEDICAL ADVISORS

**Charles Atkins, M.D.**
Medical Director, Western
Connecticut Mental Health Network;
Assistant Professor, Yale University
School of Medicine, New Haven,
Connecticut

**Jacob Bitran, M.D.**
Professor of Medicine, Finch
University of Health Sciences/The
Chicago Medical School; Section
Chief, Hematology/Oncology, Lutheran
General Hospital, ParkRidge, Illinois

**Lawrence C. Brody, Ph.D.**
Senior Investigator, Head, Molecular
Pathogenesis Section, National
Human Genome Research Institute,
National Institutes of Health,
Bethesda, Maryland (contributions
rendered as an individual, not in
the name of the U.S. government)

**Nicholas A. DiNubile, M.D.**
Orthopaedic Consultant,
Philadelphia 76ers Basketball and
Pennsylvania Ballet; Clinical Assistant
Professor, Department of Orthopaedic
Surgery, Hospital of the University of
Pennsylvania, Philadelphia

**Marygrace Elson, M.D.**
Associate Clinical Professor
of Obstetrics and Gynecology,
University of Iowa Hospital and
Clinics, Iowa City

**Bradley W. Fenton, M.D.**
General Internist, Clinical Associate
Professor, Thomas Jefferson
University Hospital, Philadelphia

**Donald R. Henderson, M.D.**
Assistant Clinical Professor of
Medicine and Gastroenterology, UCLA
School of Medicine, Los Angeles

**Joel A. Kahn, M.D.**
President, WorldCare Global Health
Plan Ltd., Boston

**Barry Make, M.D.**
Director, Emphysema Center,
National Jewish Medical and
Research Center, Denver; Professor
of Medicine, University of Colorado
School of Medicine, Denver

**Randolph P. Martin, M.D.**
Director, Emory Non-Invasive Lab,
Emory University Hospital, Atlanta,
Georgia; President of the American
Society of Echocardiography
(for 2003)

**Antoni Ribas, M.D.**
Assistant Professor of Medicine
and Surgery, Assistant Director for
Clinical Programs, UCLA Human Gene
Medicine Program, Los Angeles

**Jeffrey Schlom, Ph.D.**
Chief, Laboratory of Tumor
Immunology and Biology, Center
for Cancer Research, National
Cancer Institute, National Institutes
of Health, Bethesda, Maryland

# Contents

# PART 2 GENERAL HEALTH

# PART 3　YOUR BODY HEAD TO TOE

# About this book

Just a few decades ago, most people looked at their health as something of a game of chance. If you came down with a chronic disease, that was just the way it was – what could you do? The sort of people who exercised regularly, who were careful about what they ate and who craved medical information were just plain weird. Remember the term 'health nut'?

All of that has changed. The interest in medical information has mushroomed as health-conscious consumers take on more and more responsibility for managing their health. That's why we bring you this unique book. Medical Breakthroughs 2004 is your must-read summary of the year's most important and most interesting medical advancements.

In Part 1, The Year's Top Stories, you will find in-depth reports on the most important medical issues to touch our lives in the past year. Read about new revelations concerning the role of inflammation in heart disease (and a new way to test for risk), the lightning-quick response to the international outbreak of SARS, powerful cancer vaccines in the works and much more.

Part 2 is devoted to general health updates that affect you, your family and friends. Discover the device that appears to stop Alzheimer's disease in its tracks, the new alternative to Ritalin (it's not a stimulant), and surprising findings about high-protein diets.

Turn to Part 3 for news about specific medical concerns. Find out about the robotic heart surgery that's done through pencil-sized holes, the quicker and easier vasectomy (no snip – just a clip), and the teenager who invented a glove that translates sign language into written words.

The science behind such innovations may be mind-boggling, but we've taken great pains to give you the details in clear language. To ensure accuracy, we had every word reviewed by medical experts.

You may find this book valuable in making decisions about your own medical care or that of your loved ones. Remember, however, that many of the treatments described here are experimental and not yet widely available. Your specialist or GP may be able to help if you wish to participate in clinical trials that test the effectiveness of new treatments, or you may be advised and prefer to opt for tried and trusted conventional drugs and techniques.

Either way, Medical Breakthroughs 2004 puts you one step ahead. ' It's a great way to keep yourself informed about the latest developments in health care,' says our consultant Dr Vince Forte, a general practitioner, medical writer and expert in forensic medicine.

# PART 1

# THE YEAR'S TOP STORIES

New medical research has modified some widely held views in the past year. Dietary guidelines are being refined as we learn more about the roles of fats and carbohydrates. The new buzz acronym is RNA, as scientists research its potential for turning off troublesome genes. It was a year when health threats sprang from unusual places – with the discovery of a new risk factor for heart disease, and the previously unknown SARS virus triggering an international scare. Scientists continued to astonish us with powerful cancer vaccines, new insights into the real causes of Alzheimer's disease, and an ever-expanding list of lifesaving uses for statins. On the following pages, you'll find an in-depth look at these and other top health stories.

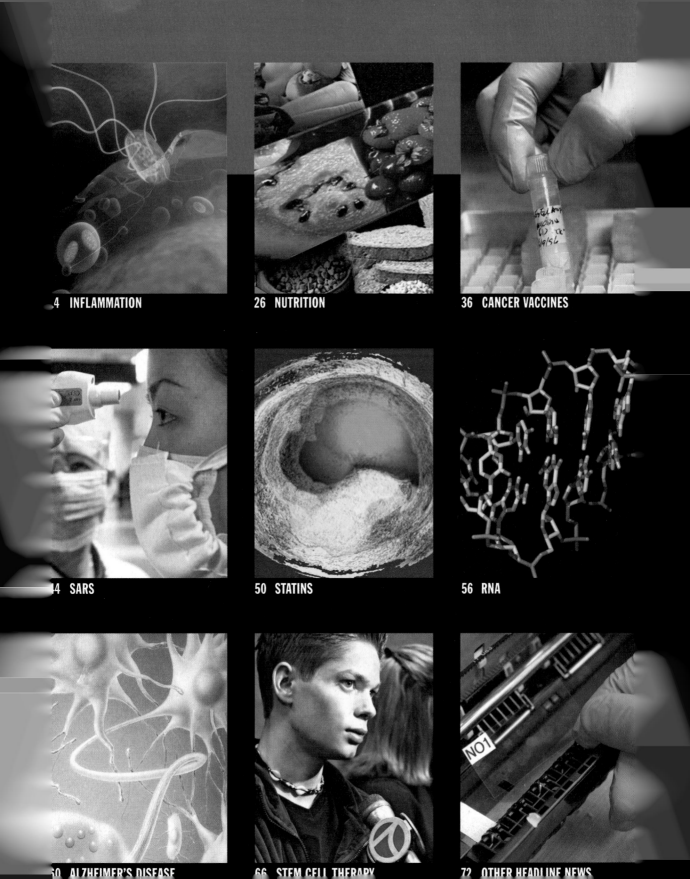

# CRP – TEST PREDICTS RISK OF HEART ATTACK

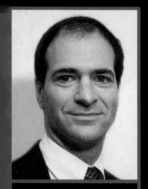

'This,' says Dr Ridker, 'is a fundamental paradigm shift in how cardiologists think about this disease.'

**Dr Paul Ridker**

Several years ago, cardiologist Paul Ridker, then a young Harvard doctor, went to a scientific meeting of heart specialists with a new finding. He had conducted a study of middle-aged men that showed that those most at risk of heart disease were not the ones affected by the well-known villains, raised blood cholesterol and high blood pressure.

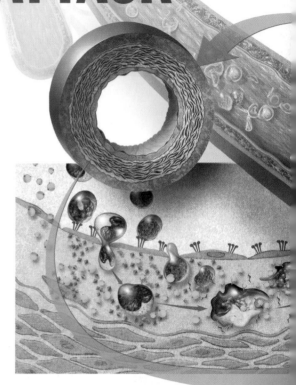

**1** Inflammation occurs when white blood cells invade the artery wall in response to an 'attack' by particles of LDL cholesterol. It is these immune cells, together with the LDL, that form fatty streaks that turn into plaque.

Instead, they were those with increased blood levels of the less familiar C-reactive protein (CRP), released by the body in response to inflammation. No one turned up to hear his findings. A few years later, in autumn 2002, at another meeting of heart specialists, there were no fewer than 100 papers discussing inflammation and heart disease. Dr Ridker was inundated with questions from colleagues and reporters, eager for the latest news on CRP.

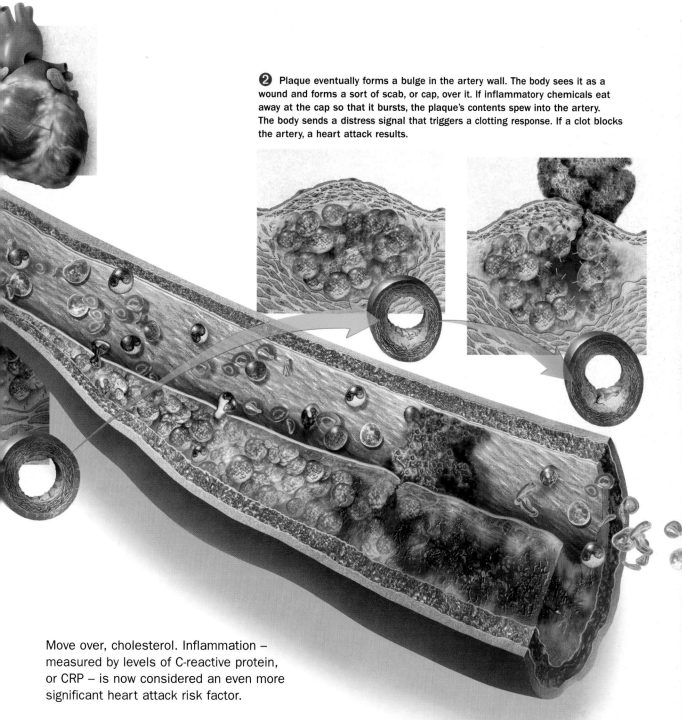

❷ Plaque eventually forms a bulge in the artery wall. The body sees it as a wound and forms a sort of scab, or cap, over it. If inflammatory chemicals eat away at the cap so that it bursts, the plaque's contents spew into the artery. The body sends a distress signal that triggers a clotting response. If a clot blocks the artery, a heart attack results.

Move over, cholesterol. Inflammation – measured by levels of C-reactive protein, or CRP – is now considered an even more significant heart attack risk factor.

15

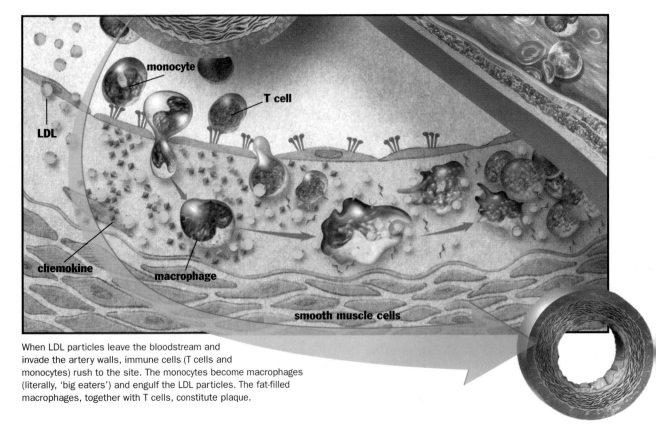

When LDL particles leave the bloodstream and invade the artery walls, immune cells (T cells and monocytes) rush to the site. The monocytes become macrophages (literally, 'big eaters') and engulf the LDL particles. The fat-filled macrophages, together with T cells, constitute plaque.

Just when we thought we knew the major culprits responsible for heart disease – cholesterol and other blood fats – comes the suggestion that our immune systems are also partly to blame for hardening our arteries. Recent research has shown that heart disease is as much about chronic inflammation – caused by overactive immune defences – as it is about cholesterol. 'This,' says Dr Ridker, 'is a fundamental paradigm shift in how cardiologists think about this disease.'

That isn't all. Chronic, low-level inflammation has also been implicated in some other major disorders, including diabetes, Alzheimer's disease and cancer.

## Our defenders attack us

You know what happens when you get a splinter. The surrounding area becomes swollen, red and hot – that is, inflamed. These are signs that your body's defences have swung into action. While you're manipulating tweezers or a needle to remove the splinter, your immune system is making its own efforts at a microscopic level. It's dispatching an army of infection-fighting white blood cells to contain the damage, destroy any bacteria that have

entered, and to start healing the wound. This system evolved thousands of years ago, when humans scrambled for food, had few defences against disease or injury – and lived 20 to 30 years at most. But what worked well in the Stone Age can cause problems in the 21st century.

Today, the average Briton's immune system is less likely to be waging pitched battles against sudden invasions than to be engaged in continual scuffles with chronic low-grade infections such as gum disease or herpes, or the self-imposed damage caused by eating too many fatty and sugary foods, taking too little exercise and smoking. The hazards of modern life don't help either – in particular the steady and unrelenting stress that affects most of us.

The result can be chronic inflammation, a situation in which, as Harvard cardiologist Peter Libby, puts it, 'our own defences bombard us with friendly fire.'

## A smouldering inflammation

The strongest evidence for the dangers of chronic inflammation shows up in studies of atherosclerosis, or hardening of the arteries. Until a few years ago, most cardiologists looked at heart disease as if it were a simple plumbing problem: globules of cholesterol and fat stick to the inner surface of an artery, just like grease in a household pipe, until the deposit gets big enough to clog the pipe and cause a heart attack or stroke. But research by Dr Ridker, Dr Libby and others has produced a more complex, more dynamic view of the process.

According to the new thinking, heart disease itself is a long, smouldering inflammation that causes plaque to accumulate not on the artery walls but within them. This process is somewhat similar to that splinter in your finger. In your cardiovascular system, the trouble starts when slivers of low-density lipoprotein (LDL) – or 'bad' cholesterol – dig into the wall of an artery.

Once inside, the fatty particles start to oxidize, a process rather like rusting that results from an attack by damaging molecules called free radicals. The cells lining the artery wall (called endothelial cells) interpret this oxidation as a sign of danger and rally the immune system. To aid the defensive action, the endothelial cells puff up and become sticky so that they can catch passing white blood cells circulating in the bloodstream.

Reinforcements follow, and a class of hormones called cytokines takes charge, orchestrating the movements of the troops. On cue, some of the white blood cells transform into cells called macrophages, which gobble up the LDL. If there's too much for them to handle, the macrophages 'ultimately become so packed with fatty droplets that they look foamy when viewed under a microscope,' as Dr Libby explained in a recent article. Those fat-filled 'foam cells' combine with other immune cells to form the fatty streak known as plaque.

Once the immune system senses that it has contained the infection, it starts to heal the 'wounds'. Perversely, though, that can create even more problems. Cells in the inflamed artery wall knit a tough, fibrous cap, much like a scab, over the plaque to seal it off. The plaque can remain stable for decades and, indeed, some people live with it into their eighties.

However, often a fresh bout of inflammation upsets the plaque, prompting the macrophages inside to secrete enzymes that chew away at the cap, creating what doctors refer to as vulnerable plaque. This plaque can rupture and spew substances into the bloodstream that trigger blood clots. The next thing you know, you're in an ambulance rushing to the nearest A&E department.

Not even Heath Robinson could have designed a system so complex. Although this new model lends itself less easily to plumbing metaphors than the old, Dr Libby and others think it explains many of the vexing riddles surrounding cardiovascular disease – such as the seemingly healthy 40 year-old who cycles from London to Brighton one weekend and drops dead of a massive heart attack the next.

A heart attack occurs when one of the coronary arteries carrying oxygen-rich blood to the heart muscle becomes blocked. When the blood supply is cut off, a part of the heart muscle dies –

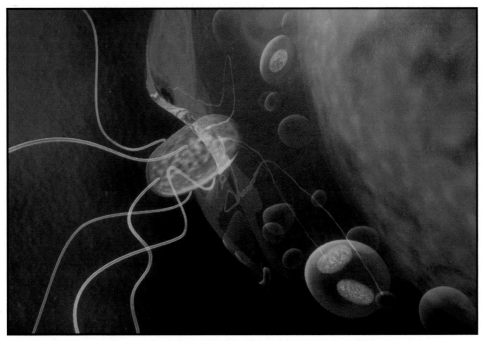

Bacterial infections are one cause of inflammation. In this image, a white blood cell is shown engulfing a bacterium. Germ-eating white blood cells also secrete inflammatory chemicals called cytokines, which direct other immune cells to the area as part of the body's immune response.

or infarcts. A heart attack is also known as a myocardial infarction (MI), a coronary thrombosis or simply a coronary. Heart attacks are the most common cause of death in the UK. Each year 300,000 new heart attacks are recorded in the population – half of which are fatal.

Cholesterol isn't the only irritant that triggers inflammation and, in turn, heart disease. Experts now believe that smoking and high blood pressure also contribute by inflaming artery walls.

Another possible inflammation trigger is germs. Researchers have begun exploring an apparent connection between heart disease and chronic (long-term) low-grade infections. For instance, studies have found that people with long-term gum disease – 15 per cent of all adults under 50 – are twice as likely to have heart disease as those with healthy gums. Another recent study showed that the risk of having a heart attack or dying of heart disease can double in people who have had cold sores, caused by the Herpes simplex type 1 virus.

One of the biggest germ threats may be *Chlamydia pneumoniae*, which causes the most common type of pneumonia. Most adults have been exposed to *C. pneumoniae* and carry antibodies to it. According to Dr Libby, traces of the bacteria are found in about 40 per cent of atherosclerotic plaque. However, prescribing more antibiotics to fight

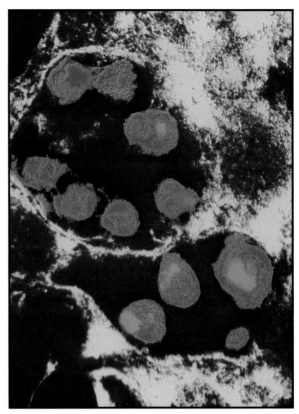

*Chlamydia pneumoniae* bacteria in a foam cell (yellow) of a coronary artery. Foam cells form plaque, and bacteria may increase plaque formation by triggering inflammation.

## ARE STATINS
# AN ANSWER?

Statin drugs were designed to lower blood cholesterol levels – specifically 'bad' LDL cholesterol. Until recently, experts thought that the reason drugs like simvastatin (Zocor) and pravastatin (Lipostat) help to prevent heart attacks is that they slow down the liver's production of LDL cholesterol. However, recent evidence suggests that statins may also work because they reduce inflammation.

Laboratory studies show that the drugs reduce the susceptibility of LDL to oxidation – the process that triggers the inflammatory response – and inhibit the enzymes that cause plaque to rupture.

Equally intriguing are studies showing that people who took statins to reduce their cholesterol also achieved, on average, a 15 to 25 per cent drop in their CRP levels in as little as six weeks. There's a catch, though – for some reason that doctors cannot yet fathom, not everyone gets that benefit.

The big question is whether reducing CRP levels in a person with low cholesterol will afford any protection against a heart attack. Dr Paul Ridker has just launched a study in the US to answer that question. His study will involve 15,000 men and women with low LDL levels but high CRP. Half will receive a statin and half will get a placebo. Researchers will then track them for five years. Until the results are in, Dr Peter Libby and others agree that there is no good reason to take these potent drugs simply to reduce your CRP.

infection is unlikely to prevent heart attacks. The largest studies to date have found no such benefits. And as the antibiotics already in use are producing drug-resistant bacteria that are increasingly hard to control, doctors are wary of over-prescribing for fear of producing even more superbugs.

## A trigger for Type 2 diabetes

Inflammation also appears to play a role in Type 2 diabetes. The incidence of this disease has rocketed in the past decade, especially among people in whom it used to be rare – children, adolescents and young adults. Nearly 1.4 million people in the UK have been diagnosed with diabetes, and doctors think that there are probably as many as a million more undiagnosed cases.

Type 2 diabetes and the less common Type 1 reflect problems with the body's use or production of insulin, the hormone that's needed to shuttle glucose from your bloodstream to your muscles and organs, which use it for fuel. When the insulin shuttle fails, blood sugar rises to dangerous levels. Type 1 diabetes is an auto-immune condition that strikes unpredictably, but there's no great mystery about the cause of Type 2: it's usually a result of years of too much food and too little exercise. Type 2 diabetes develops gradually. At first, your body is merely less responsive to insulin. But if untreated, that unresponsiveness, known as insulin resistance, forces your pancreas to churn out more and more insulin, until its insulin-producing cells burn out and stop making enough to keep blood sugar in check. At that point, you'll probably need tablets or, more rarely, insulin injections.

Inflammation has long been known to play havoc with the way in which the body regulates insulin production. When people get septicaemia – a severe blood infection – their blood sugar levels soar. And studies also show that when muscle, fat or liver tissue is inflamed, it becomes less responsive to insulin. Experts now believe that inflammation explains why the incidence of Type 2 diabetes has shot up as people's waistlines have expanded. It appears that fat tissue releases cytokines, hormones that help to stimulate the immune system cells involved in combating inflammation. Recent research suggests that cytokines can also confuse the intricate signalling process of insulin regulation. Raised cytokine levels 'create static on the line,' explains Dr Steven Shoelson, who works in a Boston-based diabetes clinic. The fatter you are, the more cytokines you produce and the less your body is attuned to the effects of insulin.

Along with obesity itself, the kinds of foods that make us fat also cause inflammation, says Paresh Dandona, professor of medicine at New York State University. In a series of studies, he measured various indicators of inflammation after feeding doses of sugar or cream or fatty foods – the basics of junk food – to volunteers with diabetes.

Dr Dandona found that all three triggered the production of free radicals, damaging oxygen molecules that activate cytokines and proteins involved in the inflammatory response. The resulting inflammation lasted for three to four hours. The way that the body reacts to a diet loaded with junk food is actually quite frightening: the immune system goes into a state of near-constant readiness, rather like firefighters repeatedly responding to a broken alarm. According to new scientific thinking, this inflammatory process may account for the fact that people with diabetes are two to four times more likely to experience a heart attack or stroke than those who have normal blood sugar levels.

'Almost everyone with diabetes ends up dying of a heart attack,' says endocrinologist John Buse, who runs a diabetes clinic at the University of North Carolina. And, he adds, a Scandinavian study published in September 2002 confirmed his gut feeling that most people with heart problems either have diabetes or exhibit early signs of the disease.

In that study, researchers tested the blood sugar of patients who had had heart attacks. Between 20 and 30 per cent were already aware that they had blood sugar problems, but another two-thirds tested positive for diabetes or pre-diabetes.

## Suspicions about Alzheimer's

Could inflammation also be at work in Alzheimer's disease? That possibility emerges from a raft of studies showing that people who take nonsteroidal anti-inflammatory drugs (NSAIDs) such as aspirin and ibuprofen regularly for many years have a 30 to 40 per cent lower risk of developing the dreaded dementia than people who don't use these drugs.

Now researchers are working backwards to determine whether there's a biological cause for that effect. In autopsies, the brains of Alzheimer's patients inevitably show two abnormalities: beta-amyloid plaques (clumps of protein and dead brain cells) and neurofibrillary tangles (twisted skeins of the same material). Scientists in recent years have also detected signs of inflammation.

Some experts speculate that when the brain's defence mechanism – immune cells known as microglia – attacks the invading plaques and tangles, it also destroys healthy neurons (nerve cells). But, says Professor John Breitner, head of geriatric psychiatry, psychiatry and behavioural sciences at the University of Washington, it's not clear whether the inflammatory response is responsible for the loss of function in Alzheimer's disease or whether it's just adding insult to injury.

## Cancer: wounds that never heal

As long ago as 1863, German pathologist Rudolf Virchow suggested that cancer might spring from sites that are chronically inflamed, but the notion was ignored until recently. Now, studies support the idea that some tumours are essentially wounds that have failed to heal. One of the strongest examples is colon cancer. People with a history of inflammatory bowel diseases have up to a 60 per cent higher risk of developing colorectal cancer than people who haven't had bowel problems. And, rheumatoid arthritis patients who regularly take NSAIDs (which fight inflammation) almost never get colon cancer, says Dr Dawn Willis, scientific adviser to the American Cancer Society.

Bacterial or viral infections may also be implicated. According to one estimate, infections cause some 15 per cent of cancers worldwide. *Helicobacter pylori*, the bug that causes stomach ulcers, is linked with gastric cancer; genital warts, caused by the human papillomavirus, are a primary cause of cervical cancer; and both hepatitis B and C raise the risk of liver cancer. As Dr Willis puts it, 'chronic inflammation sets up an environment that's very conducive to cancer'.

## Detection: the CRP test

These theories are all very well, but because chronic inflammation operates below your body's radar – it's there, but

### The cancer-inflammation link

Researchers are identifying more and more cancers associated with ongoing inflammation caused by infection, irritation (by the body's own stomach acids, for instance) or a chronic inflammatory condition. The chart below covers some of these cancers.

| CANCER | INFECTIOUS AGENT OR IRRITANT |
|---|---|
| B-cell non-Hodgkin's lymphoma | Epstein-Barr virus |
| Bladder, liver, rectal cancer | Schistosomes (parasites) |
| Colon cancer | Liver flukes (*Opisthorchis viverrini*) |
| Oesophageal cancer | Gastric acids |
| Gallbladder cancer | *Helicobacter pylori* bacteria |
| Non-Hodgkin's lymphoma | Human immunodeficiency virus human herpes virus type 8 |
| Ovarian cancer | Gonococcus (gonorrhoea), chlamydia human papillomavirus |
| Stomach cancer | *Helicobacter pylori* bacteria |

| CANCER | INFLAMMATORY CONDITION |
|---|---|
| Bladder cancer | Cystitis, bladder inflammation |
| Colorectal cancer | Inflammatory bowel disease, chronic ulcerative colitis |
| Lung cancer | Bronchitis |
| Oral squamous cell cancer | Gingivitis |

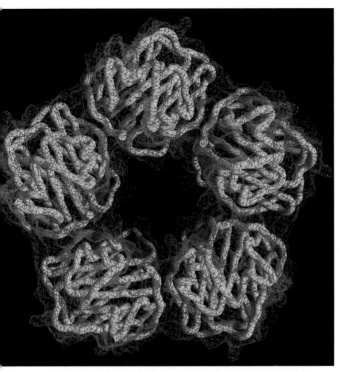

CRP is produced in the liver whenever inflammation occurs. If your arteries are under attack, your CRP level rises. People with elevated CRP levels are more likely to have a heart attack or stroke, even if their cholesterol levels are normal.

you can't feel it – so how do you know if you have something nasty brewing? This is where C-reactive protein comes in. The molecule is produced by the liver in response to inflammation. The CRP test has, in fact, been available in Britain for many years. It's a standard NHS test for suspected rheumatoid arthritis, for example. And if you have an acute infection such as flu, your blood levels of CRP shoot up.

However, as Dr Paul Ridker and others have shown in numerous studies, tiny rises in CRP are also significant because they are signs of silent inflammation. (There's even growing evidence that CRP not only indicates inflammation but also contributes to it by helping to accelerate the oxidation of LDL particles.)

The study that put CRP on the medical map was a 1997 report in which Dr Ridker and his colleagues analysed the CRP levels of 1,086 men who were being monitored over several years for their incidence of heart problems.

The researchers found that the men who had the highest CRP levels at the start of the study were three times more likely to have heart attacks and twice as likely to have strokes as those with the lowest levels.

Dr Ridker found an equally striking difference in a later study that followed 28,000 women for eight years. His results revealed that the women with the highest CRP levels were nearly 2½ times more likely than those with low levels to have heart attacks or strokes. Even if they did not smoke or have particularly high cholesterol levels or a family history of heart disease, their odds of heart disease or stroke were, nevertheless, higher.

That study also suggested that a CRP reading may predict the risk of cardiovascular disease even better than cholesterol readings. The women most likely to have heart attacks or strokes were, not surprisingly, those with high levels of both CRP and LDL. But the second highest risk occurred in women with low LDL levels and high CRP. When it comes to identifying people at risk of heart trouble, the current cholesterol-oriented guidelines completely miss this group, says Dr Ridker.

That doesn't mean that you can forget about having your cholesterol measured, however. Dr Ridker's point is that measuring CRP adds vital information to existing tests.

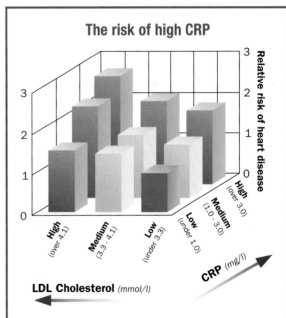

**The risk of high CRP**

Elevated levels of LDL cholesterol (purple arrow) or CRP (green arrow) raise the risk of a heart attack. A person with high CRP but normal cholesterol is still at increased risk for a heart attack, and vice versa. High levels of both cause the greatest risk.

*Source: Circulation 107: 363, 2003*

CRP may be an equally useful predictor of Type 2 diabetes. For instance, researchers in Georgia, USA measured CRP levels in 5888 healthy men and women. When they checking up on their subjects three to four years later, they found that the people with raised CRP levels were twice as likely to have developed diabetes as those with lower readings. It is still not clear whether the protein serves as a marker for Alzheimer's and cancer, however.

CRP isn't the only way to gauge inflammation. Other proteins and cytokines circulating in the blood can also indicate that something is not right. Still, many doctors now believe that CRP could be the most reliable and easily obtained marker. What has really pushed it into the limelight is that there is now a good sensitive test for CRP. It is easy (a simple blood test) and predicted to be relatively inexpensive (£12 to £15).

But the experts are urging caution. 'It's not a test for everyone,' says cardiologist Dr Thomas Pearson, chair of the department of community and preventive medicine at Rochester University in New York. Dr Pearson and a team of experts have been responsible for drafting a policy for CRP testing in the USA. They recommended that, for now, the only people who should be screened for CRP are those who already have mild cause for concern. That group includes people who, based on their current medical profile, have as little as a 10 to 20 per cent chance of having a heart attack in the next decade because they already have some of the classic risk factors. They're 20lb (9kg) overweight or their blood pressure is slightly raised; their LDL is a little high or their HDL (good cholesterol) is low.

In such borderline cases, says Dr Pearson, the CRP test can help a doctor to decide whether to treat a patient, and how. It could, for example, help to determine if the prescribing of cholesterol lowering drugs or aspirin is advisable. 'If the CRP is high, I might be more aggressive. If it's normal, I might decide not to do anything,' he says. Otherwise, a CRP test shouldn't be used for widespread screening, says Dr Pearson, and lists some reasons:

- **Too many unknowns** Participants in the CRP studies to date have been mostly white. No one knows yet what a healthy CRP level is in other ethnic groups, who may have higher or lower rates of heart disease.
- **Too many false positives** An infected tooth or a bout of bronchitis can push up CRP levels, which could lead to costly and unnecessary follow-up tests.

## A SIMPLE BLOOD TEST
# C-REACTIVE PROTEIN

Despite the current range of risk factors – age, cholesterol levels, hormones, diabetes, smoking, obesity and high blood pressure – taken into consideration by GPs, one third of heart attacks occur in patients who exhibit low or no risk factors. But one day, in the not-too-distant future, a new diagnostic technique might be used to help doctors determine your risk of heart disease or stroke.

A blood test that shows your C-reactive protein (CRP) levels could soon become as important as the universally recognized test for cholesterol.

The accurate testing of CRP levels has only recently become possible with the development of a highly sensitive technique that accurately measures CRP levels from 1 to 5 milligrams per litre (mg/l) of blood.

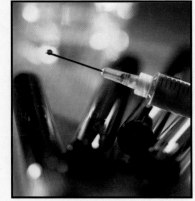

(A less sensitive CRP test has long been used to evaluate inflammation in people with rheumatoid arthritis.) A reading of 1 mg/l or less is considered low risk; 2mg/l to 3mg/l is thought to be a sign of potential trouble.

A finding of 3mg/l or higher is a warning of the sort of smouldering inflammation that doubles your risk of heart disease. Levels higher than 10mg/l suggest an acute infection – a cold, flu, a bad tooth or even a severe cut can raise CRP levels above normal, so the test needs to be repeated once the infection clears.

There is no significant difference between CRP levels in men and women, although taking hormone replacement therapy (HRT) can sometimes raise CRP levels slightly in postmenopausal women.

- **Too few solutions** A high CRP reading isn't going to change the treatment of someone who already has heart disease. And if someone has no other risk factors besides a high CRP reading, there is nothing to treat. 'If I'm not going to use the information, why collect it?,' Dr Pearson asks. What's more, as even CRP's biggest fans readily admit, no one knows yet whether reducing your CRP translates into lowering your odds of heart attack, stroke or diabetes. Studies designed to answer that question are only now getting under way.

Nehama Beer, a 52 year-old piano teacher in California, has direct experience of the test's limitations. In autumn 2002, Beer's doctor suggested that she should be tested when her cholesterol levels suddenly shot up into the danger zone, soaring to more than 6.4mmol/l. The test showed that

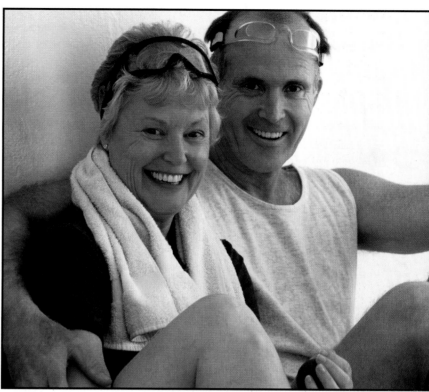

Exercise is one way that can demonstrably lower your CRP levels. One study found that the men who were the fittest tended to have the lowest levels of CRP, while those who were the least fit tended to have the highest CRP levels. Experts suggest that just 30 minutes of moderate exercise a day can boost your fitness level.

her CRP was 3.7mg/l, which was also frighteningly high (see 'A simple blood test', facing page). Beer decided to see what she could do on her own before trying medication. She rejoined her gym, changed her eating habits – no more cheese or red meat – and lost 5lb (2.25kg).

By her next check-up some three months later, her cholesterol had dropped back to a healthy level but her CRP hadn't budged. Nehama had more tests, including a heart scan, that showed her pipes were clean as a whistle.

That left Nehama, as well as her nurse practitioner, in a quandary. She did not want to start taking cholesterol-lowering statin drugs because of the risk of liver damage, and she was afraid that taking an NSAID (such as aspirin) on a regular basis would upset her stomach.

She suspects that the high CRP reading reflects her mild arthritis. Although not deeply worried, she hasn't stopped wondering about the source of her raised CRP. 'But I really don't know. I'm in an odd situation. I want to know where it comes from.'

In the meantime, she's going to keep to her diet and continue exercising regularly. '*Que sera, sera,*' she says. 'What else can I do?'

## A healthy lifestyle is still your best defence

When you listen to Dr Ridker, Dr Libby and other architects of the inflammation hypothesis, there's no mistaking the excitement in their voices. They're thrilled to be charting new scientific territory and also to see their discoveries pointing towards new ways to curb some of today's biggest killers.

A number of drugs now on the market are being looked at again for their potential in fighting inflammation. There's some evidence that the potent cholesterol-lowering drugs known as statins can soothe inflamed arteries (see 'Are statins an answer?', page 18). And it appears that the drugs now used to treat Type 2 diabetes and boost insulin sensitivity are effective because they too have anti-inflammatory effects. Researchers are exploring possible new roles for aspirin, long known as an inflammation fighter, or aspirin-related compounds, as well as their nonsteroidal anti-inflammatory kin such as ibuprofen and the newer drugs known as COX-2 inhibitors (developed to provide the same sort of painkilling and anti-inflammatory effects as NSAIDs, but without the damaging effects on the stomach lining).

Meanwhile, drug manufacturers are searching for new compounds that may short-circuit the inflammatory response in a safer and more targeted way than the medicines now available.

In the absence of any magic pills, the best way to keep internal inflammation at bay is to live healthily. That means…

**Give up smoking** Smoking is associated with higher CRP levels. The smoke particles themselves irritate your lungs and arteries, not to mention the 55 other chemicals you inhale with every puff.

**Lose weight** The heavier you are, the more likely you are to have elevated CRP, thanks to the inflammatory molecules produced by fat tissue. There's no question, says diabetes expert Dr Steven Shoelson, that someone who gains 30lb (13.5kg) is more likely to become insulin resistant than someone whose weight remains steady. When you lose the weight, your insulin resistance evaporates too.

**Exercise** The fitter you are, the lower your markers for inflammation, research has shown. For example, in a study of 3,638 healthy men and women, researchers at medical school in Atlanta found that those who exercised 22 or more times a month were 37 per cent less likely to have elevated CRP levels than those who were sedentary. Exercise helps you to lose weight, helps to keep blood vessels supple, makes muscles more sensitive to insulin and helps your body to use glucose more efficiently.

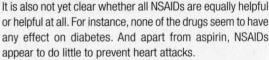

## KEEP A LID ON
# NSAIDS

If heart disease, diabetes, Alzheimer's and cancer all stem from chronic inflammation, you'd think the ideal antidote would be the over-the-counter nonsteroidal anti-inflammatory drugs (known as NSAIDs), such as aspirin and ibuprofen, that we all have in our medicine cabinets. Sadly, it is not that simple.

It's true that studies suggest NSAIDs may help to prevent these maladies. But such studies demonstrate only a correlation, not proof that the drugs' anti-inflammatory properties produce the results. Something else could be responsible. and studies to nail down a connection are only just beginning.

According to Cancer Research UK, research has shown that these drugs may help to prevent bowel and other digestive system cancers. The theory is that this type of drug stops an enzyme called COX-2 from working, and blocking this enzyme may help to stop polyps from developing. Other studies are underway for Alzheimer's; healthy middle-aged adults are being given anti-inflammatories or a placebo, while researchers watch for signs of dementia in the participants.

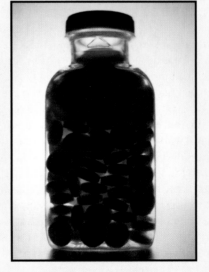

It is also not yet clear whether all NSAIDs are equally helpful or helpful at all. For instance, none of the drugs seem to have any effect on diabetes. And apart from aspirin, NSAIDs appear to do little to prevent heart attacks.

There's also some suggestion that the newer COX-2 inhibitors can make matters worse, increasing the risk of blood clots and heart attacks. And taking an NSAID every day can be damaging in other ways. The older drugs such as ibuprofen can be irritating, causing stomach upset, bleeding ulcers, and liver and kidney problems in some people.

Dr Joseph Rogers from Arizona, one of the researchers who has been investigating Alzheimer's, put himself on a daily dose of ibuprofen – acting as a guinea pig in his own experiment. However, he says: 'I started having stomach problems, so I had to stop taking it.'

The considered advice of experts is currently not to self-medicate with aspirin or other NSAIDs to ward off future health threats. Because regular daily doses of these drugs can potentially damage the lining of your stomach, it is essential to consult your doctor first.

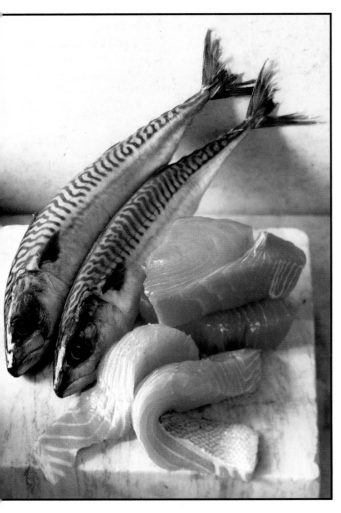

Fish rich in omega-3 fatty acids can help to lower your CRP levels, which may be one reason that people who take fish-oil supplements are less likely to die from a heart attack.

if you can move step by step towards what Dr Hu and his colleagues call the 'healthy eating pattern' – which is made up of lots of fruits and vegetables, whole grain breads and cereals, fish, poultry and low-fat dairy products.

Change one meal at a time or replace a single type of food – choosing a method that you can handle comfortably – so that it becomes a lasting improvement, not a heroic test of will.

People who fill their plates with the kinds of foods Dr Hu recommends have lower CRP levels and about a 30 per cent lower risk of heart disease and diabetes than those who follow a more traditional meat-and-two-veg diet.

Changing your eating habits may be harder and perhaps just a little more inconvenient than taking a daily pill but it's completely safe and totally free from side effects. Why not give it a try? Your body can only benefit when its hard-working immune system is given a break.

**Eat well** No single food can cure inflammation, but some nutrients help to reduce it. These include the omega-3 fatty acids in walnuts, flaxseed (linseed) and cold-water fish such as salmon and sardines; and also antioxidant vitamins C and E, which are abundant in dark-coloured fruits and vegetables.

Conversely, certain foods, such as bacon, sausages and pepperoni can exacerbate inflammation. People who eat processed meats every day have raised CRP levels, says nutritionist Professor Frank Hu, who is based at the Harvard School of Public Health.

Also, starchy, highly refined foods such as white bread, biscuits and cakes tend to push up inflammatory markers (and also triglycerides – blood fats that increase the risk of heart disease and diabetes). A diet that is high in those foods has been linked to an increased risk of insulin resistance, diabetes and heart disease.

If your diet needs a radical rethink, don't make the mistake of trying to change it overnight. Instead, see

## WHAT DOES IT MEAN TO YOU?

Inflammation, marked by raised CRP levels, can double your risk of a heart attack – even if you don't have high cholesterol – and contribute to Type 2 diabetes. A simple blood test may soon be available in the UK to measure CRP, but unless you have other risk factors for heart disease, you may not need or be offered it. There are no easy ways to reduce chronic inflammation. There are, however, ways to protect yourself.

● If your cholesterol is low but you have other risk factors for heart disease – overweight or have high blood pressure or both – talk to your doctor or practice nurse about modifying your diet.

● Exercise and lose excess weight. Both can be as effective as the best drugs for keeping your immune system fit and healthy.

● If you have a chronic inflammatory condition such as bowel disease or acid reflux, talk to your doctor about cancer screening tests.

● Take care of your teeth. Brush and floss to prevent bacteria from invading your gums – because gingivitis is linked to heart disease.

# WEIGHING UP NEW FOOD RESEARCH

Prominent nutrition experts are beginning to challenge some widely held views about healthy eating. Gone, for instance, is the old general notion that fat is 'bad' and carbohydrate is 'good'. It is now clear that there are good and bad fats, as well as good and bad carbohydrates. So dietary policies are changing as researchers produce new data on the benefits – and risks – of carbohydrates, fats, fibre and many other nutrients.

In the USA, health experts have long used a so-called 'Food Pyramid' to show the proportionate importance of different food groups in a healthy diet. This model, introduced in the 1990s, reflects general guidelines in Britain and elsewhere. At its base – the foundation of good health – were

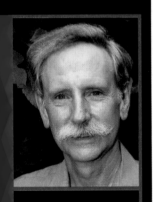

'The biggest nutritional mistake people can make is getting rid of all the fat in their diets. Not all fats are bad...'

Dr Walter C. Willett

bread, cereal, rice, pasta and other carbohydrates. Next came vegetables and fruits, then dairy foods and the group comprising meats, fish, dry beans, eggs and nuts. Perched at the top were the foods to avoid or eat sparingly – fats, oils and sweets.

The high-carbohydrate, low-fat focus seemed logical during the 1980s and 1990s. But as time passed, the model began to seem flawed. Studies started to cast doubt on the standard nutritional guidelines and some respected experts proposed a heresy: such a diet may actually promote weight gain, heart disease and diabetes.

Today, debate rages about what constitutes healthy eating, but many experts agree that the pyramid model is faulty. Researchers point to study after study showing that not all fats are bad for your health or waistline. Possibly more important, not all carbohydrates are good for you. As a result, there's a movement afoot to completely rethink nutritional guidelines, and researchers, nutrition educators and food-industry groups are clamouring to be heard.

## Fat: no longer all bad

In the forefront is Dr Walter Willett, professor of epidemiology and chair of the nutrition department at the Harvard School of Public Health in the USA. In order to encourage debate about new principles, Dr Willett unveiled his own healthy eating pyramid in his book *Eat, Drink, and Be Healthy* (see 'Will the real pyramid please stand up?' on page 34). 'There is a lot of misinformation out there', says Dr Willett. 'The Food Guide Pyramid is tremendously flawed. It says that all fats are bad and that all complex carbohydrates are good.

' That's not accurate. The biggest nutritional mistake people can make is getting rid of all the fat in their diets. Not all fats are bad, and some are required for good health.'

Dr Willett has spent much of the past 20 years researching the relationship between carbohydrates, fats and good health. He and others at Harvard have tracked the eating, exercise and lifestyle habits of thousands of health professionals and published hundreds of studies based on their data. Their research has helped to change the basic understanding of human nutrition, mostly as it pertains to fat consumption.

It appears that, rather than clogging arteries and packing on the pounds, the monounsaturated and polyunsaturated fats that are found in avocados, flaxseed, fish, soya beans, olives, olive oil, nuts and nut butters seem to improve cholesterol ratios and help with weight loss. Monounsaturated fats have been shown to help to raise levels of high-density lipoprotein (HDL, or 'good') cholesterol and lower levels of low-density lipoprotein (LDL, or 'bad') cholesterol. They also seem to be involved in the controlling of hunger and burning of fat.

This is surprising when you consider some basic facts about fat. It is a fact that 1g of fat contains 9 calories, compared with 4 calories in 1g of carbohydrate or protein. And it is also a fact that the body stores energy from fat more efficiently than from protein and carbohydrates. Thus, the overriding message of the 1990s was that you get fatter from eating fat. It seemed to follow, then, that if you wanted to lose weight, you could do it just by cutting back on fat. But, it seems that these 'facts' are less than clear-cut.

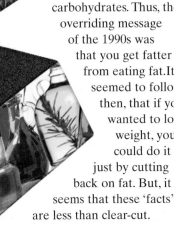

According to Liz Applegate Ph.D., professor of nutrition at the University of California-Davis, monounsaturated and polyunsaturated fats may actually help to keep blood sugar and insulin levels steady, which reduces hunger and promotes fat burning instead of fat storage. In fact, a recent investigation that compared the results of 147 different studies on nutrition and health, found that fats are absolutely essential for good health.

Even saturated fat – the kind found in steak, butter and ice cream and long considered a dietary villain – may not be quite as bad for us as we thought. Recent studies published in the *New England Journal of Medicine* and elsewhere have found that the Atkins diet, rich in protein and saturated fat, may promote more weight loss and better cholesterol levels than high-carbohydrate, low-fat diets (see 'Can research vindicate high-protein diets?' on page 116).

**The bottom line** 'Not all fats are bad, and some are absolutely essential,' says Dr. Willett. Studies of healthy populations in places such as Crete have persuaded him that you can safely get a large percentage of calories from fat – as long as nearly all of it is 'good' fat from fish, nuts, olives, avocados and soya beans. Not all experts agree, but most concede that some fats are indeed good for your heart and your waistline, so they shouldn't be eliminated from anyone's diet.

There is one kind of fat that almost everyone now agrees we should avoid: the synthetic type known as trans-unsaturated fatty acids, or trans fats. These fats, found in margarine and many packaged foods, may be especially bad for the heart. Trans fats are produced when liquid vegetable oil is hydrogenated to make it solidify. They are used to prolong the shelf life of processed foods and contribute to the taste and texture of the biscuits, crisps, pastries and fried foods so many of us enjoy.

Until the 1990s, we were told that such man-made trans fats were healthier than saturated fats, so many people switched from butter (a saturated fat) to margarine. Yet Dr Willett and his colleagues showed that trans fats raised levels of LDL and triglycerides,

# Fats

**out**

Experts agree that the trans fats in many processed and fried foods are particularly bad for you. Most also agree that the saturated fats in animal products are less beneficial than unsaturated fats.

Researchers now believe that monounsaturated and polyunsaturated fats are essential to good health.

**in**

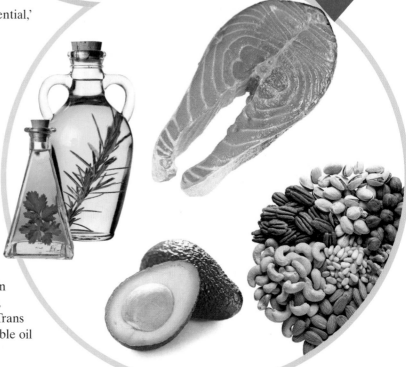

the molecules that make up fat, while lowering levels of HDL. Raising the ratio of LDL to HDL increases the risk of heart disease. Although controversial when it came out in the 1990s, the 'trans fats are bad' message is now widely accepted.

In late 2002, the US National Academy of Sciences Institute of Medicine (IOM) declared trans fats unsafe. In Britain, the advice is that trans fats should provide no more than 2 per cent of dietary energy. Nestlé has eliminated trans fats from two products; Cadbury's is considering a similar move.

## Carbohydrates: no longer all good

When people cut back on fat during the 1990s, many replaced it with carbohydrates. That would have been fine if the carbohydrate foods had been mostly fruits, vegetables and whole grains, but they weren't. Instead, a lot of people reached for processed foods such as white bread, buns, sweets, crisps, fat-free biscuits and fizzy drinks.

'It doesn't do any good to replace the fat in your diet with foods that are high in sugar or refined carbohydrates,' says Dr Willett. 'A lot of people think that a plain bagel with jam [or, in the UK, toast and marmalade] can be a healthy thing to eat in the morning, but actually that's one of the unhealthiest breakfasts you can consume. You'd be better off with scrambled eggs.'

Just as you can split fats into 'good' and 'bad', you can now do the same with carbohydrates. Unprocessed carbohydrate foods that are high in fibre – such as fruits, vegetables and whole grains – generally rate as 'good'. Those that are processed, low in fibre and are digested quickly – such as sugar, fizzy drinks, white pasta and jam on any bread made from refined flour – fall into the 'bad' category.

**Here's the reasoning** There are three main types of carbohydrate: sugars, starches and fibre. Some sugars occur naturally in fruit and sweet-tasting vegetables. Not only do they contain plant chemicals which fight disease, but most of them provide fibre as well, which is highly effective at slowing digestion. Other sugars – or 'added sugars' – such as honey, treacle, molasses and table sugar, provide no nutrition, only calories. Added sugars are are known as simple carbohydrates. They are also found in processed, vitamin-free, low-fibre carbohydrates that the body digests quickly – such as snack foods, refined-flour breads and sugary desserts – which have been shown to cause blood sugar swings that can lead to weight gain. They are absorbed rapidly and provide a fast energy boost.

The 'good' carbohydrates, usually known as complex carbohydrates, contain starches and fibre. Starchy carbohydrates, such as are found in wholemeal bread, whole-wheat pasta, brown rice, whole-grain breakfast cereal and some potatoes and yams, break down more slowly and offer a longer-term energy source.

The rate at which carbohydrates are broken down into sugar, to raise glucose levels and provide energy, is measured by the glycaemic index (GI). Foods with a high GI are quickly broken down and offer an immediate, but short-lived energy fix. In no time, you feel hungry again, and are tempted to eat more. Foods with a low GI are absorbed more slowly and make you feel full for longer. They also keep your blood sugar levels constant.

Eating processed carbohydrates is not a problem for people who are lean and fit. In these people, the hormone insulin is perfectly capable of keeping glucose (blood sugar) levels under control by

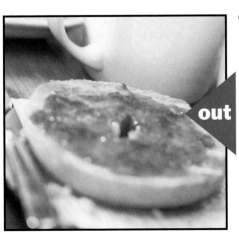

## The better breakfast?

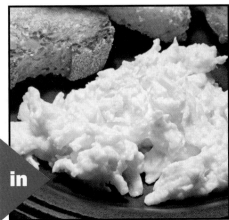

**out** A bagel with jam, or toast and marmalade are both breakfasts of sugar and refined carbohydrates, which lack fibre and lead to blood sugar swings that cause you to overeat. Protein (in scrambled eggs) and whole grains (in whole-wheat bread) don't have the same effect. **in**

shuttling it out of the bloodstream and into muscle cells, which use it for energy. Increasingly, however, the typical Briton is neither lean nor fit.

In many sedentary, overweight people, insulin can't do its job properly, so too much glucose stays in the blood, and the pancreas may respond by producing more of the hormone. High insulin levels prompt the liver to convert sugar into fat, which is eventually shuttled into fat cells. Blood sugar levels suddenly drop too low. In an attempt to bring the levels back to normal, your brain calls for food, making you feel hungry even though you don't actually need the calories.

Chronically high levels of blood sugar and insulin do more than make you fat; they've also been linked to heart disease. In one of Dr Willett's studies on thousands of nurses, those who consumed the highest amounts of quickly digested carbohydrates also had the highest incidence of heart disease. Generally, the more fibre a food contains and the less refined it is, the less it will affect blood sugar. Because foods loaded with refined carbohydrates, such as white bread, biscuits and snacks, raise blood sugar levels and lack nutrients, a growing number of nutrition experts now put them into the same category as junk food. The World Health Organization now promotes the eating of high-fibre, slow-to-digest carbohydrates such as beans, whole grains (including brown rice, whole-wheat breads and pastas, and bran or whole-wheat cereals) and many fruits and vegetables, over refined, simple carbohydrates. No one suggests that we should eat fewer carbohydrates. We should, however, eat less of some types (simple or refined) and more of other types (complex or non-processed). Since refined carbo-hydrates such as crisps, high-sugar breakfast cereals and biscuits are a major part of many people's diets, this switch may be the most important one to make.

# Carbohydrates

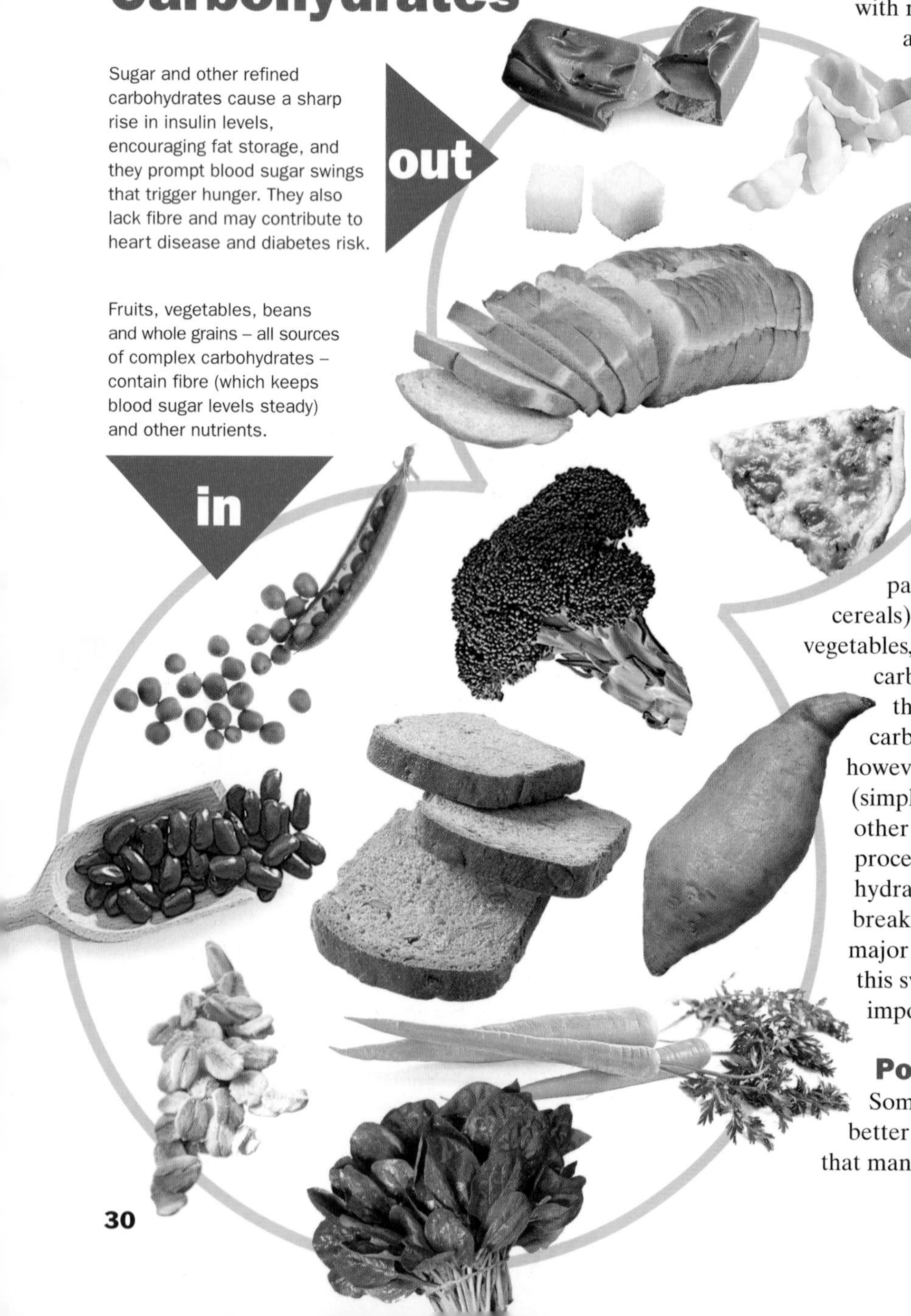

Sugar and other refined carbohydrates cause a sharp rise in insulin levels, encouraging fat storage, and they prompt blood sugar swings that trigger hunger. They also lack fibre and may contribute to heart disease and diabetes risk.

**out**

Fruits, vegetables, beans and whole grains – all sources of complex carbohydrates – contain fibre (which keeps blood sugar levels steady) and other nutrients.

**in**

## Potatoes are different
Some fats and carbohydrates are better for you than others – on that many nutrition experts agree.

But that's where the agreement stops. One of the controversial issues is about the potato and the role it should play in our diets. In the UK, potatoes are not classed as vegetables, so they don't fall into the 'eat as many as you can' group that includes fruit and vegetables. Dr Willett feels the potato should be relegated to the 'use sparingly' part of your diet. He includes it with white bread, sugar, sweets and other refined carbohydrate foods, because potatoes are digested quickly, so they tend to sharply raise blood sugar levels.

Here, Dr Applegate doesn't agree with Dr Willett. She eats potatoes almost every day. She mashes together different types – particularly the purple and blue varieties known to contain cancer-fighting chemicals – and includes the skins, which contain heart-healthy fibre and other nutrients. Also, all potatoes aren't digested at the same speed. For example, new potatoes (picked when they're young) have a low GI and break down more slowly, so their sugar hits the bloodstream less rapidly than that of mature whites and russets – and, of course, any type that's mashed or instant. Yams, sweet potatoes and red potatoes are also digested more slowly.

No one knows for sure why potatoes vary so much in terms of their effect on blood sugar, although some nutritionists suspect that the amount of starch a potato contains may be a factor. New potatoes contain less starch than more mature potatoes, and deeper-coloured varieties (yellows, reds and blues) contain less starch than white potatoes. Eating the skin can further slow the digestive process.

Dr Applegate agrees that high-sugar diets are bad for certain people, but she maintains that because potatoes are, after all, a plant food containing fibre and nutrients, they're certainly not as bad as soft drinks and other vitamin-deficient processed foods.

### Red meat: taken in small amounts

As with the potato debate, the arguments over red meat consumption can also get heated. Nutritionists often put red meat in the same category as butter, cream and other foods high in saturated fat. To fight back, the meat industry began promoting cuts of beef that rivalled chicken and turkey for leanness. Although lean red meat was enough to placate some nutritionists, Dr Willett and others say it still belongs at the pinnacle of the pyramid. Not only is heart disease a concern, he says, but there are colon and prostate cancer to consider as well.

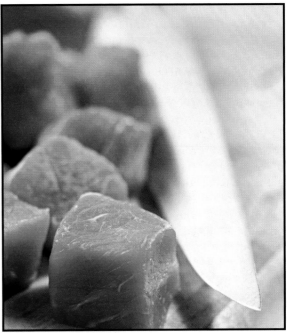

Dangerous or benign? Meat may not raise your cholesterol levels, but some experts now suspect a cancer connection.

'There are many studies indicating a higher risk of colon cancer with higher red meat consumption,' says Dr Willett. 'It doesn't just seem to be about the fat. It may be how it's cooked, usually at high temperatures, which produce a lot of carcinogens. Or it may even be the amount of iron. A lot of research suggests that high iron concentration can accelerate cell growth.'

However, red meat contains two nutrients – the antioxidant selenium and a fat called conjugated linoleic acid – that have been shown to fight cancer. Dr Willett would like to see beef put in a separate category from other high-protein foods. You don't have to ban red meat from your menu, he says, but you should limit yourself to no more than two servings a week.

### The debate on dairy products

When most of us were growing up, we were taught that dairy products are rich sources of calcium, making them essential for building strong bones. Yes, dairy products also contained a lot of artery-clogging saturated fat, but not if you switched to fat-free milk and yoghurt and low-fat cheeses.

Now it seems that, as with other foodstuffs, the dairy products story may not be quite what it originally seemed. Or so some US experts believe.

New evidence has been produced in the USA, which flies in the face of received wisdom on the subject. In a startling study on bone health, published in the *American Journal of Clinical Nutrition* in February 2003, Harvard researchers reported that they found no link between high calcium consumption, or milk consumption, and bone strength.

After tracking hip fractures and eating habits in 72,337 women for 20 years, they failed to find a correlation between consuming more than 700mg of calcium a day and stronger bones. However, they did find a link between higher intake of vitamin D and a lower risk of fractures.

'There really is no requirement for dairy products in the diet,' says Amy Lanou Ph.D., nutrition director for the Physicians Committee for Responsible Medicine in Washington, DC. 'The countries with the highest rates of osteoporosis are the ones where people drink the most milk and have the most calcium in their diets. The connection between calcium consumption and bone health is actually very weak, and the connection between dairy consumption and bone health is almost nonexistent.'

Dr Willett agrees. 'How much calcium do we need? It's probably greatly overstated by our current recommendations,' he says, referring to the US government's 1,000mg to 1,500mg daily allowance. 'The British government just reviewed their recommended daily allowance for calcium and came up with 700mg. From all the evidence I've seen, it looks as if the British number is closer to the right one.' The European Community recommended daily allowance is 800mg a day, and in the UK, extra calcium and vitamins are recommended for people who smoke, drink and or have a lifestyle which puts their health at risk. As for Dr. Lanou's statement that countries with high dairy consumption have high rates of osteoporosis, it is possible that some confounding factors are at work. For example, Asians may not drink much milk or consume a lot of calcium, but they may take more exercise than the average Westerner. And smoking, alcohol consumption, caffeine and high protein intake – all common in Western countries – have also been shown to weaken bones. Some fit non-smokers could probably get away with just 700mg of calcium daily, agrees Dr Applegate, but adds that most people need more.

Regardless of the calcium requirements, dairy opponents also point to the health risks of this food group. For example, a number of studies have linked dairy consumption with an increased risk of prostate and ovarian cancer. In Harvard's Health Professionals Follow-Up Study of 51,529 men, those who drank two or more glasses of milk a day were nearly twice as likely to develop prostate cancer as those who didn't drink milk. Although no one knows for sure why this is, Dr Willett suspects that high amounts of calcium may interfere with vitamin D's role in slowing cell division in the prostate.

Greg Miller Ph.D., senior vice president of nutrition and scientific affairs for the US National Dairy Council cautions that such population-based studies show only correlations, not cause and effect, and that some other factor could be at work. 'The clinical data that is available suggests that calcium is not a problem and that it may even be advantageous for cancer prevention,' he says.

Even Dr Willett isn't convinced that dairy should be relegated to the tip of the pyramid. His own pyramid recommends one or two calcium-rich

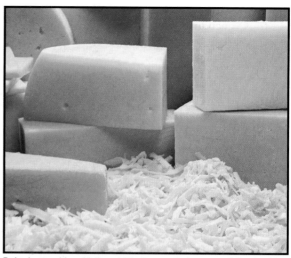

Dairy is considered by most Westerners to be essential to healthy bones. Now some US experts are beginning to challenge this view.

foods a day. 'You get different kinds of answers depending on which data you look at,' he says. 'Because there are many more studies showing harm and almost none showing benefit, it seems to me that we should be cautious about encouraging people to consume high amounts of dairy. Let's hope that in a few years we will have better data.'

In all the controversy about dairy products, it is possible to forget that there are other ways to get calcium into your diet. Many vegetables (the dark-green, leafy types), nuts and seeds are high in calcium. Fortified soya products, fruit juices and even breakfast cereals also provide calcium.

Most important for the best absorption of calcium, is an adequate amount of vitamin D, which the body makes when exposed to sufficient sunlight and is also found in some fortified foods. The vitamin helps to direct calcium into the bones and teeth.

Depressingly, the body's ability to absorb calcium starts to slow down as you age, just when osteoporosis could start to become a problem.

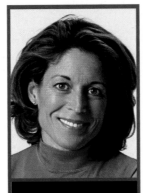

' I'm not an advocate of having dairy at every meal. You've got to look at other high-calcium food sources, too.'

**Liz Applegate Ph.D.**

Many nutrition experts in the UK recommend that older people should boost their calcium intake with a calcium supplement if their normal diet does not provide enough of this vital mineral. Many calcium supplements contain vitamin D, too.

## How flawed are the US and other dietary models?

The US pyramid recommends 6 to 11 servings a day from the grains group and 3 to 5 servings of vegetables. Surveys show that in the United States, just one person in three eats the recommended amount of grains and vegetables, and fewer than one in every five gets the minimum amount (two servings) of fruit. At the same time, Americans seriously overeat foods from the pyramid's 'use sparingly' category that includes fats, oils and sweets. That begs the question: what if they did all eat according to the pyramid? What if they actually ate five to nine servings of fruits and vegetables and followed a diet based on whole grains?

## WHITE RICE AND HEALTH
# THE CHINESE PARADOX

If refined carbohydrates are so bad, how can people in China eat white rice two or three times a day and stay as healthy as past studies have shown them to be? The answer now appears to be – they can't.

For many years, the Chinese lived in an agrarian society where, in the natural course of a day, they got plenty of exercise. Food was also scarce. Due to the regular exercise and low calorie intake, most people just didn't get fat.

Those conditions began to change in the 1950s as parts of China became more urban. This was particularly true in Beijing, where heart disease is now the number one cause of death and rates of diabetes have skyrocketed.

Life in Beijing is now similar in many ways to life in the West. People work at desk jobs and move very little during the day. During the late 1950s, the average Chinese person consumed just over 2,000 calories a day. Today, that number is closer to 2,300, yet energy expenditure has gone down. The result: weight gain.

Dr Walter Willett believes that if you're going to eat refined carbohydrates, your body handles them best when you are lean and get plenty of exercise. Exercise helps to keep muscle cells abundant and active, allowing them to mop up blood sugar more easily. As soon as you stop exercising, your metabolism undergoes complex changes that allow refined carbohydrates to push up insulin levels, raising blood cholesterol and encouraging fat storage.

'That's been a really important finding,' Dr Willett says. 'If you are sedentary and overweight, your muscle cells are probably resistant to the hormone insulin, so your metabolism won't be able to deal with these foods.'

Lack of exercise isn't the only factor in the declining health of the Chinese. As they have adopted a more urban lifestyle, they've also switched to a more Westernized diet. People in China now eat much more animal protein and saturated fat than they did many years ago, a change that could also be affecting rates of heart disease and diabetes.

'Then we would not be having some of these problems, such as our obesity epidemic. I don't care which pyramid we use,' says Jeanne Goldberg RD Ph.D., director of the Center for Nutrition Communication at Tufts University in Boston. 'The point is that we've all got to eat lots of fruits and vegetables and whole grains. The real challenge is how to move the behavioural needle and get people to change their diets.'

The UK is faced with many of the same problems. No matter how many sensible guidelines are put forward by government and health experts, changing the eating – and exercising – habits of a nation is never going to be easy.

An unbalanced, unhealthy diet is leading Britons into obesity at an alarming rate. So alarming in fact, that newspaper headlines point out the dangers to children from the way they are fed at school and at home, and the type of food advertising they are exposed to. Add to these factors the increasing trend towards computer-based activities and the 'couch-potato' mentality which keeps them slouched in front of television, and there is a generation of young people growing up whose life expectancy may be so adversely affected that there is a possibility that they could be out-lived by their parents.

## UK guidelines for healthy eating

The UK's Food Standards Agency doesn't use a pyramid, but their recommendations do place food groups in a rough pyramid shape. At the base are grains and grain products, fruits and vegetables – all the basis of a healthy diet – next, a modest amount of protein, and then small servings of sugar and fat.

The benefits of this type of eating pattern include a lower risk of major illnesses, from heart disease to diabetes. Around the world, wherever there are people with a low level of chronic disease, researchers find diets that are 'plant-based'. There are variations, of course: the Mediterranean diet, with its emphasis on olive oil, is richer than the Asian diet, but both are high in whole grains, fruits and vegetables, and low in saturated fats.

The secret of a healthy diet lies in balance, variety and moderation. And adding exercise to sensible eating is, say the experts, the real key.

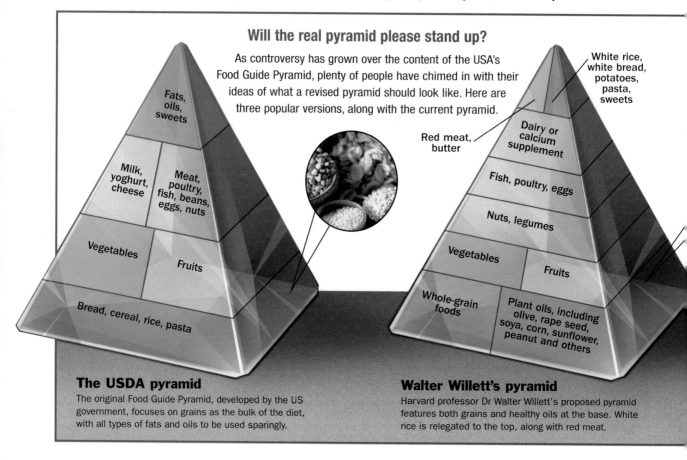

## Will the real pyramid please stand up?

As controversy has grown over the content of the USA's Food Guide Pyramid, plenty of people have chimed in with their ideas of what a revised pyramid should look like. Here are three popular versions, along with the current pyramid.

Fats, oils, sweets

Milk, yoghurt, cheese

Meat, poultry, fish, beans, eggs, nuts

Vegetables

Fruits

Bread, cereal, rice, pasta

White rice, white bread, potatoes, pasta, sweets

Red meat, butter

Dairy or calcium supplement

Fish, poultry, eggs

Nuts, legumes

Vegetables

Fruits

Whole-grain foods

Plant oils, including olive, rape seed, soya, corn, sunflower, peanut and others

### The USDA pyramid
The original Food Guide Pyramid, developed by the US government, focuses on grains as the bulk of the diet, with all types of fats and oils to be used sparingly.

### Walter Willett's pyramid
Harvard professor Dr Walter Willett's proposed pyramid features both grains and healthy oils at the base. White rice is relegated to the top, along with red meat.

# WHAT DOES IT MEAN
## TO YOU?

Although researchers and industry groups around the world may not agree on what makes up the ideal food guide, there's a strong consensus on the cornerstones of a healthy diet. They include:

● **More vegetables** Few of us eat enough. Vegetables provide fibre, vitamins and phytochemicals (plant-based compounds) that help to guard against heart disease, cancer and other serious ailments. You should aim for two, three or more portions a day.

● **A wider variety of foods** We're talking primarily about the diversity of fruits and vegetables you eat – not the types of junk food. Eating different vegetables or fruits, for example, is important because different types contain different nutrients. If you eat five servings of baby carrots a day, you're not doing your body as much good as if you had a serving of carrots (for beta-carotene, essential for good vision and resistance to infection), a helping of broccoli (for its anti-cancer

chemicals, calcium and fibre), some red or green peppers (for more beta-carotene and vitamin C for the immune system), and some dark leafy greens (for vitamin C, fibre and folate for the immune system and health in pregnancy).

● **Beans** Like vegetables, beans are one of nature's power foods. They're packed with two types of fibre that are important not only for heart health but also for bowel health. In addition, more and more research is finding that beans contain chemicals similar to those in fruits and vegetables that help to fend off disease. Add canned beans to dishes that you already eat, such as salads, soups and casseroles.

● **Whole foods** As often as possible, eat your grains unprocessed. Look for 100 per cent whole-wheat bread, for instance, and whole-grain cereals. Make switches in areas that aren't so obvious, such as choosing whole-grain pasta instead of plain.

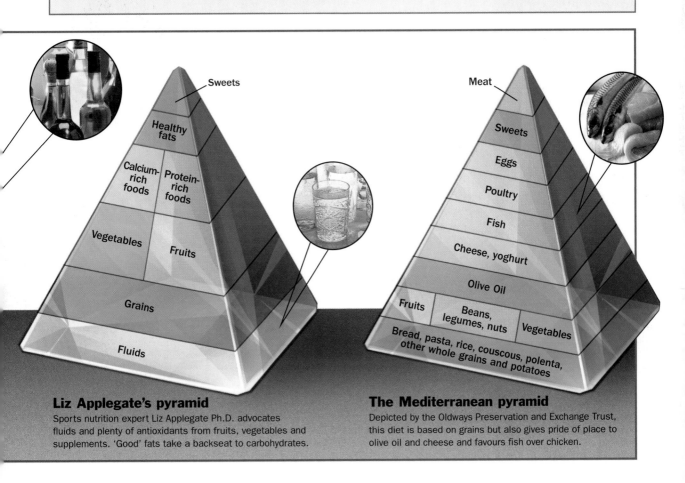

**Liz Applegate's pyramid**
Sports nutrition expert Liz Applegate Ph.D. advocates fluids and plenty of antioxidants from fruits, vegetables and supplements. 'Good' fats take a backseat to carbohydrates.

**The Mediterranean pyramid**
Depicted by the Oldways Preservation and Exchange Trust, this diet is based on grains but also gives pride of place to olive oil and cheese and favours fish over chicken.

# CANCER VACCINES

## – ON THE VERGE OF VICTORY

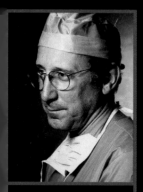

'We generated and grew in the body tumour-fighting T cells in numbers that have never before been approached.'

**Steven Rosenberg**

When John Willey joined one of the first clinical trials for the prostate cancer vaccine GVAX, at the age of 53, he had already undergone surgery, only to find that the cancer had moved into his lymph nodes. His PSA level – an indicator of how fast the cancer was growing – was rising so fast that it was giving him nosebleeds. It had increased from 3.5 to 6.4 in just a year. Levels like that, he says, 'mean that you've all of a sudden entered another realm' where life was measured in months rather than years. So when his doctor told him about the trial, he had one question: 'How do I sign up?'

Over the course of eight weeks, John Willey had 224 injections, two daily in each arm or leg. Remarkably, the only side effect was small, itchy, raised nodules where the jabs were given, similar to mosquito bites. Six months after the first injections, Willey's PSA had fallen right back to 1.2, which is just about normal for a man of his age. 'The vaccine saved my life,' says the

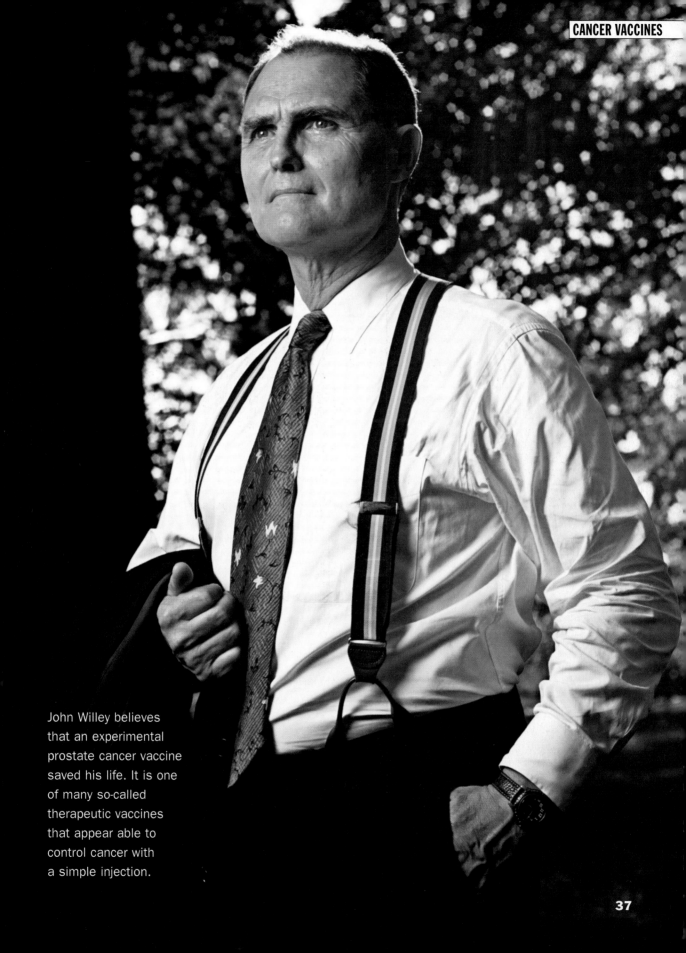

John Willey believes that an experimental prostate cancer vaccine saved his life. It is one of many so-called therapeutic vaccines that appear able to control cancer with a simple injection.

58 year-old property developer who comes from Maryland, in the USA. 'My chances of making it this far without this therapy were minimal.'

Stories like Willey's are becoming less rare as the research into the ability of cancer vaccines to limit the growth of cancers or to stop people getting them gathers pace. The vaccines are designed to stimulate

This cervical cancer vaccine uses a genetically engineered virus (*Vaccinia*) to insert a molecular tag in cancer cells to alert the immune system to kill them.

the body's own immune system to fight cancer. In the past five years, hundreds of human clinical trials of cancer vaccines have been conducted around the world and cancer conferences are dominated by presentations of the results of those trials, as well as the outcome of animal studies. But the research into this type of treatment is still at a very early stage.

Vaccines are available to people with cancer only in clinical trials because such treatment remains highly experimental. Part of the problem is that early trials designed to test the safety of vaccines can be conducted only in people with advanced cancer, for whom there is little hope. These are also the patients

who are least likely to show any benefit from the vaccine, says Jeffrey Schlom, head of the US National Cancer Institute's Laboratory of Tumor Immunology and Biology. 'The fact that we're seeing *some* clinical responses and *some* increased survival in advanced patients bodes well for the field,' he says. After years of early trials to test safety and effectiveness, some vaccines are finally moving into what are known as Phase III trials, which can be conducted with people whose cancer is not so far advanced.

## Types of vaccine

When you think of vaccines, you probably think of the injections children receive to protect them from measles, mumps and other infectious diseases. These are called prophylactic, or preventive, vaccines. They work by training the immune system to attack the disease-causing organism if it is ever detected in the body.

Some cancer vaccines are designed in this way, notably the hepatitis B vaccine, which provides protection against the virus known to cause liver cancer, and the experimental HPV vaccine, which guards against human papillomavirus that causes nearly all cases of cervical cancer. But most cancer vaccines are therapeutic in nature; this means that they're designed to bolster the immune system in its battle against existing cancers.

One major advantage of cancer vaccines is that, unlike chemotherapy or radiotherapy, which work by poisoning cancer cells and healthy cells alike, vaccines are essentially harmless to healthy cells, so side effects are practically non-existent.

Scientists do not expect these vaccines to be a magic bullet for cancer. Rather, they predict that vaccines will be used to turn an often-fatal disease – in which current treatments may produce symptoms worse than those of the disease itself – into a chronic condition that is easily controlled with a simple injection every three or four months.

To understand how cancer vaccines work, it helps to appreciate that cancer cells are very good at evading detection. Since the immune system does not recognize cancer cells as a danger, it does not try to destroy them. That is why early cancer vaccines rarely worked. In the early days, doctors simply took a piece of a patient's tumour, ground it up, subjected it to radiation so that it could not divide – then injected it back into the patient, hoping that its mere presence would stimulate the immune system to attack it. But the immune system, which had not recognized the original cancer cells, did no better with the injected cells. Cancer cells also send out signals to turn off the body's immune response – the equivalent of turning off the sprinkler system when a building catches fire.

Only a decade ago, vaccines were a minor area of cancer research. All that has changed. In the late 1990s and early 2000s, scientists found new clues about the ability of cancer cells to evade the very system that should destroy them. At the same time, they learned more about how the immune system could be prompted to pursue and destroy the cells.

## Mounting success stories

Scientists from the US Dendreon Corporation told an international conference on prostate cancer in February 2003 that they had a patient with late-stage, rapidly spreading prostate cancer who had been disease-free for 3½ years after injections of a vaccine that they had produced – a 'remarkable' response. In a study published in the February 2003 issue of the *Journal of Clinical Oncology*, doctors from Boston presented the results of their vaccine therapy on 25 patients with non-small-cell lung cancer – which accounts for 80 per cent of all cases of lung cancer. All the patients had less than six months to live when they received the vaccines; three were still alive more than four years after treatment.

One of the most dramatic stories came in September 2003, when researchers from the US National Cancer Institute (NCI), led by Steven Rosenberg, published news of their success in treating metastatic melanoma, the most deadly form of skin cancer, with a vaccine. In this case, the researchers replaced patients' entire immune systems with specially

targeted killer cells developed to attack the cancer. The treatment either stopped the cancer cells from growing or destroyed them altogether. Dr Rosenberg administered the vaccine to 13 patients, some of whom had only months to live despite previous highly aggressive treatment. One 16 year-old boy, who had been given just two months to live, was still free of disease two years later. Overall, the treatment shrank the tumours by half in six of the patients, with no growth or appearance of new tumours, while tumours disappeared completely in four patients.

In October 2003 it was announced that the first clinical trials of a vaccine treatment for melanoma would start within months in the UK. A research team at Birmingham University, led by Professor Lawrence Young, used a type of immune cell called a dendritic cell to create their vaccine. The dendritic cell plays a role in coordinating immune responses to 'foreign' invaders such as bacteria and viruses: it gathers fragments of genetic information from the invader and passes them on to other immune cells, which can then identify which cells to attack.

In this case, once dendritic cells have been extracted from the blood of the melanoma patient, genetic material from the melanoma cells themselves is added, and the dendritic cells put back into the patient. In theory, this should prompt a large-scale immune response against the tumour cells. Studies conducted in animals and on human cells in the laboratory have already shown promising results.

The growing success of the experimental use of cancer vaccines springs largely from the fact that scientists have worked out how cancer cells differ from normal cells. These differences are often too small for the immune system to notice, says cancer researcher Dr Antoni Ribas of the University

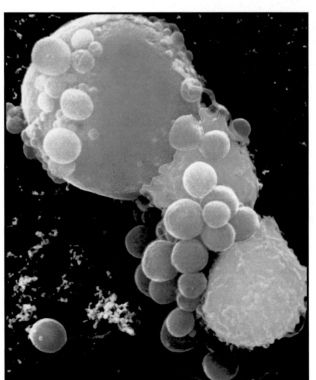

Immune cells (orange) called T lymphocytes attach themselves to a cancer cell (pink) to induce it to undergo cell death. Cancer vaccines aim to help the body to recognize cancer cells.

of California at Los Angeles (UCLA). For instance, cancer cells make certain proteins that normal cells don't make – or they make more of the proteins than normal cells do. These proteins should have the same effect on the immune system as waving a red flag at a bull – if only there were a way to get the immune system to realize the danger.

Therefore, the goal of much of today's cancer vaccine therapy is about 'breaking tolerance', that is, teaching the immune system to recognize these chemical markers as foreign – to stop tolerating cancer cells – rather than attacking them.

Researchers are focusing on three main types of cancer vaccines: as well as dendritic vaccines, there are also heat shock protein and viral vector vaccines.

● Dendritic vaccines use immune cells called dendritic cells that have been made to carry proteins from a tumour. These cells then train other immune cells to recognize the protein – and therefore the cancer cells – as bad.

● In the case of heat shock protein vaccines, doctors isolate 'red flag' proteins called heat shock proteins from a patient's cancer cells. These proteins are then injected back into the patient after the tumour has been removed to stimulate the immune system to attack any tumour cells that might remain.

● Viral vector vaccines use a harmless virus to carry tumour proteins into the patient in a kind of biological 'Trojan horse'.

## Arming the generals

Professor Lawrence Young uses a military analogy to explain the dendritic cell vaccine that he will be testing in the Birmingham University clinical study involving people with melanoma. He says that dendritic cells are like the generals of the immune system, giving orders to other immune cells. Their job is to tell the army of fighter cells (called T lymphocytes or T cells) what to attack. By loading dendritic cells with a protein that the tumour cells make, scientists make the generals 'command' the T cells to recognize this protein, or antigen, as bad, and then to attack it. 'We take the dendritic cells out of the body, educate them about melanoma, then put them back,' says Professor Young. He believes that this approach to creating a cancer vaccine could potentially be used to combat other cancers, such as prostate, lymphoma and kidney cancer.

To make the vaccine, researchers grow a patient's own dendritic cells in the laboratory. Then they either insert the cancer antigen into the cells or fuse it to them using electricity. Sometimes they insert the gene responsible for making the cancer protein into the dendritic cell so that the cell itself becomes an antigen-making factory, creating future generations of dendritic cells that also carry the cancer protein.

And it works – sometimes. 'We have occasional, rather spectacular, responses with dendritic cells, where we have patients with late-stage melanoma cancer in whom the cancers just disappear,' says Dr Ribas of UCLA. Some of those patients are still free of cancer three years after treatment. Given that every other treatment for these patients has failed, saving one out of ten or one out of five is no small feat. 'It proves that we can rationally design vaccines tailored to the patient's tumour antigens using the body's system to fight these bad things,' says Dr Ribas.

More important, in most trials, patients have an immune response to the cancer. In other words, the dendritic cells are doing their job. The big question is why can't the immune system destroy the tumours? Dr Ribas thinks one reason may be the

Dendrites are white blood cells that alert other immune cells to launch an attack. Dendritic cell vaccines use dendrites, which have been loaded with a tumour antigen, to prompt the immune system to seek and destroy cancer cells.

cancer cells themselves. 'Cancer cells make a huge array of proteins that try to turn off the immune system and they evade the immune system by turning off the dendritic cells so they don't pick up the antigens.' Researchers are looking for ways to prevent immune system cells from being 'turned off'.

## 'Shocking' the immune system into action

A second type of vaccine targets heat shock proteins (HSPs), also called stress proteins, which are present in all cells. HSPs are made when a cell undergoes any of various types of environmental stresses, such as heat, cold and oxygen deprivation. They are also made by healthy cells to 'chaperone' other proteins in the cell so that they end up in the right place. HSPs are normally found inside cells, but in a diseased cell they move outside to the cell's surface, where they act as red flags, triggering an immune response. HSP vaccines mimic the 'danger signal' sent by these extracellular HSPs.

The American company Antigenics is developing a vaccine called Oncophage by extracting HSPs from the patient's cancer cells and capturing from them the cancer's unique 'fingerprint', made of peptides, or pieces of proteins attached to the HSPs. The peptides are then injected back into the patient's bloodstream – where the immune system can find them – after the tumour is removed. The hope is that they will prompt the immune system to pursue and destroy any remaining tumour cells, which contain the same peptides.

Oncophage is one of the few cancer vaccines to have reached Phase III clinical trials in the USA – the last phase before approval by the Food and Drug Administration (FDA). At the University of Texas MD Anderson Cancer Center, where the vaccine is being tested in patients with kidney cancer, earlier trials stopped the growth of tumours in patients in advanced stages of the disease. 'That's significant,' says Dr Christopher Woods, an assistant professor at Anderson, 'because although the cancer didn't go away, it didn't grow either.' He presented the results at the May 2003 meeting of the American

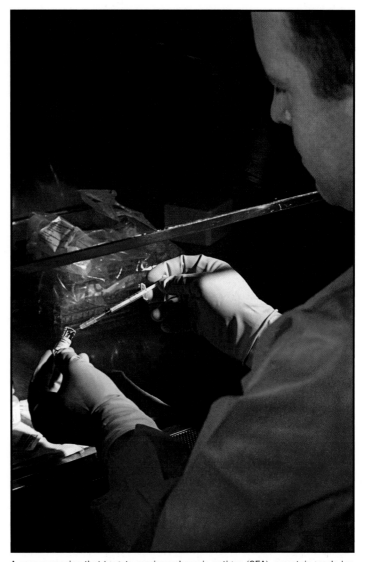

A cancer vaccine that targets carcinoembryonic antigen (CEA), a protein made by many different cancer cells, goes through one stage of preparation. The vaccine marks for destruction any cancer cells that express CEA.

Society of Clinical Oncologists. Antigenics is also conducting Phase III trials of Oncophage for the treatment of metastatic melanoma.

Researchers from the Memorial Sloan-Kettering Center in New York obtained promising results from an initial study of the effects of an HSP vaccine on ten patients with pancreatic cancer. Virtually all people who develop this form of cancer die, most within two years of diagnosis. The pancreas makes digestive enzymes that destroy proteins, so the tumour cells initially destroyed the HSP vaccine – but the scientists found a way to purify the vaccine so that it could be used, and all the patients were

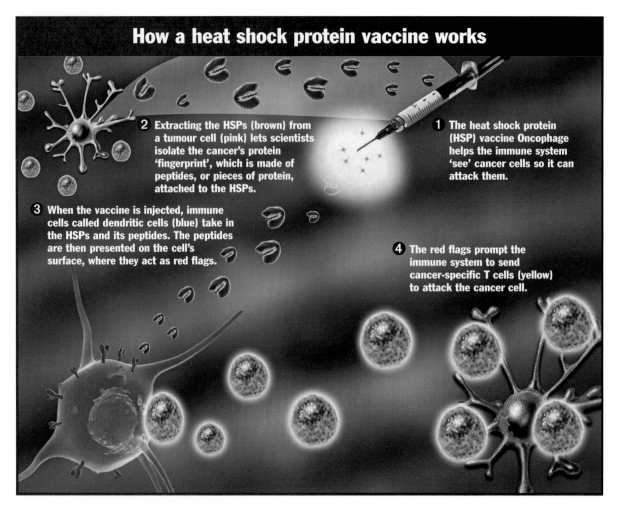

# How a heat shock protein vaccine works

**1** The heat shock protein (HSP) vaccine Oncophage helps the immune system 'see' cancer cells so it can attack them.

**2** Extracting the HSPs (brown) from a tumour cell (pink) lets scientists isolate the cancer's protein 'fingerprint', which is made of peptides, or pieces of protein, attached to the HSPs.

**3** When the vaccine is injected, immune cells called dendritic cells (blue) take in the HSPs and its peptides. The peptides are then presented on the cell's surface, where they act as red flags.

**4** The red flags prompt the immune system to send cancer-specific T cells (yellow) to attack the cancer cell.

vaccinated within eight weeks of having surgery to remove their tumours. Two were alive and disease-free two years after being vaccinated and one more was alive and well after five years. Dr Robert Maki, who led the research, says that, given the high mortality rate associated with pancreatic cancer: 'The finding of even a few patients surviving two years or more is promising regarding the usefulness of this vaccine after removal of the cancer.'

## The Trojan horse vaccine

Another type of cancer vaccine, called a viral vector vaccine, is similar to the dendritic cell vaccine, but instead of the antigen (tumour protein) being put into the patient's dendritic cells – a time-consuming, expensive and labour-intensive process – it is put into a carrier, also known as a vector. This is the approach taken by the pharmaceutical company Aventis Pasteur with its ALVAC colo-rectal vaccine, which has reached Phase II testing at several sites in the USA and Canada. The vector is a virus called canarypox, which is found only in canaries and is harmless in humans. The antigen is a protein called carcinoembryonic antigen (CEA), found in about 95 per cent of colon cancers.

In one trial, the vaccine stabilized the disease in 40 per cent of colon cancer patients in whom it was tested – a result that pleased Neil Berinstein, one of the leaders of the Aventis vaccine programme, who is a professor in the department of medicine at the University of Toronto. Several current trials in Canada and the USA combine the vaccine with chemotherapy, in the hope that the two together will have a stronger effect than either one alone. 'We're so optimistic that we're already designing Phase III trials,' says Dr Berinstein.

## Other promising vaccines

Other vaccines that have reached, or nearly reached, late-stage trials include treatments for the following:

**Breast cancer** Theratope, from the Canadian Biomira Corporation, combines an immune system enhancer, interleukin-2, with cancer-associated antigens. Phase III trials, now completed, involved 1,030 women at more than 120 clinical sites around the world. The company expects to submit its data to the FDA for approval in 2004.

**Cervical cancer**
GlaxoSmithKline plans to start advanced international trials of its vaccine to protect against the human papillomavirus (HPV), the main cause of cervical cancer, this year. The first vaccine could be ready in around three years, and it will be targeted at thousands of women aged 15 to 25. Early trials of an HPV vaccine from Merck Sharp & Dohme, involving 2,400 women between 16 and 23 in the USA, showed that the vaccine reduced the incidence of the virus by 100 per cent after one year; Phase III trials of this vaccine, involving 6,000 women worldwide, including recruits from Glasgow, London and Nottingham, are getting under way.

**Melanoma** Canvaxin, produced by CancerVax in California, is undergoing Phase III trials in patients with advanced melanoma. Earlier studies found that

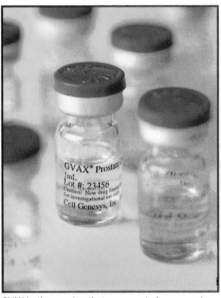
GVAX is the vaccine that appears to have cured property developer John Willey of prostate cancer.

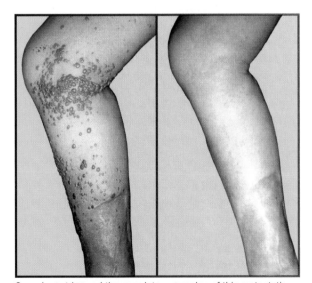
Oncophage triggered the complete regression of this metastatic melanoma 32 months after treatment with the vaccine.

the vaccine significantly increased overall survival in these patients. Another melanoma vaccine, called Melacine, is already being used in Canada.

**Pancreatic cancer** Avicine, produced by Avi Bio-pharma, was due to begin Phase III trials for pancreatic cancer in late 2003. The vaccine spurs the immune system to attack cells that express human chorionic gonadotropin (hCG), a hormone associated with pregnancy and foetal development that is also expressed in most cancer cells.

**Prostate cancer**
A dendritic cell vaccine called Provenge, produced by Dendreon, completed a Phase III clinical trial that showed that the drug significantly slowed down progression of prostate cancer and delayed onset of pain from the disease. At least one participant in the earlier, Phase II trials, who had advanced, progressive, metastatic cancer, experienced a complete remission after treatment and was still free of the disease 3½ years later.

Another vaccine aimed at prostate cancer, GVAX, from Cell Genesys, was due to enter Phase III trials in late 2003. This is the vaccine that John Willey credits with saving his life.

## What the future holds

For every cancer vaccine that reaches a Phase III clinical trial, a dozen or more begin Phase I trials, so this area of research will clearly continue to grow. Already, scientists are exploring a 'generic' cancer vaccine – one that could be used on all cancers because it targets the telomerase protein, an enzyme that helps prevent natural cell death and is thought to be involved in cancer.

'The field is moving very, very rapidly, and building on itself in terms of what is right and not right,' says Dr Jeffrey Schlom of the US National Cancer Institute.

'That is why I'm fairly optimistic that there are going to be some cancer vaccines that will be used early on in the management of a whole range of human cancers.'

# SARS A RACE AGAINST TIME

The doctor from Singapore did what doctors have to do: he treated sick patients. In this instance, the patients were sick with a mysterious form of pneumonia, but when the doctor flew to New York City in early March with his pregnant wife and his mother-in-law, he thought nothing more about it. Then the doctor began to experience the same symptoms as his patients had suffered: high fever, shortness of breath and coughing. Just before he boarded a flight back to his home country on March 15, 2003, the doctor told a colleague just how sick he felt.

The fellow health care worker alerted officials at the World Health Organization (WHO), who were already mobilized to identify and attack an unknown illness responsible for the deaths of at least four people since it first began to claim international attention in late February.

The plane had about 300 passengers and crew who were bound for 15 countries. After much debate, WHO officials grounded the plane in Frankfurt, Germany, quarantining the doctor and his family. (All of them eventually recovered.) Within hours, the agency had issued a rare global travel alert, calling the newly named severe acute respiratory syndrome (SARS) 'a worldwide health threat'.

'We not only had a disease with an unknown causative agent but we had no treatment, no diagnostic test, and we had an international outbreak that was spreading over continents in a short period of time,' says Klaus Stöhr Ph.D., who is coordinating global research on the SARS virus for the WHO.

What started off as a localized emergency had quickly become a crisis that had global implications. Dr Stöhr knew that there was not a moment to waste. He picked up the telephone to make the first of what would be 12 critical calls –

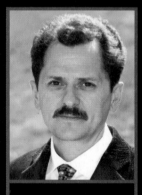

'We had an international outbreak which was spreading over continents in a short period of time.'

Klaus Stöhr Ph.D.

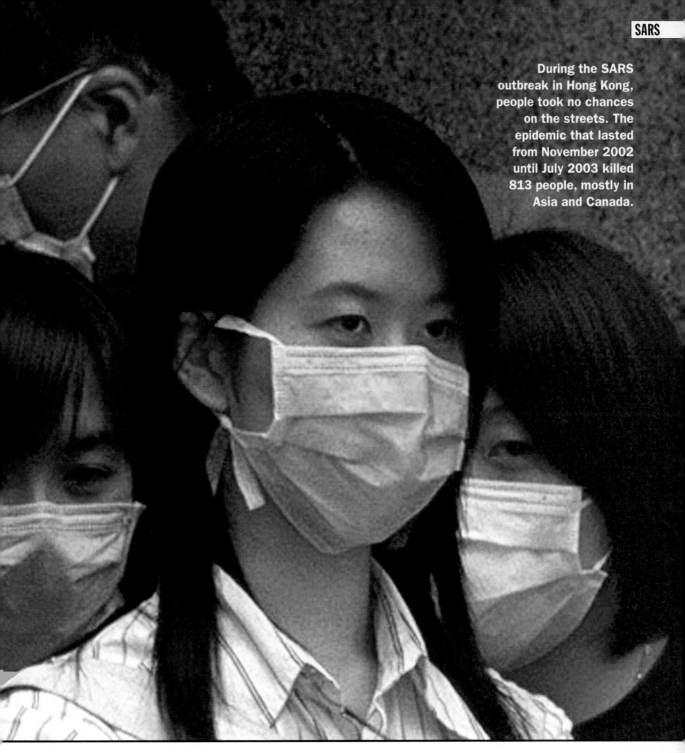

During the SARS outbreak in Hong Kong, people took no chances on the streets. The epidemic that lasted from November 2002 until July 2003 killed 813 people, mostly in Asia and Canada.

each one to a member of the WHO's global influenza network laboratories. 'We need your help,' Dr Stöhr told laboratory officials.

## The incredible shrinking timescale

Anyone frustrated by the snail's pace at which medical research often seems to move should consider the story of the SARS virus, responsible for the deadly disease that terrified much of the world in early 2003. Just 23 days after the first confirmed case of the unknown disease and 8 days after the first WHO medical alert, researchers identified a new strain of coronavirus as the cause. Three weeks later, the virus's entire genome – the genetic code that defines it – had been sequenced and posted on the internet for scientists around the world to use. Only three months after the first confirmed case, the Centers for Disease Control and Prevention (CDC) in Atlanta, USA had already submitted a diagnostic test to the US Food and Drug Administration (FDA) for approval.

Compare that with the two years it took to identify the human immuno-deficiency virus (HIV) after AIDS was first recognized in 1981. The HIV genome wasn't sequenced until the mid-1980s, a commercially available blood test didn't exist until 1985 and the first treatment wasn't approved until 1987.

With SARS, researchers responded rapidly, collaborating across different laboratories and countries. They had little choice. Today, we live in a global environment, where a single passenger on a packed aeroplane can spread a virus to nearly every continent within a few hours.

The unprecedented speed in identifying the virus and sequencing its genome was possible, say those familiar with the process, because of a confluence of technology, new communication techniques (web pages, list servers and email didn't exist in 1981, when AIDS first struck) and a greater appreciation of the risks posed by new infections in a global environment. 'It shows that complementary work in a competitive environment, knowing a public health emergency exists, can propel research much better than working in a closed, confined laboratory and doing these things all by oneself,' says Dr Stöhr.

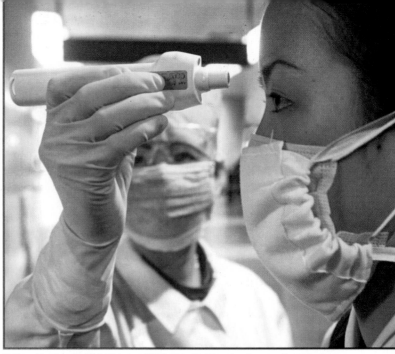

At the airport in Beijing, China, a flight attendant has her temperature checked. Airlines also screened passengers for SARS symptoms.

That's a good thing, for although officials deemed the crisis over by the early summer of 2003, they knew the reprieve was most likely temporary. SARS is expected to roar back to life, like the conventional flu, sometime in early 2004.

## Hunting down the mystery virus

The first inkling that something might be wrong came in early February 2003, when Chinese officials reported an outbreak of some form of virulent flu in the southern province Guangdong, with several hundred cases and five deaths. They assured WHO officials that the outbreak was under control, but by February 20 reports of atypical pneumonia began coming out of Hong Kong. WHO officials initially believed that the illnesses were caused by a form of the influenza virus called H5N1, an avian flu that had supposedly struck the Chinese in Guangdong as early as November 2002.

As reports of more cases began trickling into the WHO, however, along with blood and saliva samples that showed no evidence of flu, worry mounted. WHO labs in Hong Kong, the United States, and Japan began testing the samples, to no avail. 'We looked for haemorrhagic fevers, for every possible virus we could think of,' says Dr Stöhr, 'and we could not find any of them.'

Until then, officials thought the outbreak was regional, confined to the Chinese mainland and Hong Kong. But on March 10, 2003, a WHO doctor

## SARS
# THE FACTS

- By the end of July 2003, SARS had been reported in 32 countries and affected 8,437 people, 813 of whom died, according to WHO figures. In the UK, there was one confirmed and three probable cases.

- The cause is a new form of coronavirus, which belongs to the family of viruses that cause colds. It may have crossed over to humans from wild animals — probably civets, which are sold in southern China.

- Symptoms include fever, headache and muscle aches, cough and shortness of breath.

reported a cluster of similar cases in Vietnam, most affecting health care officials who had treated a patient there with the disease. The next day, officials in Hong Kong reported that their own health care workers were falling ill. Cases also began turning up in Singapore and Canada. On March 12, the WHO issued a global health alert, warning of an outbreak of atypical pneumonia and urging medical officials to report cases to authorities in their countries.

Then came the Singapore Airlines flight and Dr Stöhr's phone calls. The day after the calls, he followed up with emails, and the network of influenza laboratories held its first conference call on March 17. To get the laboratories working together and sharing information, Dr Stöhr set up a web site and arranged twice-daily conference calls.

By March 24 – barely a week after they started working on the problem – a huge international effort had resulted in the identification of the probable culprit: a mutated form of the common coronavirus, the second leading cause of colds in humans.

Sure enough, antibodies found in patient samples were able to neutralize the suspect virus. Like calling cards, the antibodies represented the immune system's past response to the virus, proving that the patients' bodies had done battle with it before. However, further tests were needed to complete the multi-step checklist that researchers use to definitively identify a virus as the cause of an illness.

That same day in March, members of the CDC team sent samples of the virus to researchers at the University of California, San Francisco (UCSF), who had recently developed a sophisticated gene chip that could quickly identify viruses. It took just one day to verify that this one was indeed a coronavirus that had never been seen before, and the UCSF researchers emailed CDC officials coded sequences of genetic material confirming the identification.

As stretches of the virus's genome were sequenced the results were continually posted on the WHO web site so that other laboratories could use it. The genome centre at the British Columbia Cancer Agency in Vancouver pulled nearly half of its 90 staff off other projects to work on SARS, and soon they hit gold. At 2.25 am on April 12 Canadian researchers announced that they had completely sequenced the genome for the SARS coronavirus. They posted the virus's genetic map on the web site later that day. On April 16, the WHO confirmed that SARS was caused by the new coronavirus.

There were several reasons for the unprecedented teamwork on this investigation and the speed with which it occurred, says Dr Stöhr. First, all the laboratories had worked together before, so they trusted each other and the WHO. Also, the WHO has the neutrality necessary to lead such a project because it wasn't competing to find the virus, it was merely coordinating the effort. Perhaps most importantly, the WHO insisted that credit would go to whichever laboratory found the virus.

'Of course we played a catalyzing role,' says Dr Stöhr. 'We gave strategic direction and initiated certain research which the laboratories might not

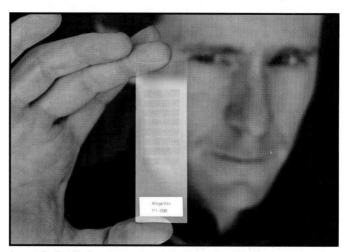

Joseph DeRisi Ph.D., a researcher at the University of California, San Francisco, holds a slide containing every known viral sequence. His laboratory identified the virus behind the SARS outbreak.

have started on their own. But we felt it was important that the laboratories saw themselves as equal partners, with no one trying to dominate their efforts or impose opinions.'

## Now for the hard part: treatment

However, the same approach is unlikely to work as well in the search for treatments and a vaccine for SARS, says Dr Stöhr. 'Drugs are commodities that cost money to produce and which will have a price. That changes the whole ball game.' But the WHO still has a critical role to play. For instance, it has created a repository of virus samples from people who were infected, from which researchers may draw. It also negotiated with the Genomic Institute in Singapore, which created one of the first diagnostic tests for the virus, to provide 25,000 free test kits to China. The WHO will continue to use this bargaining power, providing free viral samples in return for a guarantee that tests, treatments and vaccines will be provided at reduced cost to developing countries, Dr Stöhr says.

In the USA, the National Institutes of Health (NIH) has taken a leading role in coordinating the search for treatment and a vaccine. It awards grants to researchers working with coronaviruses to find drugs to combat the virus and is working with private industry to develop genetically engineered antibodies for potential use in a SARS vaccine. By early June, thousands of compounds had been screened for potential use in fighting the virus. The NIH plans to screen as many as 100,000 compounds.

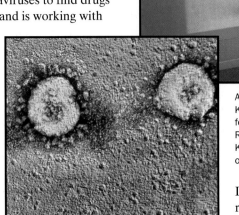

This search for a treatment wouldn't be possible without the genetic sequencing of the virus, says Earl G. Brown Ph.D., professor at the University of Ottawa in Canada and an expert on viruses. With the genetic code in hand, scientists can compare it with that of other viruses, including coronaviruses, looking for similarities. If an existing drug already works on a virus with a similar genetic code, that drug could be modified to work against the SARS virus. That way, researchers aren't starting from scratch.

At a press conference in Hong Kong, a University of Hong Kong pathologist talks about a rapid new diagnostic test for SARS. The test checks for the presence of the virus's RNA in a nasal swab or throat culture. University of Hong Kong scientists were among those who identified a strain of the coronavirus (left) as the cause of SARS.

In September 2003, Canadian researchers reported a promising breakthrough: SARS patients who were treated with interferon – an anti-viral protein – showed dramatic improvement, and 15 out of 19 of the seriously ill patients who were treated with the drug survived. The doctors used a highly potent version of interferon called Infergen.

Earlier studies conducted by researchers at Frankfurt University Medical School in Germany on the multiple sclerosis drug beta-interferon found that it can help to stop the virus from spreading and may even provide patients with some immunity against a second attack. This research was published in *The Lancet* in July 2003.

# SARS TIMELINE

**March 10–11** The disease is reported in Hong Kong and Canada as well as mainland China.

**March 15** The WHO issues a heightened global alert about atypical pneumonia, now called SARS. The alert includes a rare emergency travel warning to international travellers, health care professionals and health authorities. An international network of laboratories is established to find the cause of SARS and develop potential treatments.

**2002** **2003**

**Nov 16** A mysterious illness strikes the southern Chinese province of Guangdong. By early February 2003, five people have died and more than 800 are infected.

**March 12** The WHO issues a global alert about a new infectious disease of unknown origin in both Vietnam and Hong Kong.

**March 24** An international effort, coordinated by WHO, results in the first evidence that a new strain of the coronavirus, a virus most frequently associated with upper respiratory infections and the common cold in humans, may be the likely cause of SARS.

The CDC and the NIH are planning to conduct a large clinical trial of interferon during the next SARS outbreak. If it is indeed effective against the virus, the treatment could be available immediately.

## The holy grail: a vaccine

The best defence against an infectious disease is a vaccine because the effects are global, says Gary Nabel Ph.D., chief of the Vaccine Research Center at the USA's National Institute of Allergy and Infectious Diseases (NIAID).

Consequently, NIAID is now spearheading a campaign to produce a vaccine in a groundbreaking time-frame of three to five years – instead of the 10 to 15 years it normally takes. It's doing that by using a form of research called parallel tracking, in which animal and human studies are conducted simultaneously once the vaccine is deemed safe. (Drug companies typically take an experimental compound through animal studies first, determining its effectiveness before putting the time and money into human studies.)

Researchers at NIAID, as well as private companies such as vaccine-maker Aventis, are also pursuing two different lines of research simultaneously: they're developing an old-fashioned virus vaccine, such as the ones used for polio and smallpox, as well as a cutting-edge, gene-based vaccine in which pieces of the SARS virus are inserted into harmless viruses or other carriers, then injected into people in the hope that it will stimulate an immune response.

Dr Nabel thinks the latter approach may be the winner. Genetic vaccines, he says, tend to induce both a cellular response, helping cells resist the virus, and an antibody response, creating antibodies that attack it. Overall, he says, he's cautiously optimistic about the eventual development of a vaccine, even though more than 20 years after the identification of HIV, there is still no vaccine to combat that virus. SARS has two things going for it that HIV doesn't, he says: many patients recover from SARS, so scientists can study their immune responses and compare them with the responses triggered by experimental vaccines. Also, the SARS outbreak was contained fairly quickly, unlike HIV, which meant that the virus had less chance to mutate.

As with the early efforts to identify the SARS virus, the campaign to develop a vaccine is also taking place globally. There are collaborators in mainland China, Hong Kong and Singapore, among other countries. France's important research institute, the Institut Pasteur, and more than a dozen US and European drug manufacturers, including GlaxoSmithKline, have agreed to put aside rivalries and work together to find a vaccine.

In the UK, much concern has been voiced about the lack of measures in place to prepare for disease outbreaks. A report released by the House of Lords science and technology committee in July 2003 claimed that the NHS is ill equipped to deal with epidemics. It called for extra funding and the establishment of infection centres, responsible for disease surveillance. It also suggested key vaccines should be manufactured in the UK to ensure there are adequate supplies in the event of an epidemic.

There are also plans to create a European Centre for Disease Control (ECDC) by 2005, which would help the EU to respond more quickly and effectively to epidemics.

David Byrne, from the European Health Commission said: 'In terms of communicable diseases, we find ourselves with 19th century instruments to deal with threats of the 21st century … SARS was a wake-up call for Europe to get better prepared and to substantially enforce cooperation at an EU level.'

**April 12** Canadian researchers announce completion of the first successful sequencing of the genome of the coronavirus believed to cause SARS.

**April 16** A new form of coronavirus never before seen in humans is confirmed as the cause of SARS. (In order for any new pathogen to be confirmed as the cause of a disease, it must meet four specific conditions, called Koch's postulates.)

**April 14** CDC officials announce that their laboratories have sequenced a nearly identical strain of the SARS-related coronavirus.

**June 12** Just seven new SARS cases are reported worldwide, and the WHO says the outbreak may be coming to an end.

# STATINS
## – THE NEXT ASPIRIN

Statins have reaped plenty of glory in the past few years. After all, millions of people worldwide are taking these drugs to lower artery-clogging cholesterol and prevent heart attacks. Now experts believe that millions of other people – even those who don't have high cholesterol – should be taking them to prevent heart attacks.

But the story doesn't end there. In 2003, statins were elevated to star status as new research revealed a host of other potential benefits, including protection from diabetes, cancer, osteoporosis and Alzheimer's disease.

Currently, about one million people in the UK are using statins, which have been found to reduce the risk of heart attacks and strokes by up to 15 per cent for every year they are taken. Moreover, in the past year dozens of studies have been published in major journals or presented at major scientific meetings suggesting medical uses for statins far beyond the original objective of lowering cholesterol levels. In June 2003, diabetes experts began proclaiming that most people with diabetes, regardless of their cholesterol levels, should take statins to protect against heart disease.

With all this new evidence of statins' potential, it's no wonder that doctors around the world are calling them 'the next aspirin' and jokingly suggesting that they be added to the drinking water. It seems that, one day, statins may even surpass the ubiquitous white tablets in usefulness.

Like aspirin, statins have wide-ranging effects. They block an enzyme called HMG-CoA, which the liver uses to form cholesterol. And although cholesterol has a reputation as the 'bad boy' of modern lifestyles, it's required by every cell in the body. That's why statins' exploding potential is not surprising to

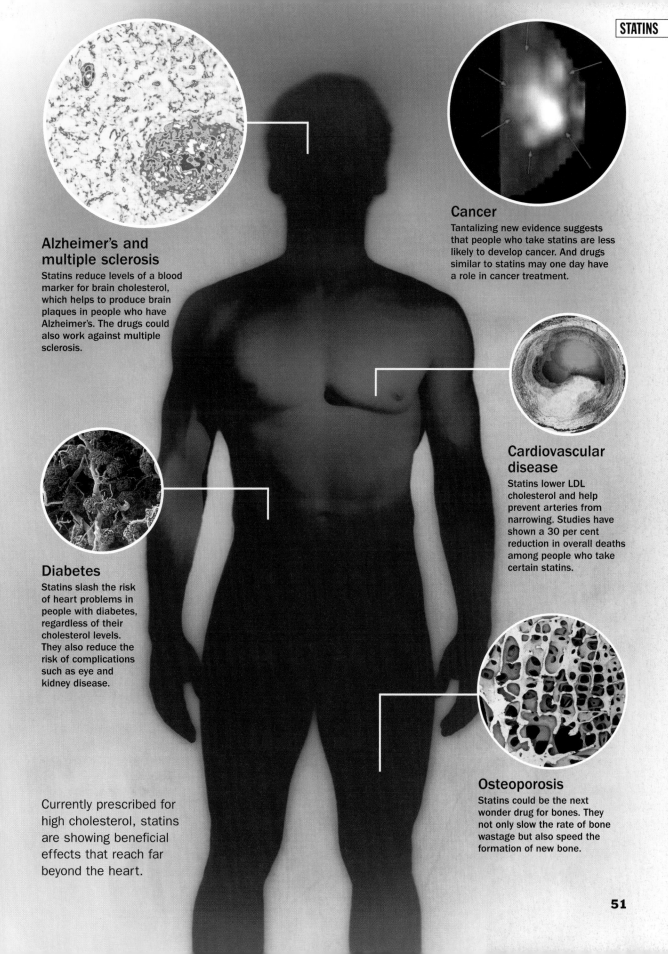

## Alzheimer's and multiple sclerosis

Statins reduce levels of a blood marker for brain cholesterol, which helps to produce brain plaques in people who have Alzheimer's. The drugs could also work against multiple sclerosis.

## Cancer

Tantalizing new evidence suggests that people who take statins are less likely to develop cancer. And drugs similar to statins may one day have a role in cancer treatment.

## Cardiovascular disease

Statins lower LDL cholesterol and help prevent arteries from narrowing. Studies have shown a 30 per cent reduction in overall deaths among people who take certain statins.

## Diabetes

Statins slash the risk of heart problems in people with diabetes, regardless of their cholesterol levels. They also reduce the risk of complications such as eye and kidney disease.

## Osteoporosis

Statins could be the next wonder drug for bones. They not only slow the rate of bone wastage but also speed the formation of new bone.

Currently prescribed for high cholesterol, statins are showing beneficial effects that reach far beyond the heart.

researcher Gloria L. Vega Ph.D, professor of clinical nutrition at the University of Texas Southwestern Medical Center at Dallas, who is examining their role in preventing Alzheimer's. 'Statins appear to be a wonder drug simply because their target is a key molecule in the life of cells.'

## Arresting Alzheimer's

Scientists weren't actually looking for a cure for Alzheimer's when they studied the effects of statins on cholesterol, but they couldn't ignore tantalizing clues that suggested that people taking the drugs were less likely to develop the debilitating brain disease. Researchers began publishing articles about their observations as early as

> ### 'Statins appear to be a wonder drug simply because their target is a key molecule in the life of cells.'

2000, but it was too early to draw any direct links. Then, in April 2003, Dr Vega and her colleagues published the first major study to show clearly that statins reduced levels of a blood marker for brain cholesterol. Brain cholesterol is thought to drive the production of beta-amyloid protein, which is implicated in the development of the characteristic brain plaques found in people with Alzheimer's.

In Dr Vega's study, researchers gave 44 people with Alzheimer's either one of three different statin drugs or a dose of extended-release niacin, which also lowers cholesterol. After six weeks, those taking the statins saw a 20 per cent decrease in the markers for brain cholesterol, compared with 10 per cent for those taking niacin. Rebecca Wood, chief executive of the UK Alzheimer's Research Trust, said 'This interesting research backs up previous results showing the protective effects of statins. It is early stages but it is certainly a promising area of research.' The study was published in the *Archives of Neurology*.

Exercise, antioxidants and now statins are thought to help stave off the development of Alzheimer's.

## Growing bone

With the news on hormone replacement therapy getting worse by the minute, doctors are on the lookout for other ways to protect bones. Now they may have found one in statins.

In an Italian study of 60 postmenopausal women, researchers gave 30 women with high cholesterol 40mg a day of simvastatin (Zocor). Another group of 30 women, who had normal cholesterol, weren't given the drug. After a year, the researchers found that bone density in the spines, legs and hips of the women taking Zocor had significantly increased, while bone density in the other women had significantly decreased. The study was published in the April 2003 issue of the journal *Bone*.

It seems that statins not only slow the rate at which bone breaks down (as shown in animal studies) but also actually increase bone density. That's critical because, until early 2003, all drugs approved for osteoporosis worked by preventing further breakdown of bone and were of little use to women who already had fragile bones. A new drug, teriparatide (Forteo) – which is currently awaiting approval by the European Union – does build bone, but it's very expensive, has significant side effects, and requires regular injections.

No one really knows how statins help to build bone, but animal studies suggest two possibilities, says Dr Douglas Bauer, associate professor of medicine, epidemiology and biostatistics at the University of California-San Francisco. One idea is that it may promote the production of a protein called BMP2, which stimulates bone-building cells called osteoblasts, and the other is that it could rein in bone-destroying cells called osteoclasts.

Similar research has been carried out both in the USA and in Britain as far back as 1999. A National Osteoporosis Society (NOS) spokesman said: 'The NOS looks forward to further studies investigating the effect of statins on bone formation and a potential role in the management of the disease.'

## Statin drug stimulates bone formation

After 14 days of treatment with the drug cerivastatin, cultures of small pieces of bone showed remarkable growth compared with untreated bone.

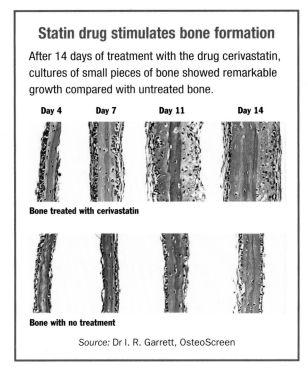

Day 4    Day 7    Day 11    Day 14

Bone treated with cerivastatin

Bone with no treatment

*Source: Dr I. R. Garrett, OsteoScreen*

## Conquering cancer

Cancer specialists are accustomed to using cancer drugs that are essentially poisons, with side effects that sometimes kill the patient before the cancer can. However, at the American Society of Clinical Oncology meeting in May 2003, the specialty's largest conference, statins took a starring role as Dutch researchers presented a study showing that people who used statins were 20 per cent less likely to develop cancer.

The greatest risk reduction occurred for prostate and kidney cancer, according to the study, which compared medical records of 3,219 people with heart disease who took statins with those of 16,976 who didn't. The connection was also strongest in people who had been taking the drugs for at least four years. Six months after they stopped taking statins, their cancer risk returned to what it had been prior to taking the drugs. Dr Matthijs Graaf from the University of Amsterdam, who carried out the research, commented: 'Given the huge prevalence of statin use, the impact on public health may be considerable.'

One theory about how statins may reduce cancer risk stems from their effect on the enzyme HMG-CoA. In addition to helping the liver form cholesterol, this enzyme reduces production of a protein called mevalonate, which in turn lowers the activity of genes that play a role in cancer development. Statins also appear to block epidermal and blood vessel growth factors, which are critical in creating the blood vessels that feed tumours.

Two studies published in the spring of 2003 looked at a statin's action on breast cancer cells. In one, French researchers found that cerivastatin (Baycol) impeded mechanisms that cause breast cancer cells to divide aggressively. Although Baycol is no longer on the market because it was linked to a rare muscle disorder, it is likely that other statins would have similar effects on cancer cells.

In another study, scientists from the University of Texas MD Anderson Cancer Center in Houston discovered that Zocor and lovastatin (Mevacor) – the latter is not available in the UK – have a unique side effect. Namely, the drugs allowed cells to maintain high levels of proteins that stop cancer cells from growing.

Interestingly, researchers noted that it was the 'inactive' part of a statin, which remains in the body after most of the drug has been taken up by the liver, that seems to have the anti-cancer effect.

'Because these statins have the ability to kill tumour cells, they have a potential role in the future treatment of a number of cancers when used in combination with other drugs,' says Khandan Keyomarsi Ph.D., lead author of the study.

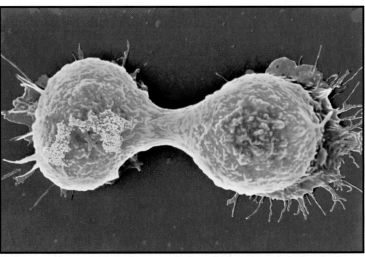

Statins seem to prevent breast cancer cells from dividing aggressively. People who take the drugs may also be less likely to develop cancer in the first place.

## Defeating diabetes

Statin drugs work so well at preventing heart disease in people with diabetes – regardless of their cholesterol levels – that, in June 2003, experts began to recommend that all diabetics take them.

The remarkable pro-statin stance came about after a major Medical Research Council/British Heart Foundation study, involving 6,000 people with diabetes, found that a daily dose of the statin simvastatin cut the risk of cardiovascular problems by about a third, even in those with normal cholesterol levels.

These findings are especially important because people with diabetes are two to four times more likely to develop heart disease than people who don't have the disease. Dr Jane Armitage, clinical coordinator of the multi-centre Heart Protection Study, said that statins could prevent a major cardiovascular problem, such as angina or a heart attack, in 45 out of every 1,000 people who have diabetes. The results were reported in *The Lancet* in June 2003.

Around one million people in the UK suffer from diabetes and experts claim that if diabetic patients are given cholesterol-lowering statins, this could prevent at least 10,000 heart attacks, strokes and other cardiovascular problems in the UK every year.

Simon O'Neill, Head of Care Developments at Diabetes UK, comments: 'We hope that all health care professionals will take this research into account when treating people with diabetes. Many people could benefit greatly if offered statins as an integral part of their diabetes care programme.'

Other research on diabetes and statins found that the drugs reduced the risk of leg ulcers, kidney disease and the eye disease diabetic maculopathy, all of which are common complications of diabetes. One of the most intriguing findings of the year was the discovery that statins may actually prevent the development of diabetes in high-risk people.

Statins prevent diabetes by increasing the body's production of nitric oxide. Without sufficient levels of this important chemical, your risk of diabetes, as well as diabetes complications, increases. Studies have found that people with Type 1 and Type 2 diabetes have a decreased ability to generate nitric oxide from food.

It is thought that an increase in the body's production of the chemical reduces the risk of insulin resistance, a precursor of diabetes. That's just what happened when Swiss researchers fed a high-fat diet to mice that lacked part of a gene necessary to make nitric oxide (and were insulin resistant) and then gave them Zocor. The levels of nitric oxide increased significantly in the mice, thus reducing their insulin resistance.

'One potential mechanism behind this effect,' says Dr Peter Vollenweider, the lead author of the study, 'is that nitric oxide increases blood vessel dilation partly in response to insulin. This increased blood flow (particularly in muscles) probably plays a role in insulin sensitivity, as it increases delivery of insulin and glucose to target tissues, thereby increasing the amount of glucose cells can take up.'

So if you're not making enough nitric oxide, this will result in insulin resistance, a major risk factor for diabetes.

The results of the study, carried out at the Institute of Cellular Biology and Morphology in Lausanne, were presented at the April 2003 American Physiological Society meeting.

> One of the most intriguing findings of the year was the discovery that statins may actually prevent the development of diabetes in high-risk people.

Narrowed coronary arteries like this one are heart attacks waiting to happen. Statins reduce heart attacks and heart disease deaths mainly by lowering levels of LDL cholesterol.

## Managing multiple sclerosis

Early studies on statins suggested that the drugs may be able to tone down an overactive immune system, leading hopeful researchers to conduct a plethora of studies on their effects on a variety of autoimmune diseases. In a study carried out in early 2003 by the Institute of Ophthalmology and University College London, researchers discovered that statins could tackle the development of multiple sclerosis at a very early stage. In laboratory and animal tests, they found that statins appear to block the immune cells that attack myelin, a protective sheath that covers many nerves in the brain and spinal cord and is damaged in multiple sclerosis (MS).

Mike O'Donovan, chief executive of the Multiple Sclerosis Society, said: 'These encouraging results in a model of MS show that statins might play an important role in the control and treatment of the disease. We hope it will not be too long before trials involving patients can be conducted.' This research was published in the *FASEB* (Federation of American Societies for Experimental Biology) journal and reinforces two separate studies carried out in the USA in late 2002.

Scientists also think that statins may help organ transplant recipients, who require huge doses of immune-suppressing drugs to prevent their bodies from rejecting donor organs. In one recent study, researchers found that lung transplant patients who took statins after their operations had a six-year survival rate of 91 per cent, compared with a rate of 54 per cent for those who didn't take the drugs.

## The future of statins

These research findings are set to revolutionize the way statin drugs are prescribed. In the UK, statins are currently only used to treat people who have heart disease and high cholesterol levels, but the results of the Heart Protection Study (HPS) are changing that. Professor Sir Charles George, medical director of the British Heart Foundation, has called for a complete review of guidelines on the use of statins. The HPS team believe that if 10 million more high-risk people were to be put on the drug, it would save 50,000 lives a year – that's 10,000 lives in the UK alone. Further research into statins' other benefits may bring even an wider use for the drugs.

In response to these calls, in October 2003 the UK government was considering whether statins might be reclassed as an over-the-counter pharmacy drug rather than being available only on prescription.

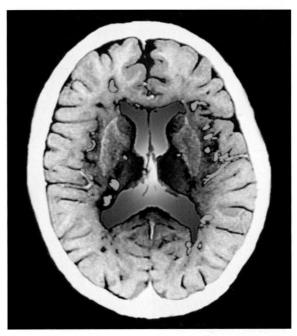

Statins could help reverse or prevent multiple sclerosis. One study found that the drugs reduced brain plaques caused by the disease (shown above in pink) by 40 per cent.

## WHAT DOES IT MEAN TO YOU?

Researchers are now discovering unexpected applications for statins, typically prescribed to lower cholesterol. One day they may be used to prevent or treat many diseases, such as Alzheimer's and other dementias, cancer, osteoporosis, and multiple sclerosis. Meanwhile, keep these tips in mind.

● If you have diabetes, ask your doctor whether you should consider taking a statin drug to lower your risk of heart disease, even if your cholesterol levels are normal.

● Don't start taking your spouse's statins. You need to talk to your doctor first about whether they're right for you. After all, no drug is without risks. Your doctor will consider your health history, your family's health history, and any risk factors for heart disease, including smoking, high blood pressure, low levels of 'good' HDL cholesterol and your age. Men aged 45 and over and women of 55 and over are at increased risk.

● Whether you have heart disease or diabetes, you cannot rely on medication to resolve the disease for you. Diet and exercise will still play a very important role.

# RNA BIOLOGY'S NEW SUPERSTAR

Most people are familiar with the idea of DNA, the strands of matter found in every cell that carry the blueprint for life. But few have heard much, if anything, about RNA, its humbler cousin. It used to be thought that RNA amounted to little more than a chemical messenger whose job was to carry instructions from the DNA to another part of the cell, where it could be turned into proteins. Now it is being touted as the key to a possible cure for cancer and other serious diseases.

A groundbreaking new approach to unravelling the mysteries of our genes has recently been hailed by *Science* magazine as 'the breakthrough of the year'. Scientists involved in the research are being talked about as candidates for a Nobel prize, and more than 50,000 researchers around the world are now using a technique called RNA interference to work out what the 30,000 or so genes mapped in the Human Genome Project actually do.

RNA interference is a natural process discovered from observing the way in which some plants and worms use tiny pieces of double-stranded RNA ('small RNAs') to 'switch off' certain genes. If scientists can use small RNAs to turn off individual genes, they can better understand the role of those genes in the body. But far more tantalizing is the theory that – by using small RNA to turn off the genes responsible for certain diseases, such as HIV, hepatitis C or a particular type of cancer – we may be able to cure them.

'Despite the massive advances in sequencing the DNA in the human genome, the function of most of our genes remains a mystery,' says Sir Paul Nurse, chief executive of Cancer Research UK. 'The next big challenge is to work out which of them are playing an important role in cancer and other diseases. Thanks to the incredible discovery of RNA interference, we should now be able to crack the problem.' In February 2003, Cancer Research UK

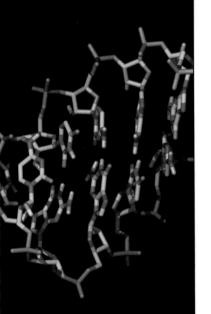

Molecules of small RNA like this one can be used to 'turn off' individual genes.

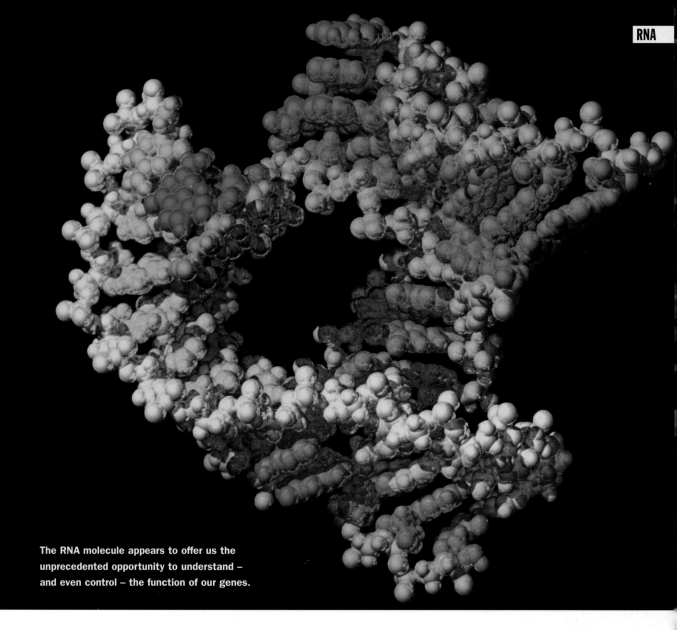

The RNA molecule appears to offer us the unprecedented opportunity to understand – and even control – the function of our genes.

launched an international initiative to use RNA interference (the ability to switch off individual genes) to systematically explore gene function.

## The workings of RNA

To appreciate what the breakthrough means, it helps to recall some basic biology. We all have 23 pairs of chromosomes – one set from each parent. Each pair contains DNA, which holds the genetic instructions for eye colour, height and everything else about us. DNA is essentially a code for making proteins, the worker bees of cells. Turning that code into proteins involves a type of RNA called messenger RNA, which makes a copy of the code and delivers it to cellular 'protein factories' called ribosomes. Scientists have long sought a way to interfere with

this information transmission to keep faulty, disease-causing genes from being translated into proteins. Enter small RNA. It appears that this RNA can ambush and interfere with 'complementary' bits of messenger RNA, inhibiting the function of a gene – hence the name RNA interference. Biologists think that in plants, and probably also in animals, the interference is an organism's way of blocking bad DNA or viruses that threaten the genome.

What's so exciting about RNA interference, says one of its pioneers, Andrew Fire, of the Carnegie Institute of Washington in Baltimore, is that it's a totally natural cellular function that scientists can manipulate for their own purposes. Because it is natural, it could be easier to work with than the artificial methods that researchers previously used.

## The case of the purple petunias

RNA's new role was discovered by accident in 1989, when plant researcher Richard Jorgensen tried to make purple petunias more purple by adding an extra copy of the purple pigment gene. In the event, the flowers came out white or purple streaked with white. Somehow, the extra gene had managed to turn off the colour-making genes. Dr Jorgensen didn't know it at the time, but the gene he had inserted into his flowers triggered the plant to make small RNA that interfered with the very process he was trying to enhance.

A few years later, Andrew Fire and Craig Mello of the University of Massachusetts Medical School, with several of their colleagues, injected double-stranded RNA into worms. (RNA is typically single-stranded, but sometimes it develops kinks that put complementary sequences of the 'letters' that 'spell' the RNA beside each other.) They found that the double-stranded RNA dramatically inhibited the genes the scientists were targeting. In that way, RNA interference was born.

The only problem was that the double-stranded RNA did not work in humans and other mammals. Other researchers trimmed the double-stranded RNA molecules, creating their own small RNA and enabling the use of RNA interference in human and other mammalian cells. A patent on the use of the technique was issued in January 2003, and has since been widely licensed in the USA, Europe and Japan to address a broad range of research questions.

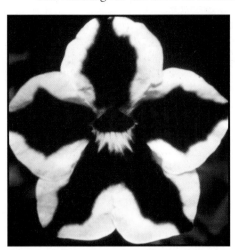
This petunia flower is streaked with white because small RNA interfered with its purple-making gene.

By allowing scientists to turn off genes, RNA interference may help them to work out what specific genes do.

Until now, explains Dr Fire, researchers who wanted to determine the role of a gene had to breed 'knockout' organisms – that is, organisms (usually mice) with that particular gene 'knocked out', or

disabled. The process took a year or more, and if the disabled gene was critical for development, the mouse would never grow properly. Also, once the animal was born, other genes couldn't be turned off.

As reported in the January 2003 issue of the journal *Nature*, scientists are now taking bits of RNA, modifying them to turn off specific genes, and setting them loose in cells, Gary Ruvkun, professor of genetics at Harvard Medical school, and his colleagues, along with collaborators in the UK, used the RNA interference technique to turn off almost all a worm's genes, one at a time, to discover those linked to obesity.

**If you work out the genes responsible for obesity in humans, the argument goes, you could develop drugs to interfere with the actions of those genes.**

If you work out the genes responsible for obesity in humans, the argument goes, you could develop drugs to interfere with the actions of those genes. Even better, you could send a modified form of RNA into human cells to turn them off.

## A future cure for cancer?

Researchers are already considering ways to use RNA interference technology to treat diseases, many of which are caused when genes produce too much of the protein they are designed to make – a phenomenon called 'gene over-expression'. The beauty of the technique is that it is not an all-or-nothing approach. Instead of turning off a gene completely, RNA can act as a dimmer switch, reducing the gene's expression a little or a lot.

Researchers have used the technology to turn off just one copy of a disease-causing gene and leave the healthy gene alone. (Remember, everyone has two copies, one from mother and one from father.) Such efforts have great potential in treating diseases such as Huntington's chorea and some cancers.

This is the approach planned in the project by Cancer Research UK, which will be undertaken in collaboration with the Netherlands Cancer Research Institute. Scientists working on the initiative will genetically engineer cells with DNA coding for a specific piece of interference RNA, permanently blocking a particular gene. They will also bombard cancer cells with 30,000 pieces of interference RNA in order to determine the genetic essence of a cancer cell. Treated cells will then be screened to

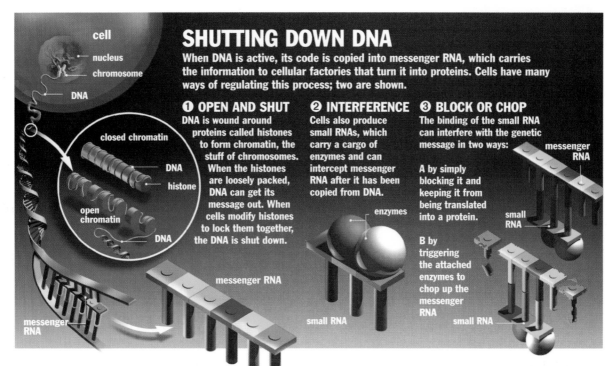

# SHUTTING DOWN DNA

When DNA is active, its code is copied into messenger RNA, which carries the information to cellular factories that turn it into proteins. Cells have many ways of regulating this process; two are shown.

### ❶ OPEN AND SHUT
DNA is wound around proteins called histones to form chromatin, the stuff of chromosomes. When the histones are loosely packed, DNA can get its message out. When cells modify histones to lock them together, the DNA is shut down.

### ❷ INTERFERENCE
Cells also produce small RNAs, which carry a cargo of enzymes and can intercept messenger RNA after it has been copied from DNA.

### ❸ BLOCK OR CHOP
The binding of the small RNA can interfere with the genetic message in two ways:

A by simply blocking it and keeping it from being translated into a protein.

B by triggering the attached enzymes to chop up the messenger RNA

find the few that have reverted to type and become normal again. The set of genes switched off by RNA interference in these cells may represent the most crucial group of cancer genes in the human genome and are likely to be very good targets of future anticancer drugs.

'Using RNA interference, we should be able to find out precisely what we need to take away from a cancerous cell in order to make it normal again,' says Dr Julian Downward of Cancer Research UK, one of the leaders of the project. 'Essentially, we will be dismantling cancer at the level of its genes.'

However, clinical applications of the technique are still a long way off, according to Professor Gary Ruvkun of Harvard Medical School. 'Medicine takes a long time,' he says. 'It's like turning around a giant aircraft carrier.' He compares the RNA revolution to the molecular biology movement, which began more than 25 years ago but is only now producing certain anticancer drugs and other practical applications.

So far, all experiments on RNA interference have been conducted on small animals or in petri dishes, with human trials not expected to begin until at least 2006. One challenge will be finding a way to stabilize RNA in the laboratory, since it is fragile and breaks apart quickly in solution. Another problem, says Dr Andrew Fire, will be working out how to get the relatively large RNA molecule into

human cells and how to get it into the right cells. 'Delivering even small molecules to cells is an art form in itself,' he says. Pharmacologists are working on the technique. Meanwhile, medical scientists are concentrating their RNA interference research on specific diseases, as described below.

- **HIV** Several groups of researchers have coaxed human cells to produce double-stranded RNA that matches RNA sequences from the HIV virus. The strands prevent infected cells from making HIV proteins.
- **Hepatitis C** Researchers at Harvard reported that they had successfully cured hepatitis C in mice by using injected small RNA.
- **RNA-linked chromosomal defects** Scientists have found that Prader-Willi and Fragile X syndromes (chromosomal abnormalities that result in mental retardation) and chronic lymphocytic leukaemia may be linked to RNA defects. The finding suggests that, if researchers can work out what goes wrong genetically and fix it early in a foetus's development, it may be possible to avoid the defects altogether.

Dr Fire describes the mood among researchers as 'cautiously optimistic': cautious because of the false hopes often raised in the past about the potential of genetic biology, and optimistic because, if RNA interference lives up to its promise, they will have the power to control the very seed of life.

# IDENTIFYING THE REAL ALZHEIMER'S CULPRIT

For nearly a century, medical researchers have been trying to unravel a mystery first described in 1907 by the German doctor Alois Alzheimer. They have recently made enormous strides – and their new understanding about the nature of the mind-robbing disease that bears Alzheimer's name may have brought effective treatments within reach for the first time. Just as promising are advances in screening that may soon allow doctors to diagnose the disease much earlier, even before any mental decline is evident, and start treatment at the time when it can be of the most benefit.

In 1901, a 51 year-old woman named Auguste D. was taken to a psychiatric hospital in the German town of Frankfurt by family members alarmed by how disoriented and forgetful she had become. She was put in the care of Dr Alois Alzheimer, who could do little but watch as her condition steadily deteriorated. Auguste D. spent five years at the hospital, unable to remember her husband's name or to care for herself. After her death, Dr Alzheimer examined her brain and found there was what he described as a 'peculiar substance' in her cerebral cortex – thick clumps of fibres lodged between

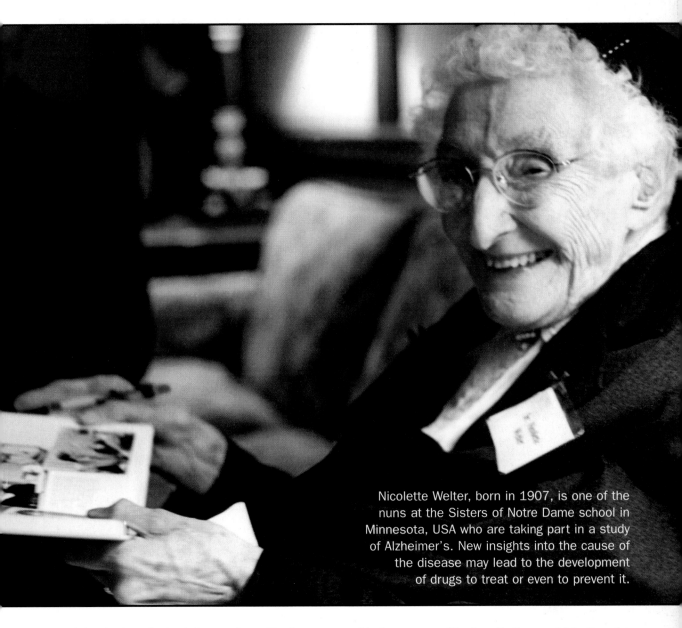

Nicolette Welter, born in 1907, is one of the nuns at the Sisters of Notre Dame school in Minnesota, USA who are taking part in a study of Alzheimer's. New insights into the cause of the disease may lead to the development of drugs to treat or even to prevent it.

remaining brain cells. And the number of brain cells was far fewer than what would have been expected in a healthy brain.

In the years since Auguste D.'s death, the fibre clumps and marked lack of brain cells have been recognized as the defining anatomical features of Alzheimer's disease, and they have been seen in the brain autopsies of many thousands of patients.

Medical detectives around the world have worked to understand what causes them and their link with the ravages of Alzheimer's. To pathologists peering through microscopes, these clumps, called plaques, look like the smoking guns in a crime scene littered with the corpses of brain cells. It was widely thought that the death of brain cells must be the problem, and the unwelcome plaques the underlying cause.

## Nasty stuff in the brain

'You see that gunk lying there between the neurons, and you think: "That must be bad for your brain," says Eliezer Masliah, a neuropathologist at the University of California in San Diego. 'It looks pretty nasty. So, for years, based on what Dr Alzheimer had found and subsequent research, people thought: "That's the toxic agent. That's the bad thing in the brain."'

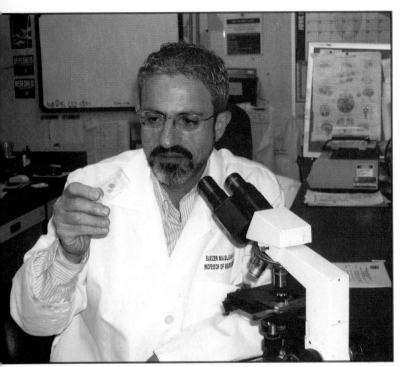

Dr Eliezer Masliah has studied the brain autopsies of hundreds of Alzheimer's patients. He is currently investigating how fragments of amyloid-beta protein in the brain may rob people of precious memory stores.

However, a few years ago, Dr Masliah and a colleague, Robert Terry, noticed that the number of plaques in the brains of patients who had had autopsies did not appear to bear much relation to the severity of their dementia. Some patients whose memory impairment had been mild had extensive plaques, while some whose dementia had been severe had few. 'There was really no correlation,' Dr Masliah says. Subsequent studies in mice have supported these findings.

Over time, the lack of a direct correlation between plaques and dementia has helped to change theories about the cause of Alzheimer's disease. Today, mounting evidence suggests that loss of memory may actually begin long before plaques ever form – even, many experts think, before brain cells start to perish. According to David Teplow, associate professor of neurology at Harvard, writing in the September 2002 issue of the *Journal of Neuroscience Research*, the 'paradigm shift' in thinking about Alzheimer's disease is that the infamous plaques may not be the real culprits at all.

## Interrupted brain signals

Dr Masliah explains that the real culprits are believed to be the sticky fragments of a protein called amyloid-beta (or A-beta) that are produced and secreted by brain cells. Over time, these tiny fragments join, forming the large clumps, or plaques, first seen by Dr Alzheimer.

It is thought that, in the early stages of the disease, the fragments interfere with communication across the synapses, the tiny gaps between neurons that must be bridged for brain signals to be transmitted. Amyloid-beta does this from both inside and outside the neurons. 'It's like a double whammy,' says Dr Masliah. He believes that mini-clusters of amyloid-beta molecules accumulate inside the neurons, in the borders of the synaptic membranes and prevent the exchange of neurotransmitters, the brain chemicals that help signals to cross the gap.

Outside the cell, says Lennart Mucke, director of the Gladstone Institute of Neurological Disease at the University of California at San Francisco, 'small assemblies of these amyloid-beta proteins float around like cruise missiles, disrupting the complex networks of neurons in which our memories are formed and stored.' Dr Mucke and other

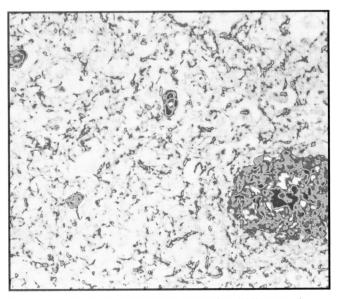

Brain plaques like the five shown above, made of amyloid-beta protein, are the hallmark of Alzheimer's disease, but scientists think they may not be what actually causes the disease.

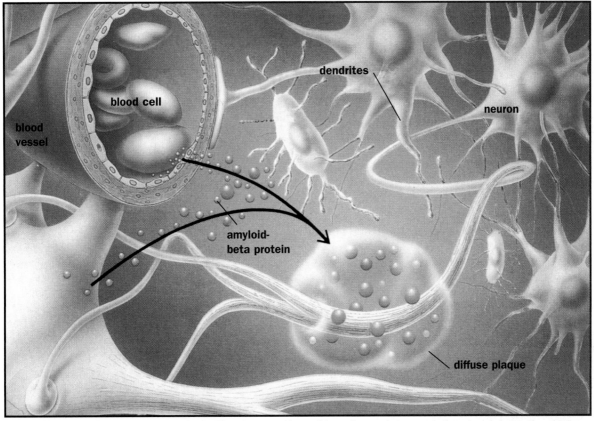

Amyloid-beta proteins are secreted by brain cells. They clump together and form plaques, but – even before plaques form – the proteins disrupt communication between nerve cells (neurons).

researchers are still not certain exactly how these floating missiles attack, but they believe that, within five to ten years, new treatments may be able to prevent or even reverse the devastating effects of Alzheimer's disease. Drug companies, eyeing a huge potential market, are pouring billions of dollars into the effort to develop effective treatments.

The treatments could take various forms. One approach is to try to prevent the production of amyloid-beta by using a drug, similar to those used against HIV, to inhibit the enzymes that help make the protein. Another strategy, says Dr Mucke, is to take advantage of the body's immune system by triggering antibodies to devour and degrade the toxic proteins that exist in the brain.

## The big tease

In 1999, Elan Pharmaceuticals announced successful tests of a vaccine that greatly reduced the creation of amyloid plaques in mice that had been genetically altered to produce human amyloid-beta. Even more astonishing was the fact that the mice, which had

developed a form of Alzheimer's, showed rapid improvement in memory and learning ability. Elan researchers tried the vaccine on 300 people with Alzheimer's. To their great disappointment, they had to call off the study in early 2002 after 15 of the patients developed brain inflammation.

Despite the setback, the experiment was not a complete failure. It provided extra evidence that amyloid-beta is the primary agent of brain damage in Alzheimer's. If the vaccine can be re-engineered, it may still prove to be a useful treatment. (For more about vaccine-like strategies, see page 87.)

Another exciting advance is the development by scientists at University College London (UCL) of a drug to treat amyloidosis, a disorder that claims the lives of 1,000 people in the UK every year. In amyloidosis, the body's own proteins accumulate as abnormal fibres that damage organs and tissues, leading to disease.

Professor Mark Pepys and his team at UCL have managed for the first time to remove from the human body a naturally occurring blood protein known as SAP that is linked to development of the disease. They first showed that SAP from the blood contributes to amyloid deposition by sticking to amyloid fibres. Then they worked with Roche to produce a drug called CPHPC that blocks SAP from sticking to amyloid. Disappearance of SAP from the blood greatly speeds up the removal of SAP from the amyloid deposits in the tissues.

Importantly, the research means that CPHPC can also be used to remove SAP from amyloid deposits in the brain in Alzheimer's disease. The first clinical studies in Alzheimer patients are about to start.

## New hopes for early detection

While some investigators explore treatment options, others are working on new screening techniques. In an April 2003 issue of the *Journal of the American Medical Association,* researchers from the National Institute of Mental Health (NIMH) reported that they could distinguish people with Alzheimer's from healthy volunteers with 90 per cent accuracy by looking at levels of two markers in cerebrospinal fluid (found in the brain and spinal cord). One of the markers, called tau, is the key element in another sign of Alzheimer's disease, the twisted strands of protein found inside neurons and known as neurofibrillary tangles. The other marker was amyloid-beta. The surprise was that the Alzheimer's patients had much lower levels of amyloid-beta in their spinal fluid than the volunteers.

Trey Sunderland, head of geriatric psychiatry at NIMH, who led the research, speculates that the amyloid-beta may get stuck in cellular membranes in the brain rather than escaping, as it should, into the cerebrospinal fluid. The same pattern was also found in 14 of 17 other studies reviewed by Dr Sunderland and his colleagues. (For news on surgery that may help to flush harmful proteins from the brain, see 'Washing away memory loss', page 84.)

A new NIMH study now under way will look at the levels of these same markers in people who have a family history of Alzheimer's disease but do not yet have any symptoms themselves. By tracking the levels of these proteins, Dr Sunderland and his colleagues hope to detect the very beginnings of Alzheimer's – before people start losing their memory. 'Our goal is to develop the equivalent of a cholesterol test for people at risk of Alzheimer's,' he says. For the moment, such a test would be of little use, since the drugs presently available to people

## THE RACE FOR A
# BREAKTHROUGH TREATMENT

University scientists such as Mark Pepys in London and Eliezer Masliah in San Diego have carried out research that has helped to identify the path to a more effective treatment for Alzheimer's disease. Now, Dr Masliah says, it is up to the drug companies.

'These companies have hundreds of chemists working on the problem,' he explains. 'They'll figure it out – probably within five to ten years.' The progress of some of the leaders in the field is described below.

● **Pfizer Inc.** dominates the existing Alzheimer's market with Aricept, one of four drugs designed to maintain brain levels of acetylcholine, a neurotransmitter involved in learning and memory. The company is also working to identify a compound that could interfere with the enzymes that produce amyloid-beta protein.

● **Elan Pharmaceuticals** suffered a major setback when the clinical trial of its Alzheimer's vaccine was halted in early 2002 after 15 patients developed brain inflammation. One of them, a 72-year-old woman, ultimately died, but an autopsy showed that the vaccine had actually succeeded in clearing amyloid-beta from her brain. Elan researchers believe their approach still holds promise and are testing two new formulations of the vaccine in the laboratory. The company has filed applications with the US Food and Drug Administration (FDA) to begin human testing.

● **GlaxoSmithKline** is searching for compounds that can inhibit enzymes involved in the production of amyloid-beta. Researchers are investigating a protein called Nogo, which may be involved in inhibiting regeneration of nerve cells. They hope that blocking the action of Nogo may allow damaged neurons to regrow.

● **Ceregene Inc.,** a San Diego biotech company, is trying a different approach: injecting into the brain a harmless virus that has been genetically modified to spur the production of nerve growth factor. The hope is that the growth factor will help keep neurons alive. Researchers are investigating two different techniques. One is now in a Phase I trial – in the USA, the earliest phase of human testing, to gauge safety – with eight people. The company has filed an application with the FDA to begin trials on the other method.

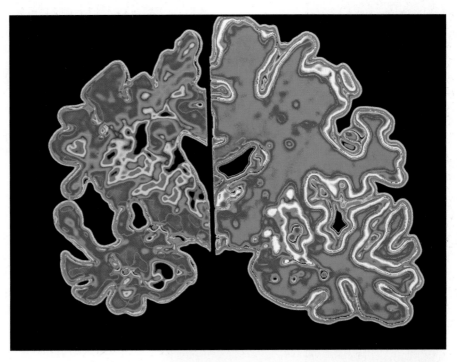

The brain of an Alzheimer's patient, shown on the left, is shrunken as a result of the death and degeneration of nerve cells. The brain shown on the right is healthy.

with Alzheimer's can't do much more than slightly slow down the progress of the disease. In fact, it could create ethical problems, says Dr Sunderland. 'It becomes a dilemma because, if you have information on who's going to get Alzheimer's disease, that can only be used today to hurt people.' Insurance companies might decline to cover them, for example, and employers might be reluctant to hire them.

Dr Sunderland hopes that this problem will be solved by good timing in the pace of medical research. 'There is a race going on between the drug companies that are developing medicines and those of us who do diagnostic testing,' he says. 'In the perfect scenario, we'd develop a marker to identify people who might get this illness at the same time as a drug company is developing a preventative agent that could be tested in them.'

One thing Alzheimer's researchers are not likely to develop is a 'cure' for the disease. The most probable scenario is that widespread screening will let people know they are at risk well before they develop a problem, allowing them to take some precautions and to manage their condition – in the same way that people suffering from diabetes or high cholesterol can do.

People who are identified as vulnerable can cut down on their cholesterol, since high levels are thought to increase risk. They can consume plenty of antioxidants, since an emerging – though unproven – theory is that oxidative damage to the brain can also increase the risk of Alzheimer's. And some will need to take the new treatments believed to be in the pipeline – and they will have to take them for life. What people will gain in the process is the ability to grow old with their minds and their memories intact.

## WHAT DOES IT MEAN
## TO YOU?

It is estimated by the Alzheimer's Society that by 2010 there will be about 840,000 people in the UK with dementia – and, if nothing changes, that number is expected to rise to 1.5 million by the year 2050. More than 50 per cent of people with dementia have Alzheimer's disease. But today's researchers are optimistic that effective treatments and tests may be just a few years away.

● Most Alzheimer's experts now agree that a protein called amyloid-beta, which is made in the brain, is the real culprit that injures the brain.

● With amyloid-beta squarely in their sights, drug companies are scrambling to develop treatments that can either block the brain from producing the protein or help brain cells to get rid of it.

● A test that could identify people who are on the way to developing the disease may also be close at hand. If the test has the hoped-for results, future Alzheimer's patients could learn what lies in store in time to do something about it.

● Lifestyle has a bearing on Alzheimer's disease. For example, high cholesterol seems to increase the risk of the disease and lipid-lowering drugs such as statins seem to help control it.

# A PUNCTURED HEART
## A DARING REPAIR

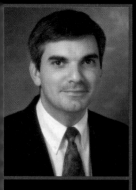

In the American town of Almont, Michigan, Dimitri Bonnville spent the summer of 2003 doing the usual things that teenagers like to do in the summer: messing around with friends, going to parties, playing basketball and generally having a good time. There was nothing special about that – except that, a few months earlier, the 16-year-old boy had been shot through the heart in a gun attack on a construction site, leading to a massive heart attack that destroyed a third of his cardiac cells. His heart was left pumping so weakly that it looked most unlikely that he would survive into adulthood.

Convinced that the condition of the boy's heart would only grow worse, the surgeons at Beaumont Hospital in Royal Oak, Michigan, made the bold decision to use an experimental procedure.

They took millions of stem cells – immature cells that can transform themselves into almost any kind of tissue cell – from Dimitri's blood and injected them into his heart to stimulate its repair. 'This treatment was the boy's only option, aside from a heart transplant,' Beaumont's chief of cardiology, William O'Neill, told the press afterwards.

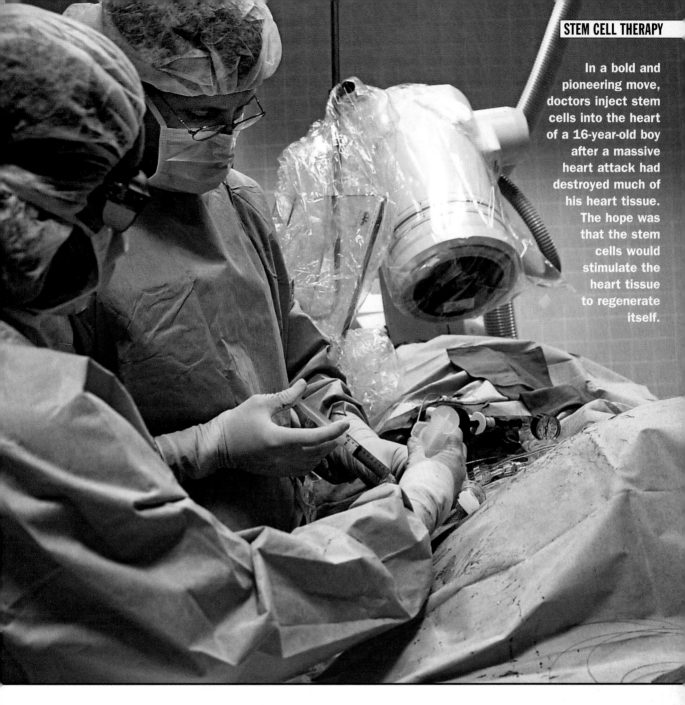

Four months later, it looked as if the surgeons had made the right decision, since Dimitri's heart function had improved enough for him to play baseball again. In the intervening period, what was described as his 'ejection fraction' – the percentage of blood pumped out of the left ventricle, the heart's main pumping chamber – had risen to 40 per cent from a low of 25 per cent after his heart attack.

Although still lower than a healthy person's ejection fraction of 50 per cent or higher, the improvement was far greater than would have been expected without the stem cell treatment, according to Dimitri's doctors. The positive outcome of the operation confirmed the potential of stem cell therapy to repair damaged heart tissue in humans.

## Progress with adult stem cells

The success of Dimitri's treatment represents the crest of a two-year wave of progress in heart repair using stem cells. In the USA and Europe, several research studies are under way into the capacity of stem cells to restore efficient cardiac function in

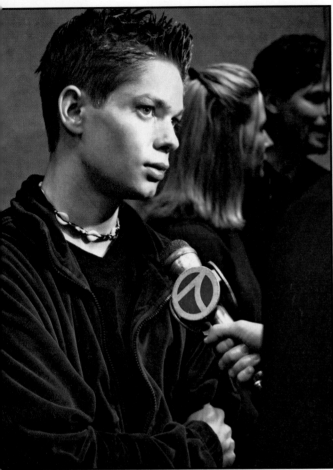

On 5 March 2003, Dimitri Bonnville wins fame as the subject of the USA's first stem-cell transplant to treat a heart attack.

people with heart failure. In 2003, reports of successful procedures using stem cells, which had resulted in measurable improvements in blood-pumping power, proliferated across the globe, notably in Germany, France, Brazil and the USA.

This followed the announcement in September 2002 of plans to build the world's first national stem cell bank north of London, which will put Britain at the forefront of research into the therapy. 'Stem cell research opens up the possibility of repairing tissue damaged or destroyed by a range of devastating conditions,' says Sir John Pattison, executive director of research at the Department of Health.

The potential of stem cell therapy to improve the condition of heart attack victims was demonstrated by scientists at Rostock University in Germany, who used stem cells from patients' own bone marrow in the treatment. The German team injected these cells into the hearts of six people who had suffered

attacks. The patients were also given conventional procedures, such as heart-bypass surgery, but all of them did well after surgery – and five had unusually good blood flow to the heart. Similar results were obtained by a team in Hong Kong who injected stem cells into eight patients, all of whom had improved heart function three months later. 'Stem cells are going to have an impact on treating heart disease, says James Willerson, the medical director and head of cardiology, at the Texas Heart Institute, reflecting general optimism among cardiologists.

That is a big change from a few years ago, when it first became widely known that days-old human embryos contain 'master cells', or stem cells, that are capable of becoming any kind of cell. At the time, scientists in some countries were already able to harvest the stem cells from embryos left over from in vitro fertilization (IVF). The goal was to treat certain diseases by manipulating the stem cells to re-create destroyed cells or tissue – to grow new nerve cells for people with Alzheimer's disease or Parkinson's disease, for example, or develop new kidney tissue for people with kidney disease.

Using stem cells to repair damaged heart tissue seemed a distant dream. For one thing, it was not known for sure whether the heart was capable of regenerating itself under any circumstances. Then, in 2001, President George Bush severely restricted stem cell research in the USA, responding to anti-abortion campaigners who opposed the medical use of any part of an embryo – even 'spare' laboratory embryos that would never be implanted into a uterus – on the grounds that it was a destruction of human life. In Britain, the use of stem cells from embryos is allowed in research, but the Human Fertilisation and Embryology Act bans their use as a source of spare body tissues for transplants.

One avenue left open for the development of stem cell therapy was adult stem cells, similarly adaptive, early-stage cells whose use was uncontroversial. There was little indication that any of these adult stem cells were capable of turning into heart cells. But diligent laboratory work and animal research revealed that the heart can indeed regenerate itself – with the help of stem cells. It also turned out that adult stem cells, especially those from bone marrow and muscle tissue, could be used, thereby avoiding ethical issues, research restrictions and any danger of rejection of 'foreign' cells by the immune system.

'Embryonic stem cells might be more potent, but adult cells are pretty good. I've never been let down by them,' says Emerson Perin, a cardiologist at the Texas Heart Institute, who has personally injected adult stem cells into human hearts.

Pure necessity is also helping to turn stem cell therapy into a reality. For example, in the UK more than 878,000 people suffer from heart failure, a deadly condition marked by the inability of the heart to pump enough blood. Even if you are lucky enough to survive a heart attack, the damaged heart tissue you are left with makes you vulnerable to advancing heart failure. Unfortunately, the best existing treatment for severe heart failure is a heart transplant. The British Heart Foundation hopes that, in future, stem cell research may allow hearts and other tissues to be grown for transplantation, ending the current system whereby patients die because of a lack of donated organs.

## Encouraging results in Rio

While Dimitri Bonnville's transplanted cells were beginning to multiply in his heart, another amazing stem cell story was unfolding in Brazil. Cardiologists from the Texas Heart Institute, including Dr Perin and Dr Willerson, had tested the transplant of stem cells on 14 people at the Hospital Procardiaco in Rio de Janeiro. All had had heart attacks and suffered from heart failure so severe that stem cell therapy was to them a great deal more than just a clinical experiment; it was their last chance.

The results were extremely encouraging. 'I saw what bad shape the patients were in before the procedure, and it's unbelievable to see how well they're doing now,' Dr Perin says. 'They were

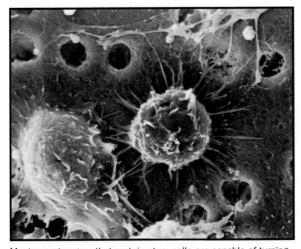
Most experts agree that certain stem cells are capable of turning into heart muscle cells, but it is not known whether that was exactly what happened in the case of Dimitri Bonnville.

## CELTIC MYTH REVIVED IN
## MASTER GENE

Imagine a not-too-distant future with an endless supply of powerful, heart-healing embryonic stem cells – which do not come from embryos. Instead of harvesting the cells from embryos, scientists have learned how to reprogramme normal body cells in the laboratory to function in the way embryonic stem cells do, and how to direct them to create precisely the kind of tissue your heart needs to be healthy.

Such a medical marvel became possible in May 2003, when researchers in Scotland and Japan said that they had identified the gene that gives stem cells their extraordinary power to transform themselves into any kind of cell in the body. Now that this master gene has been found – it was named Nanog, after a mythical land of eternal youth in Celtic folklore – the next step is to understand the conditions that activate and deactivate it. Once researchers are armed with that knowledge, they will be within reach of a Holy Grail of medical science – the ability to duplicate stem cells' regenerative powers to cure disease.

bedridden and couldn't even walk outside the house – and now these guys are jumping around, going in the water, and climbing stairs.'

On the day of the procedure, surgeons sucked out a bit of bone marrow with a needle and sent it to a nearby laboratory to filter out what was not needed (red blood cells and fat cells, among other things), keeping the mononuclear cells, a class of bone marrow cells that includes the stem cells. Within a few hours, the stem cells were ready. 'We only used the fresh stuff,' says Dr Perin. 'We didn't culture them up or grow a colony or even isolate specific types of mononuclear cells. All we did was filter and purify.' (Dimitri's doctors, some 8,000 miles to the north, varied this technique by using a drug to coax the desired cells out of the bone marrow into the bloodstream, from which they were extracted.)

Before they transferred the cells, the surgeons threaded a special 3-D camera through a catheter (a long, narrow tube) up an artery to the heart. This allowed them to identify which areas of the heart muscle were healthy, damaged or dead. Using the same catheter, Dr Perin aimed the stem cell solution at the damaged (but not dead) tissue and

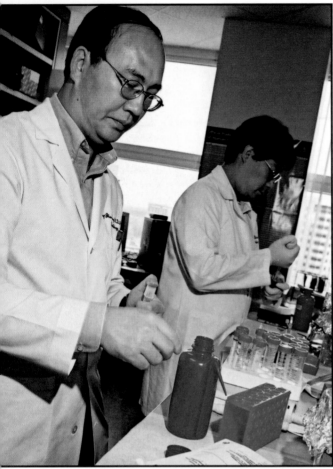

Dr Yong-Jian Geng of the Texas Heart Institute took part in the stem cell research that led to a new treatment for heart failure.

## New blood to power the heart

Dimitri Bonnville's surgeons in Michigan and the cardiologists involved in the Brazilian study doubt that the transplanted stem cells from the blood or bone marrow actually turned into heart cells. 'The reason we're putting those stem cells in there is to stimulate the growth of new blood vessels in the heart itself, not necessarily to create new heart muscle tissue,' Dr Perin says. 'That's why we insist on planting a colony of stem cells on what we call hibernating myocardium – heart muscle that's damaged but not dead. Get that hibernating heart muscle tissue a better blood supply, and it will wake up and start working again. That's what these bone marrow cells have done.' It seems that the mere presence of the cells stimulates processes in the heart that recruit other circulating cells to become blood vessel cells.

Other scientists, though, are doing research into a version of stem cell heart therapy that does seek to transform stem cells into heart cells and grow new heart muscle tissue. Rather than filtering out adult stem cells from bone marrow, these scientists are culling adult stem cells out of skeletal muscle. Unlike embryonic stem cells or bone marrow stem cells, these young skeletal muscle cells, called myoblasts, are already committed to being a certain kind of cell: a muscle cell. But – and this is the exciting breakthrough – they are not necessarily committed to being skeletal muscle cells. Recent research indicates that myoblasts can adapt to become a different kind of muscle: heart muscle. German tests in 2001 showed that myoblasts injected directly into the heart during open-heart surgery improved the pumping power of the patients' weakened hearts. In 2002, researchers at the Arizona Heart Institute transplanted myoblasts into more than a dozen people with failing hearts and also saw the desired improvements in pumping power. Imaging equipment used in the tests picked up indications of tissue regeneration – that is, new, live tissue was seen in the area of dead tissue. The hearts were apparently regrowing.

The scientists who transplant myoblasts follow a different procedure from bone marrow researchers. They take a tiny piece of calf or thigh muscle, tease out

injected 0.2cc – a couple of drops – containing about 2 million stem cells. Each Rio subject received 15 injections, for a total of 30 million stem cells.

According to results published in the May 2003 issue of the journal *Circulation*, in just two months, the subjects' 'ejection fraction' improved on average by a huge 31 per cent. Their scores in a treadmill test improved, their incidence of angina (chest pain) decreased and their blood flow improved. The gains were maintained for the following two months. Dr Willerson was confident that there would be no regression in the first year and remained hopeful that there would be even more improvement.

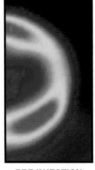
**PRE-INJECTION**

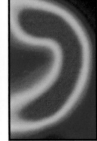
**POST-INJECTION**

A PET scan shows scar tissue becoming living tissue after a stem-cell transplant.

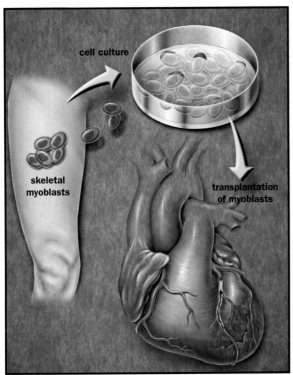

cell culture

skeletal myoblasts

transplantation of myoblasts

Skeletal muscle stem cells (myoblasts) are being used to revitalize damaged heart tissue to save patients with severe heart failure.

the myoblasts, and grow them in a culture for a few days. Once enough myoblasts have been grown, they are injected into and around dead heart tissue, the 'scar' tissue formed after a heart attack. The idea is to replace that tissue with new, live, heart muscle.

## A promising future

Dimitri Bonnville's case, the Rio results and several successful myoblast treatments indicate that stem cell therapy already exists as a viable option for people with heart failure.

To win official support for the treatment from the American government, in 2003 the Texas Heart Institute started a second study at the Procardiaco Hospital in Rio. This time, they doubled the number of heart patients receiving stem cells and refined the selection of bone marrow cells by picking the specific kinds of mononuclear cells that they suspect will be most effective for heart repair.

The results from the second Rio study should be announced some time in 2004, followed closely by results from a similar study by the same team in Houston. Plans are already being laid for a much bigger study that will involve hundreds of patients in various medical centres across the USA. With many other institutions preparing themselves for similar studies, it is possible that the US government could approve some form of cell therapy for heart repair as early as 2005.

Dimitri Bonnville and the patients in Brazil have brought real hope for heart patients around the world. As Dr Perin points out, adult stem cells are a remarkable source of renewable life that lies within us. The medical community's new-found ability to take advantage of that force to save failing hearts cannot but help to stimulate optimism about conquering heart disease.

## WHAT DOES IT MEAN
## TO YOU?

The unique ability of stem cells to transform themselves into any kind of body tissue will deliver powerful treatments for failing hearts. If the current successes in the use of stem cell therapy to repair the heart are repeated in future studies, heart patients can start taking advantage of stem cells in a number of ways.

● Stem cells transplanted from your bone marrow can stimulate the formation of new blood vessels inside the heart, reactivating damaged cardiac tissue to improve your heart's pumping capacity.

● Adult stem cells from your own thigh or calf muscles can turn into heart cells and grow into new heart muscle, replacing dead scar tissue caused by a heart attack, improving heart function and reversing heart failure.

● Cardiologists are now attempting to develop a technique for sending selected genes inside stem cells to hearts that are failing. This clever combination of cell therapy and gene therapy would build blood vessels or new tissue in the heart. The combination would also either replace damaged genes or deliver new genes that have been specially altered to improve heart function.

● In the more distant future, scientists may be able to manipulate stem cells in the laboratory to create an exact replica of your own heart (as well as other organs). If you need a heart transplant, there will be no need to wait for a compatible donor – there will be a perfect heart waiting for you.

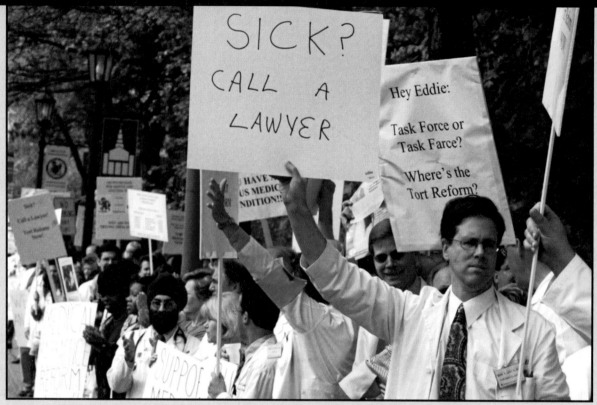

Doctors in Pennsylvania, USA protest about the dramatically rising cost of malpractice insurance premiums; in Britain, the NHS foots the bill for successful claims against hospital doctors, who enjoy crown indemnity, but premiums are rising for GPs and private consultants.

# Medical negligence claims – new government proposals

Patients whose treatment goes wrong could receive up to £30,000 compensation without cases going to court under government proposals for dealing with cases of alleged medical negligence. The new system, outlined in June 2003, also suggests 'no-fault' compensation for babies born with severe brain damage. In addition, health service staff will be obliged to inform patients if errors occur during treatment. 'Patients deserve to be told what has happened when things go wrong, and to be compensated if appropriate,' says Britain's chief medical officer, Sir Liam Donaldson.

But his report, 'Making Amends', does not suggest a universal no-fault scheme, a position criticised by the British Medical Association, which has called for measures to end 'the blame culture within the NHS'.

The reforms have been put forward against a background of crisis in the NHS over the question of alleged negligence and suspension of doctors. Annual NHS clinical negligence expenditure rose from £1 million in 1974-75 to £446 million in 2001-2. Every year NHS trusts also spend £50 million on suspending hospital staff, and at any one time some 100 doctors and consultants are prevented from working – sometimes for more than a year – while complaints against them are investigated. Yet only a small proportion of suspensions follow complaints from patients; most seem to be punishments for 'whistle-blowing' or related to rows with colleagues.

Under the new scheme, whistle-blowers who report incidents in order to improve patient safety would be given immunity from disciplinary action.

The government is aware that at present much of its clinical negligence expenditure – rather than benefiting patients – is being spent on legal and administrative costs which in most claims under £45,000 exceed the money actually paid to victims. The report also reveals that claimants' legal costs outweigh defendants' legal costs by as much as 88 per cent.

Under the new scheme, patients retain the right to sue in court, but the government aims to avoid the need for litigation. Negligence claims would be investigated by experts and payments of up to £30,000 would be awarded where serious shortcomings in the standards of care are identified and it is decided that the harm could have been avoided. Redress for people whose treatment has gone wrong might also include the provision of remedial treatment, care and rehabilitation.

Families of babies born under NHS care with severe neurological damage will also be able to claim compensation, without having to prove a hospital's negligence. As well as medical care for the child, they would be entitled to payments for other care of up to £100,000 a year, lump sums for home adaptations of up to £50,000, and compensation for pain and suffering of up to £50,000.

Under the proposals, the redress scheme will initially be applied to NHS hospitals. If successful, it will be extended to primary care. The scheme is currently limited to England but could be extended to the whole of the UK.

The medical negligence cost crisis, which sparked the proposed reforms, mirrors the situation in the USA, where compensation awards of $1 million or more are growing ever more common. Doctors in several US states have downed tools and taken to the streets to protest at the consequent spiralling costs of malpractice insurance.

# Genetic census will track 500,000 Britons

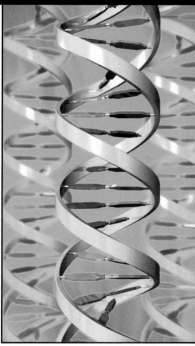

Genetic information on hundreds of thousands of people will be stored at the groundbreaking Biobank.

Easily administered gene therapy to cure Alzheimer's disease and cancer … a DNA-based early warning system for heart disease … 'personalized' medicine based on an individual's genetic traits. When will ordinary people reap these and other health benefits promised by the publication in 2001 of the rough draft of the human genome? Half a million people in Britain are volunteering to make certain that it happens sooner rather than later.

The completion of the human genome – a blueprint of the genetic information that goes to make up a human being – was a breathtaking achievement. But the human body is not a blueprint. Genetically speaking, it is a messy affair whose well-being and destiny are complicated by lifestyle choices, environmental factors, genetic differences among individuals and genes that don't appear to fit in with the plan. For us to reap the full practical benefits of the genome, researchers need to observe the influence and interaction of all these factors over time. And they need to observe the process taking place in plenty of different people.

These considerations are what British researchers had in mind when they announced a staggeringly ambitious project that will follow for decades – at the most intimate, molecular level – the health of 500,000 middle-aged Britons. Launched in 2003 and dubbed UK Biobank, the mega-project is a 'prospective' study, which will observe a group of people over time to determine correlations between what they do (or what's done to them) and how healthy they are.

What gives this study an edge over other research in the field is that the precise genetic make-up of each of the subjects will be known. Not only will environmental influences such as smoking, medication, exercise, diet and

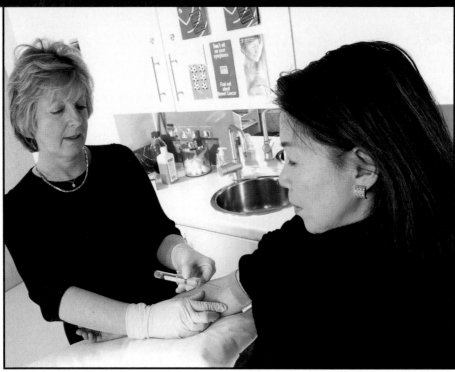

Blood samples given by Biobank volunteers may eventually reveal how individual gene variations contribute to certain diseases.

yoga every day … well, you've always wanted to give yoga a try, haven't you?

Other 'genetic censuses' are planned or under way around the world – notably in Iceland and at the Mayo Clinic in Minnesota, USA – but none matches the scope of Biobank or focuses as broadly on both nature (genetics) and nurture (lifestyle and environment).

The 500,000 people taking part in the study will be chosen from more than a million volunteers aged 45 to 69 who started signing up early in 2003. People in this age range were chosen because they are the ones most likely to develop serious illnesses in the next 10 to 20 years. The participants will give blood samples to reveal their DNA. They will also answer all sorts of questions, ranging from what they normally eat and drink to how much they earn. Then they will continue with their lives as anyone else would, except that all their subsequent health records – visits to the doctor, diagnoses, medications and so on – will be added to the Biobank database.

The availability of personal genetic information is a double-edged sword. In the hands of your doctor, it may be a blessing, but you might not want it to be accessible by your employer, for example. Such concerns have surrounded Biobank from the start, but the project organizers say they have taken the necessary precautions to safeguard privacy, at least for the study volunteers. Unlike similar projects, Biobank is a public sector initiative, conducted under the auspices of the Department of Health and two fund-raising charities, the Medical Research Council and the Wellcome Trust. By law, it must operate only for the public benefit. A monitoring body will make sure that access to the data is limited to scientists and medical researchers – and that even they won't know the names of the participants.

stress be tracked, but every individual gene variation or other personal genetic trait will be collected, evaluated and stored to create an enormous databank to help scientists answer vexing questions about the origins of disease.

For example, what combination of gene variations predisposes an individual to develop heart disease or cancer? How do those variations combine with environmental and lifestyle factors to cause disease – and how can those elements be manipulated to prevent or cure it? These big questions require study on the huge scale envisaged by UK Biobank.

How will individuals benefit once the Biobank has gathered enough information to be useful – some time around the year 2014? By then, it should be more practical and economical, if not yet routine, for ordinary people to have their personal genomes 'read'. If so, your doctor may be able to match your particular gene variations with study results made possible by the Biobank. For example, if 80 per cent of Biobank volunteers with the same variations as you developed heart disease over the course of the study, it would strongly indicate that aggressive preventive treatment is a good idea for you. If almost all of the remaining 20 per cent practised

# Live tissue hot off the presses

In an exciting advance in the engineering of animal cells, the technology that drives desktop computer printers is being used to create three-dimensional living tissue. The technique may eventually be used to create 'mini' human organs, which could be useful in testing drugs. Scientists even hope that it might one day be used to create complete organs for people who require transplants. 'The printing technology has a lot of promise,' says Professor Tim Hardingham, director of the UK Centre for Tissue Engineering, 'but there's much work to be done before we know how we can actually apply it.'

A report published in the April 2003 issue of the US journal *Trends in Biotechnology* explains how a modified ink-jet printer can produce tubes made of hamster ovary cells. Thomas Boland, one of the authors of the paper, who is assistant professor of bio-engineering at Clemson University in South Carolina, says that he and his fellow researchers are the first to print living cells in this way, although other scientists have printed more basic substances, such as proteins and DNA.

The researchers start by cleaning out an ink-jet cartridge and filling it with the living cells. Another clean cartridge is filled with a liquid that turns into a gel when sprayed onto a surface. Scientists cannot simply print cells onto any surface and expect them to stay in place, Dr Boland explains, so they use the gel to hold the cells together in a particular shape.

Using special software on the computer that is linked to the printer, they print a thin layer of the gel onto a glass or plastic slide, then print a ring of cells on top of the gel. Then they repeat the process, printing another layer of gel and another ring of

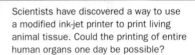

Scientists have discovered a way to use a modified ink-jet printer to print living animal tissue. Could the printing of entire human organs one day be possible?

cells, and so on. Eventually, they have many layers of stacked rings in the shape of a tube, which is embedded in the gel. The printers that are used in the procedure have been specially modified to work in three dimensions. The cartridge moves back and forth across a surface like a normal cartridge, but it also moves up and away from the surface as the printed object grows taller.

Once the stack of rings has been printed, it is put in an incubator for up to 72 hours. The incubator feeds the cells the nutrients they need to stay alive, such as protein and sugar. The rings fuse, and the researchers then wash away the supporting gel, leaving a tiny tube of living cells. Currently, the cells can be kept alive for several weeks.

The scientists have been working on this process for more than two years. 'While we have made good progress, we are still at the beginning of the research,' Dr Boland says. His next step is to print out a mouse blood vessel, which is more complex since it requires two types of cells.

This technology could some day be a boon to pharmaceutical companies, which could print out large amounts of complicated tissues to use while testing new drugs. Even farther down the road – at least 10 years, Dr Boland estimates – doctors may be able to use printers to create entire organs.

# Hydrogenated fat warning

The giant food manufacturer Nestlé announced in July 2003 that it would be removing hydrogenated vegetable fat from its Rolo and Toffee Crisp brands and investigating how it could be removed from other products. Hydrogenated vegetable fat and oil – also known as trans fatty acids, TFAs or trans fats – have been linked to clogging of the arteries and heart disease. Cadbury Schweppes said that it, too, was considering removing the fats from some of its products. 'Although the evidence is inconclusive, we are aware of rising levels of public concern:'said a spokesman for Cadbury. 'We are looking at the available options to remove partially hydrogenated fat from the limited number of our products which are a source of TFAs.'

Trans fats are most widely found in snack foods such as chips, crisps, confectionery and biscuits, and in some margarines. They are created by a process called hydrogenation, in which hydrogen is added to vegetable oil used in foods. This solidifies the oil, increasing its shelf life, and contributes to the food's flavour stability and texture, but provides no nutritional benefits. The Food Standards Agency (FSA), an independent food safety watchdog, advises people to cut down on foods containing hydrogenated or saturated fats, as well as reducing the total amount of fat they eat. 'Because of the effect they have on blood cholesterol, trans fats increase the risk of coronary heart disease,' says the FSA. 'Evidence suggests that the effects of trans fats are worse than those of saturated fats.' Trans fats raise levels of 'bad' cholesterol (LDL) in the blood without giving a similar boost to 'good' cholesterol (HDL). LDL is the chief culprit in the formation of dangerous plaques inside the artery walls that cause heart attacks and strokes. HDL, on the other hand, is believed to protect against cardiovascular disease by stopping plaques from accumulating.

In the USA, hydrogenated vegetable oil has been the subject of warnings by the Food and Drug Administration (FDA) and the National Academy of Sciences. In 2003 the FDA ordered food makers to include in the Nutrition Facts information that appears on product labels the amount of trans fats that foods contain. Until then, the only way for US consumers to know that trans fats were present in a food was to look for a phrase such as 'partially hydrogenated vegetable oil' in the ingredients list. The FDA urges Americans to consume as little trans fat as possible, while the National Academy of Sciences says that no amount of trans fat is safe.

**Evidence suggests that trans fats are worse for your health than saturated fats, according to the Food Standards Agency.**

In Britain, trans fats do not have to be included in a food's ingredients list, but hydrogenated fats are usually declared in the list – and foods that contain hydrogenated or partially hydrogenated fats will also contain trans fats.

Trans fats were already in the news in America well before the FDA ruling. In September 2002, McDonald's said that it would reduce the amount of trans fats in its chips, but later held up the proposed change, citing product quality issues.

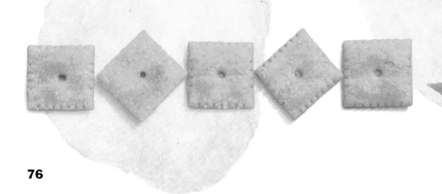

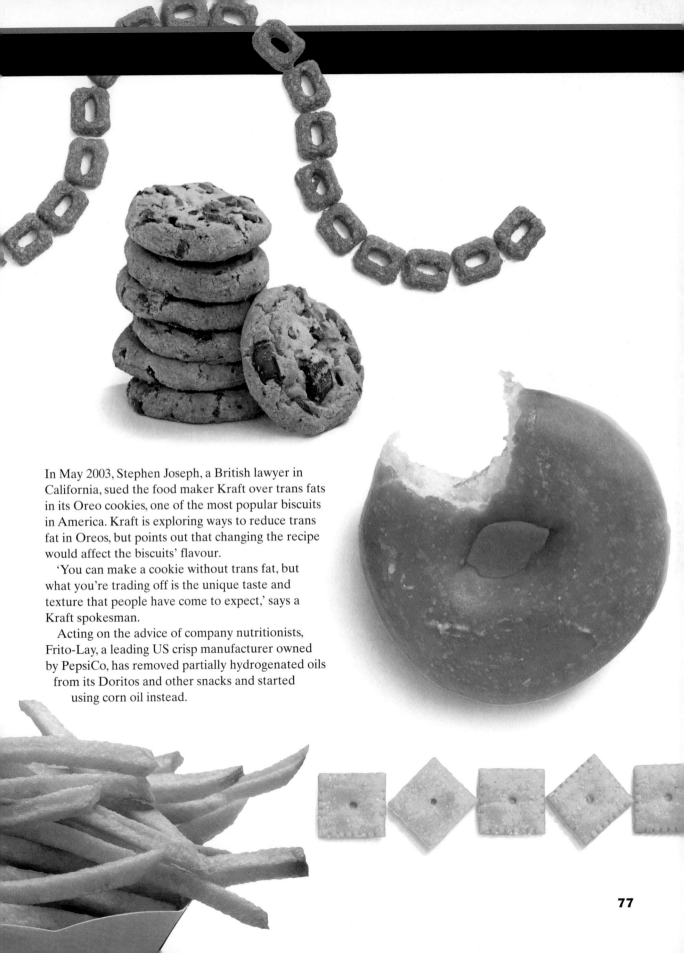

In May 2003, Stephen Joseph, a British lawyer in California, sued the food maker Kraft over trans fats in its Oreo cookies, one of the most popular biscuits in America. Kraft is exploring ways to reduce trans fat in Oreos, but points out that changing the recipe would affect the biscuits' flavour.

'You can make a cookie without trans fat, but what you're trading off is the unique taste and texture that people have come to expect,' says a Kraft spokesman.

Acting on the advice of company nutritionists, Frito-Lay, a leading US crisp manufacturer owned by PepsiCo, has removed partially hydrogenated oils from its Doritos and other snacks and started using corn oil instead.

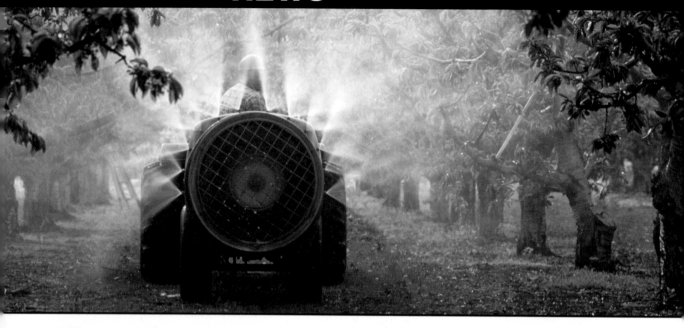

# Human body – or toxic dump?

How safe are we in our homes? Environmental campaigners fear our surroundings are much more dangerous than most people realize. A huge range of household items, from fire retardants to insecticides, contain man-made chemicals that are potentially hazardous to health, yet no one knows the precise extent of the danger.

What is known is that our bodies absorb and accumulate chemicals from the world around us and there is increasing concern about the potential effects on health. Environmental pressure groups such as Friends of the Earth (FoE) and Greenpeace have long campaigned for increased testing and banning of dangerous substances – to little avail. However, this could be about to change if proposals put forward by the European Commission in October 2003 become law.

Many of these chemicals were first produced in the 1960s and 1970s, when manufacturers were not obliged to perform even basic safety tests. None had been tested on humans, and no one knew how the chemicals might react together

– nor could anyone predict whether the chemicals might together or individually eventually lead to serious illnesses.

It is estimated that more than 100,000 chemicals that have never been tested are currently used in consumer goods ranging from cleaning products to children's toys. Some of them are suspected of causing birth defects, serious allergies, lowered sperm counts and cancer, while others are thought to be seriously harmful to the natural environment. Many of these chemicals can accumulate in body fat and are easily passed on to babies by mothers. Some are substances used in flame retardants, which are suspected of being detrimental to health, yet these are used extensively in textiles and plastics, in polyurethane foam for furniture, and in electrical appliances. Only since 1981 have chemical companies been obliged to ensure that new substances are safe before bringing them to market, and in

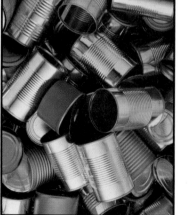

Surveys have found around 300 different synthetic chemicals in human bodies, some of which may be harmful. These include bisphenol A, found in tin can linings.

A farmer sprays pesticide over fruit trees, a requirement of modern intensive agriculture but also a potential hazard to human health.

recent years concerns have been growing about the long-term effects of chemical cocktails.

'Given our understanding of the way chemicals interact with the environment,' says the Royal Commission on Environmental Pollution, 'you could say we are running a gigantic experiment with humans and all other living things as the subject.'

Despite increasing awareness, the legacy of the early years is impossible to escape. Researchers have found traces in the human body of dangerous chemicals long since banned from commercial use, such as PCBs (polychlorinated biphenyls), once widely used in the manufacture of electrical goods, and organo-chlorine pesticides such as DDT, DDE, Lindane and HCB.

HCB has been banned in Britain since 1975 and in the European Union since 1988, but it is still used in manufacturing in some places. It has been found in air, water and organisms as far away as the Arctic, as well as in amniotic fluid, human placentas, foetuses and human milk.

Chemicals found in many household items will be more tightly regulated if the European Commission proposals put forward in October 2003 are adopted. The new environmental legislation, known as Reach (Registration, Evaluation and Authorisation of Chemicals), has been hailed as the most important development in the field in 20 years and will totally change the way chemicals are controlled.

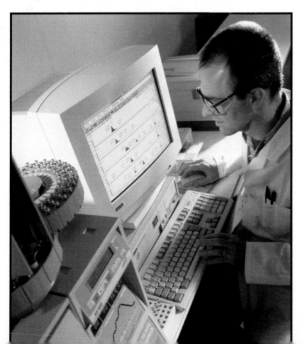

For the first time chemical companies will have to subject each substance to official screening before it can be licensed for use. The Reach process will identify potentially harmful chemicals – such as those which cause cancer or damage genetic material – and classify them as 'substances of very high concern'. One of the goals is to ensure such chemicals are phased out and replaced with safer alternatives. Although companies will have to disclose basic data on all the chemicals they produce, some campaigners insist that the regulations do not go far enough. While 30,000 chemicals would need to be registered on a new European Union database, only 6,000 of those would be subjected to testing. Just 1,500 substances 'of very high concern' would need licensing, and it is estimated that only around 2 per cent of chemicals currently on the market would have to be withdrawn. Companies could also be able to continue using known hazardous and carcinogenic chemicals even if safer alternatives exist.

'Hazardous chemicals might even be allowed to remain in everyday items such as shampoo, deodorant and toys if manufacturers can claim "adequate control",' says Friends of the Earth.

FoE is among those organizations who believe that the European Commission has capitulated to intense lobbying from commercial and political interests in Britain, France, Germany and the USA. Together with other pressure groups, it is anxious to see the enforcement of 'mandatory substitution', which would oblige companies to replace dangerous chemicals with safe ones. Manufacturers respond that such a provision could have a devastating effect on the economy in the countries affected and cause a large rise in unemployment.

One serious flaw in the legislation, according to campaigners, is that, when a substance of very high concern has been identified, it will not automatically be banned. Instead, the company producing it will have to demonstrate 'adequate control' over its circulation. 'Our concern is that it will be business as usual and companies will just carry on producing dangerous chemicals,' comments Oliver Knowles, a spokesman for Greenpeace. 'This is because the proposals do not define what they mean by "adequate" controls.'

Using a gas chromatograph, a pesticide pollution control scientist measures pesticide levels in food and analyses his results.

# PART 2

# GENERAL HEALTH

The good news just keeps coming in for health-conscious people of all ages. In the Ageing chapter, find out about a new device, a new vaccine and a new drug to fight Alzheimer's disease. And in Children's Health, read about an effective non-drug treatment approach for ADHD. The Wellness chapter is filled with surprises, including some evidence that seems to favour the controversial, high-protein Atkins diet and a warning about the potential risks of consuming certain types of fish.

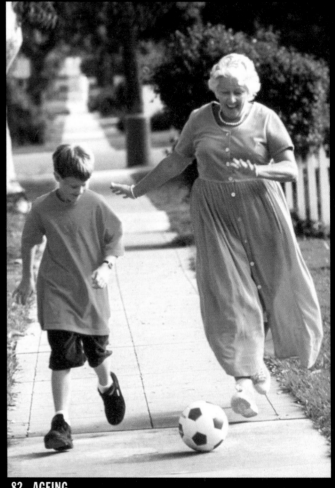

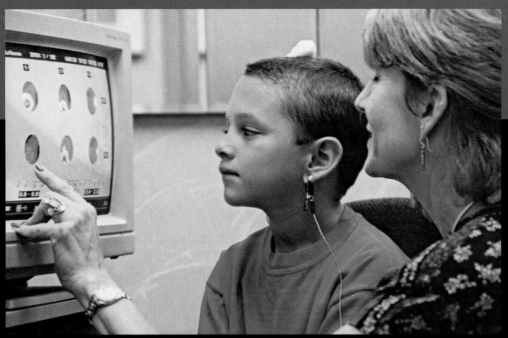

92 CHILDREN'S HEALTH

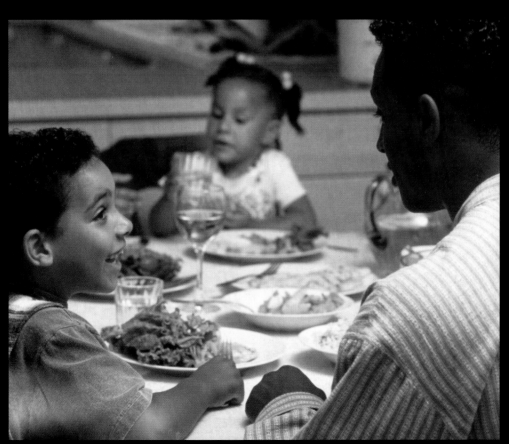

104 WELLNESS

# AGEING

## RESEARCH INTO THE DISEASES OF AGEING IS PROGRESSING BUT MANY STILL FEAR MEMORY LOSS

If you are seeking to safeguard your mind and memory, try to do some aerobic exercise (a new study links it to mental fitness) and keep your blood sugar at a stable level. One way to control blood sugar is to make sure your diet includes plenty of healthy fats – the same kind of fats that help to prevent Alzheimer's disease, according to new research.

Also on the Alzheimer's front, a new procedure that literally flushes out proteins linked to the disease from the fluid surrounding the brain may help to preserve mental capacity for people in the early stages. For those in the advanced stages of the disease, a new drug may soon be available on the NHS that should help many people to dress and feed themselves for the first time in years.

People looking to human growth hormone as an antidote to ageing have embraced new evidence that the injections boost muscle mass and reduce body fat in older people – but some experts are sceptical and worried.

## Progress in prevention

# For a healthy brain, choose fats wisely

If you are trying to do all you can to avoid Alzheimer's disease as you get older, new research points to a clear strategy: eat the right kind of fats. A US study of more than 800 older men and women found that those who ate mostly healthy fats were noticeably less likely eventually to develop Alzheimer's than those whose diets were loaded with unhealthy forms of fat. Careful choices at the supermarket today may help to keep you sharp and active for the rest of your life.

Fats linked to a lower risk of Alzheimer's include those found in vegetable oils (such as olive and corn oils), fatty fish (such as salmon and mackerel), nuts and avocados. The fats to avoid – because they increase your risk – are animal fats (from meat and dairy products), foods that are fried (in any kind of fat) and trans fats, the hydrogenated fats found in margarine and many processed foods, especially snack foods and packaged baked foods.

**How they found out** The researchers based their study on 815 people aged 65 or older, none of whom were affected by Alzheimer's. About four years later, 131 of them had developed the disease. From examining information about the subjects' diets during the study, the researchers were able to conclude that those who ate the most animal-derived or hydrogenated fats had more than twice the risk of Alzheimer's compared with those who ate the least amounts of these fats. They also found that the more of the 'good' fats the subjects ate, the lower their Alzheimer's risk. What mattered was the kind of fat they ate, not how much.

### Good for your heart, too

Although recent research in Sweden has shown a clear link between obesity and Alzheimer's disease, other studies linking diet and Alzheimer's risk have been inconclusive, so there is still no generally accepted 'anti-Alzheimer's diet'. The US 'fat' study, published in February 2003 in the *Archives of Neurology*, is promising because it parallels current thinking on the ideal fat intake necessary to avoid heart disease and promote general health. Despite the belief that all fat is bad in any amount, it is only saturated (usually animal-derived) fat and trans fats that should be kept to a minimum. These are the types that boost the level of artery-clogging cholesterol in the bloodstream. High cholesterol is a known heart disease risk and it is also thought to increase the build-up of harmful proteins in the brain that are linked to Alzheimer's.

On the other hand, unsaturated, unhydrogenated fats – the same vegetable, nut and fish fats that were demonstrated in the study to lower the risk of Alzheimer's – have been shown to be beneficial for overall health. It appears that by substituting unsaturated fats for saturated and hydrogenated fats, we have nothing to lose and everything to gain.

## Surgical solution
# Washing away memory loss

Is it possible that a tiny implanted device might be able to preserve memory in Alzheimer's patients? A neurosurgeon at Stanford University and his research team in the USA believe it is.

They have invented a special shunt – essentially a drainage tube – that appears to halt the progress of Alzheimer's disease by speeding up the natural 'flushing' of the liquid in the space between the brain and the skull.

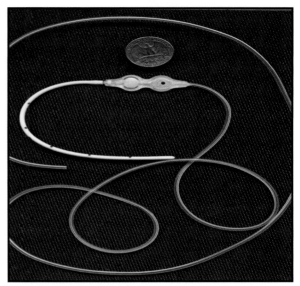

The shunt device is shown next to a small coin to illustrate its size. It is attached to a catheter that drains fluid from the brain.

BEHIND THE BREAKTHROUGHS

## Inventor of shunt says he'd use it himself - if necessary

Anyone who pioneers a ground-breaking medical treatment needs, some might argue, much the same skills as a person who commits a crime; the three important elements are: motive, means and opportunity. As the leader of the research team developing a new shunt implant to stop Alzheimer's disease, Gerald Silverberg, a neurosurgeon at Stanford University in California, has the strongest of motives.

'It's self-preservation,' he says. 'My grandmother died of what was then called senile dementia but may have been Alzheimer's. Anybody with a relative who develops Alzheimer's has a higher likelihood of getting it himself. And that might be me.'

Dr Silverberg created the means to achieve a medical breakthrough by becoming a neurosurgeon with expertise in cerebrospinal fluid (CSF), the fluid surrounding the brain. The opportunity came in the mid-1990s, when it was noticed that people with hydrocephaly, a brain disease caused by an overaccumulation of CSF, often had Alzheimer's too.

'A group of us sat down to think about what the common denominator of those two diseases could be,' Dr Silverberg says. The theoretical culprit: poor circulation of the CSF and a failure to wash away the tau and amyloid proteins that clump together in the brain. Says Dr Silverberg, 'We did some experiments and, sure enough, it turned out to be true.' A shunt to drain excess fluid from around the brain was already an accepted treatment for hydrocephaly. Dr Silverberg's team set out to adapt the shunt, turning a pressure-relieving drainage device into a constant, low-flow circulation booster.

Anti-dementia shunting had been tried as long ago as the 1960s, but it was abandoned because of mixed results and dangerous side effects. To avoid the same pitfalls, Dr Silverberg and his colleagues created a product development company and worked with engineers to build a safe shunt system designed specifically for Alzheimer's treatment. The company, appropriately enough, is called Eunoe after the 'river of returning memory' in Dante's *Divine Comedy*.

Dr Silverberg points out that the treatments available now provide only temporary memory improvement by inhibiting enzymes that break down a chemical that is crucial to memory. They do nothing to halt the progress of Alzheimer's disease and the death of brain cells that goes with it. 'If the shunt is as successful as we expect it to be, it will be the first treatment that actually alters the course of the disease,' he says.

Does that mean Dr Silverberg would consider having a shunt implant himself? 'I'm 65,' he says. 'If I start losing my memory, you bet I would.'

Like many drug treatments under study, this surgical approach seeks to prevent proteins called tau and beta-amyloid from clumping together in the brain to form the plaque deposits, which have been associated with dementia in Alzheimer's patients. But, instead of getting rid of the proteins by chemical means, the shunt literally washes them away before they can enter the brain, much as the circulating water in a fish tank keeps scum off the glass.

To test the shunt, the research team assembled 29 people who were all at a similar early stage of Alzheimer's disease. From this group, 12 were fitted with the device. After a year, they all underwent mental capacity tests and the 12 fitted with the device scored better than those who did not have the drains. The results of this pilot study were published in the October 2002 issue of the journal *Neurology*.

**How it works** Ageing normally slows down the rate at which cerebrospinal fluid (CSF), the liquid surrounding the brain, refreshes itself. In the same way that stagnant water can turn into a breeding ground for mosquitoes, the sluggish circulation makes it easy for tau and amyloid proteins to mass outside the brain and eventually enter it to do their damage.

The shunt effectively gets the flow going again by draining fluid through a tiny catheter, or tube, threaded down from the implant site in the skull, through the neck and chest and into the abdomen, where the fluid is easily absorbed. A specially engineered valve at the top of the shunt and the natural pressure difference between the head and the abdomen maintain a controlled flow that constantly removes old CSF, making way for fresh fluid produced by the body.

**Availability** Gerald Silverberg, the principal author of the research, thinks that the successful pilot study represents a promising start for two new approaches to treating Alzheimer's: preventing formation of tau and amyloid plaque by boosting the circulation of CSF, and using a shunt to do it.

A much larger study is now under way to ensure that the positive results were not a fluke. The new study will test the shunt in more than 250 Alzheimer's patients at about 25 sites across the USA. Results are expected in 2005.

## Shunt treatment for Alzheimer's

The device allows fluid from the brain to drain all the way to the abdomen, where it can be easily absorbed.

Shunt is implanted below the skin

Catheter continues under the skin to the abdominal cavity

CSF is reabsorbed in the abdominal cavity

**RESEARCH ROUND-UP**

## Silly walks could mean dementia 10 years down the road

Almost half of all cases of dementia, or mental impairment, in the elderly have nothing to do with Alzheimer's. Researchers into these disorders have now detected one indicator of future risk.

According to the results of a study published in November 2002 in the *New England Journal of Medicine*, certain abnormal gaits are reliable predictors that a person will develop dementia 10 years or more in the future. Such odd walks are almost never associated with Alzheimer's, only with non-Alzheimer's dementia.

The researchers discovered the connection by evaluating the walking styles of 422 people aged 75 and older who did not have dementia. Over the next 10 years, 55 of them developed non-Alzheimer's dementia and those identified with abnormal gaits at the start were more than twice as likely to be among those 55.

Three specific varieties of gait were the best predictors. One unsteady gait was marked by swaying, loss of balance or placing one foot directly in front of the other, as in a sobriety test. The second (called the frontal gait) was characterized by taking short steps with the feet wide apart and without lifting them off the ground. The third (hemiparetic gait) involved swinging the legs outwards in a semicircle.

The researchers hope their discovery can be used to provide an early warning of dementia and spur development of ways to prevent it.

## Drug development
# Relief at last for advanced Alzheimer's symptoms

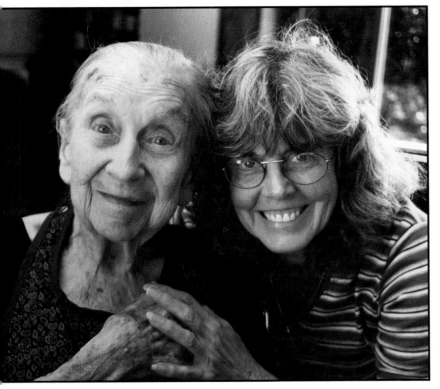

Picture a 76-year-old woman in the advanced stages of Alzheimer's disease. She looks reasonably normal, she can walk (with difficulty) and she can communicate at a basic level. However, her memory is weak, and the mechanics of everyday life, such as dressing, bathing, eating, are beyond her. What can modern medicine do for this woman? And what hope can it offer to those who love her and take care of her?

To date, very little. Existing treatments such as donepezil (Aricept) and rivastigmine (Exelon) target only mild to moderate Alzheimer's, while most experimental drugs are aimed at preventing the early stages of the disease from advancing. There is currently no approved medication for moderate to severe Alzheimer's, but that could soon change, thanks to the promising performance of a new drug called memantine (Ebixa).

In a study published in an April 2003 issue of the *New England Journal of Medicine*, the 97 volunteers with moderate to severe Alzheimer's who took memantine daily for 28 weeks scored better in tests of mental and physical function than the 84 who took placebos. More importantly, the researchers noted marked improvement in the behaviour of those taking memantine. Generally, they showed less agitation, their reasoning abilities increased and their memories improved. Many were more capable of dressing, bathing and feeding themselves and attending to their bathroom needs. Carers were able to spend fewer hours with them. While none of this means a cure is at hand, the drug's ability to offer these improvements answers many prayers from Alzheimer's patients and their loved ones.

**How it works** Memantine is being hailed as a breakthrough for two reasons. One is its application for people in more advanced stages of Alzheimer's. But the drug also works in an unprecedented way. Typical drugs for mild Alzheimer's increase the supply of a memory-aiding brain chemical called acetylcholine by limiting the enzymes that break it down. Memantine, however, quells the action of another brain chemical called glutamate, which is so overproduced in people with Alzheimer's that it damages nerve cells (neurons). Less damage means milder symptoms.

**Availability** Memantine was launched in the UK in 2002 as Ebixa. If it meets government criteria, it should be available on NHS prescription in 2005, but it may be easier to obtain in some areas of the country than in others. By that time, a treatment that combines memantine with one of the existing medications now used for milder Alzheimer's symptoms may be available for late-stage patients. Results of a newer study announced in April 2003 indicated that advanced Alzheimer's patients who took both memantine and Aricept showed marked improvement in cognitive (mental) functioning.

## Drug development

# Vaccine offers new approach to treatment of Alzheimer's

A promising vaccine for Alzheimer's disease had to be abandoned abruptly in February 2002, when test participants started showing signs of damage to the nervous system. But, fortunately for Alzheimer's patients, scientists seldom gives up.

A year later, researchers sponsored by the US National Institutes of Health and the Alzheimer's Association put forward a possible new way to achieve the same positive results as the ill-fated vaccine – without the dangerous consequences.

The potential treatment is not what would normally be thought of as a typical vaccine, such as a flu injection, which is intended to prevent an ailment. Rather, it is designed to treat existing Alzheimer's. It is called a vaccine because – like a vaccine – it triggers an immune system response to activate defender cells known as antibodies.

The failed vaccine worked from within the brain to help antibodies to remove proteins called beta-amyloids, which form the clumps, or plaques, in the brain that are associated with Alzheimer's. Researchers now think it was that activity in the brain that caused the negative reactions.

**How it works** On experiments with mice, the researchers found that two compounds, gelsolin and GM1 (substances extracted from cow brains), can reduce amyloid build-up by attaching to the proteins and ushering them away from the brain before they can enter. By working in the area surrounding the brain, gelsolin and GM1 act like nightclub bouncers, keeping the riffraff – the amyloids – from entering the premises. That approach is safer than trying to kick out the troublemakers after they have gone inside, which was what the old vaccine did.

The researchers injected gelsolin, GM1 or a placebo (dummy drug) into mice with Alzheimer's every other day for three weeks. The ones who had the gelsolin or GM1 had less beta-amyloid in their brains than the others, as well as fewer brain plaques.

**Availability** No one is suggesting that gelsolin or GM1 should be tested in humans based solely on the findings of the mouse experiments. But the authors of the study, published in January 2003 in the *Journal of Neuroscience*, say their results clearly demonstrate that beta-amyloids in the brain and the plaques they form can be reduced by drug compounds that work safely outside the brain.

Such a 'proof of concept', as it is described in scientific circles, brings us one step closer to the day when a new Alzheimer's treatment or even a preventive drug will be available.

# ALSO in the NEWS

## Strong bones for a strong mind

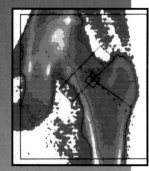

A new study establishes a much firmer link between bone loss and loss of mental function in older women. US researchers studying more than 4,000 women over the age of 70 in various US cities have found that those who experience rapid loss of bone density in the hip area are more likely to lose some mental function than those who lose bone more slowly.

Earlier research had indicated a link but the new study, published in the *Journal of American Geriatrics* in January 2003, went further, finding that the connection exists regardless of whether a woman carries the ApoE gene, the so-called Alzheimer's gene. Ruling out the gene as a factor more firmly establishes the correlation between bone loss and memory loss.

The researchers do not consider osteoporosis to be a likely cause of mental decline, nor do they foresee using bone-strengthening treatments to prevent it. But bone loss, they say, may one day serve as a warning of accelerated ageing processes or problems, such as inflammation, that promote mental decline. A doctor who thinks you are at risk of osteoporosis will probably suggest that you have a bone mineral density scan, a test that is quick and painless.

Drug development

# Debate about growth hormone gets hotter

Giving older people injections of human growth hormone (HGH) boosts their muscle mass as well as reducing their body fat, a new study confirms. The results have aroused intense interest among the growing legions of Americans dedicated to fighting the ageing process by taking supplements. But more cautious experts in the medical establishment warn that the supposed anti-ageing benefits of the hormone are unproven and its potential risks unknown.

**Who's right?** The study, published in the *Journal of the American Medical Association* in November 2002, offers something for both sides. After injecting 27 women and 34 men aged between 68 and 88 with either growth hormone or a placebo (dummy drug) for 6 1/2 months, the researchers confirmed what was first revealed in a study published in 1990 in the *New England Journal of Medicine* – that growth hormone treatment does indeed firm up older bodies, adding muscle mass and noticeably reducing body fat.

When stomachs shrink without diet or exercise, the world takes notice, and the results of this study have fuelled what was already a growing demand in the USA for growth hormone treatment. HGH therapy is approved in America for younger people who are deficient in naturally occurring growth hormone, but physicians can (and some do) prescribe it for anti-ageing purposes.

Other people, including the editors of the two journals where the research was published in 1990 and 2002, have sounded a warning shot. They point out that the improvements in body composition caused by HGH treatment have not been shown to translate into better aerobic fitness or muscle strength. The people in the study got the packaging without the contents, so to speak. More importantly, the risks of cancer and other possible complications of the treatment in the elderly won't be known until larger, long-term safety studies are carried out.

**A risky proposition** The authors of the new study were worried by higher incidences of diabetes and glucose intolerance among the people who were given HGH. They explicitly warn against the use of growth hormone for anti-ageing purposes except by elderly people who are participating in approved clinical studies.

The two journal editors criticized internet-based purveyors of HGH 'supplements' for claiming that the medical literature supports their use for anti-ageing purposes, which it doesn't. Most of those products are oral forms of HGH, which are useless – since growth hormone that is swallowed is broken down by stomach acid before it can have any effect. Other popular supplements contain no HGH but rather substances that supposedly encourage the body to use more of its own HGH. There is no evidence that these 'HGH releasers' work.

**Awaiting answers** More studies are needed to look at HGH treatment in the long term. But the treatment's supporters point out that Americans in their sixties don't want to wait. The question then becomes: is it worth spending as much as £7,000 a year for a treatment that may not work and may have side effects? Judging by the recent increase in the number of physicians prescribing HGH, plenty of hopeful people are saying yes. But countless studies point to a better anti-ageing strategy: exercise.

# ALSO in the NEWS

## Male hormones for memory?

Ageing men may experience a decline in two things they value most: the male hormone testosterone and cognitive ability, including memory, reasoning and learning. A study of men between ages 51 and 91 has now confirmed a long-suspected link between the two.

Scientists working on a research programme known as the Baltimore Longitudinal Study of Aging followed some 400 men for 10 years, analysing their blood levels of testosterone and their scores on a series of cognition tests. The results were clear: more testosterone in the blood meant better mental function. However, larger studies are needed to show whether testosterone replacement actually protects mental function. Testosterone replacement therapy, like oestrogen replacement therapy for women, raises serious health concerns.

## Key discovery

# One secret of longevity revealed

Tiny bits of genetic material found in all cells may reveal our chances of surviving well into old age. These 'telomeres', which cap the strands of gene-bearing chromosomes like the plastic tip at the end of a shoelace, have caught the attention of longevity researchers, who have now identified a connection between their length and the risk of premature death.

Until recently, no one had actually compared the survival rates of older people with varying telomere lengths. But the results of a study published in *The Lancet* in February 2003 are exactly what anyone interested in a long, healthy life wants to hear. In the study, researchers at the University of Utah found that people over 60 with longer telomeres are much less likely to die from age-related killers such as heart disease and infectious diseases than people of the same age who have shorter telomeres. The finding is exciting because

it points to a way in which human beings might be able to delay death. If shorter telomeres mean a shorter life span, why not make them longer? The researchers think this is a real possibility. 'Medical interventions that lengthen telomeres may help people stay healthy longer and live longer,' says Richard Cawthon, the study's leading author.

Exactly what interventions may successfully elongate the tips of trillions of chromosomes will have to be revealed by future research. Gene therapy? Hormones? Perhaps – but the answer may even be found in something as simple as diet or exercise, Dr Cawthon suggests.

**A short-cut to long life** Telomeres shorten naturally with age, losing a bit of length each time a cell divides, but they shrink at different rates in different people. Knowing that, the researchers measured telomere lengths from blood samples given in the 1980s by 143 people over the age of 60.

Analysis of the donors' subsequent medical records revealed that those whose telomeres were among the longest were three times less likely to die from heart disease and eight times less likely to die from infectious diseases. On average, they lived four to five years longer than those in the bottom half of rankings of telomere length.

The link between shorter telomeres and increased risk of age-related disease may have something to do with the telomeres' effect on overall cell health. It is possible that, once a telomere shortens to a certain point, the cell that encases it essentially commits suicide. When that happens often enough, a cell-depleted body lacks the resources to fight off disease and eventually even to stay alive.

It is also possible, however, that shortened telomeres only predict a shorter life span rather than cause it. Even if that is the case, the conclusions of the new study suggest a line of research that could result in treatments to help to fend off age-related disease and death. Since the difference in telomere length between age-matched people is largely hereditary, researchers could try to identify the genes that influence it. It is highly likely that some of those genes are 'longevity genes', which influence the rate of ageing. Such a discovery would bring us closer to finding life-extending treatments.

A computer illustration of a human X chromosome shows the telomeres at the ends in green.

## Key discovery
# High blood sugar may be the cause of memory lapses

Can't remember the name of the book you read last week? Forgot what you needed at the corner shop? For some people, noticeable memory lapses are the bane of middle age. While they are less serious than true dementia, they can be very annoying. Medical scientists have been searching hard for causes of age-related memory loss, and new research from the New York University School of Medicine has uncovered a likely culprit: high blood sugar. The discovery may mean that the key to maintaining a sharp memory throughout life is as simple as watching your diet, keeping your weight down, and exercising regularly – all proven ways to avoid blood sugar complications, including diabetes.

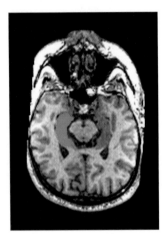

The brain of a 63-year-old man with normal glucose tolerance: the hippocampus is highlighted in red.

**The problem of glucose intolerance** Food converted by the digestive system to glucose (blood sugar) is the main fuel that powers the cells of all organs in the body, including the brain. But many people, especially older people, have poor glucose tolerance, meaning they have trouble processing glucose out of the bloodstream and into their cells. People with diabetes have seriously impaired glucose tolerance – and as a result, high blood sugar – and studies show that they often experience some degree of memory impairment, whatever their age.

What the latest research found, however, is that even mild, non-diabetic glucose intolerance appears to reduce short-term memory in middle age and

beyond. That opens up the possibility that, by taking steps to keep your blood sugar at a healthy level, you will not only reduce your risk of diabetes but also protect your memory.

**How they found out** The researchers assembled 30 healthy men and women aged between 53 and 89 and measured their blood sugar metabolism by injecting glucose into their blood and measuring how long it took to reach their organs. They also gauged the subjects' short-term memory by a series of recall tests and by measuring a brain structure called the hippocampus, which is responsible for short-term memory.

The results of the study, which were published in the *Proceedings of the National Academy of Sciences* in February 2003, showed a clear connection between blood sugar and memory loss. The participants with the poorest glucose tolerance scored worse on the memory tests and had smaller hippocampuses.

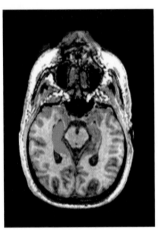

A brain of a 63-year-old man with impaired glucose tolerance has a smaller hippocampus.

**What it means** Does glucose intolerance literally starve the brain into memory impairment by depriving it of the glucose it needs? One 30-person study is not enough to provide a definitive answer, so the same team is conducting further experiments. In the meantime, the finding is good news if you want to protect your memory, as the more effective ways to maintain proper blood sugar metabolism are already well known.

The top priorities are to get your weight down to where it should be (and keep it there) and to exercise regularly, whether you are overweight or not. Also, eat reasonably sized meals at regular intervals, choosing vegetables and fibre-rich whole grains rather than 'white' carbohydrates such as pasta, white bread, potatoes and white rice. Finally, choose the good fats – the kind found in vegetable oils, nuts, seeds, avocados and fish – rather than the bad saturated fats in meat and whole-fat dairy products and the even worse hydrogenated fats in margarine and many other processed foods.

**Key discovery**

# Exercise will keep the brain in good shape

For years now, 'use it or lose it' has been wise advice for older men and women hoping to keep their memory sharp. But when you are not challenging your intellect by solving crossword puzzles or mastering a foreign language, set aside some time for another mind-preserving activity: exercise. A six-year study of 349 adults aged 55 and over has provided convincing new evidence that staying physically fit as you age keeps your brain as well as your body in shape.

The new findings should be enough to get most people out of their comfortable chairs and onto the exercise bike or into the swimming pool. Simply put, those in the study who were most physically fit maintained more of their mental acuity over the course of the study than those who were less fit. The fittest had the best scores in mental function tests (such as remembering words), while the least fit scored the worst.

Poor physical fitness had been linked with poor mental fitness in earlier studies, but the latest research, published in April 2003 in the *Journal of the American Geriatrics Society*, gives a big boost to the theory of a connection between body and mind, according to the authors, who cite two reasons for their claim.

One is that this was the first well-designed study that looked exclusively at older people (aged 55 and up). The other is that, instead of relying on the participants' own reports of their fitness activity (in other words, taking their word for how much they exercised), the researchers measured their fitness levels by putting them through treadmill tests – which never lie. As far as healthy people were concerned, the more cardio-respiratory

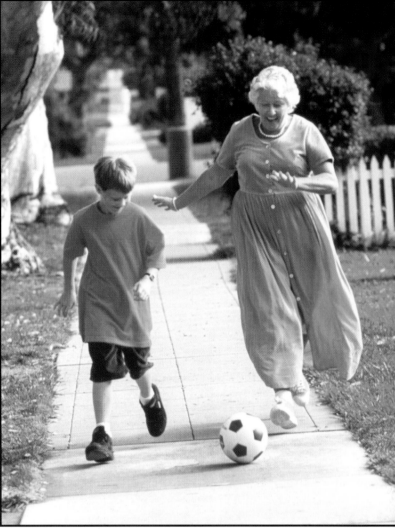

Exercise is a well-established way to overcome physical problems. Now it seems that staying active may help to keep your brain healthy as well as your body.

exercise they did (meaning endurance activities such as swimming, jogging, biking and stair climbing), the better they did on the treadmill test.

**How it works** The American researchers are not yet sure why regular exercise keeps the old grey matter performing well. However, their findings are backed up by Age Concern in the UK, which emphasizes the strong connection between physical and mental well-being, and the fact that oxygen flow to the brain is increased through exercise, improving mental alertness. 'Regular participation in aerobic exercise is associated with greater mental well-being (i.e. less depression) and more efficient mental activity,' says Age Concern. 'The regularity of the exercise seems to be the key.'

# CHILDREN'S HEALTH

## TALK ABOUT TURNING CONVENTIONAL WISDOM ON ITS HEAD

This is the year we learned that divorce does not have to mean damaged children (just a few hours of parental training makes a difference), that owning a household pet can actually prevent allergies and that many more people – though not teenage boys – are now wearing protective cycle helmets. On the medicines front, there may soon be a new nonstimulant alternative to Ritalin for treating attention deficit hyperactivity disorder (ADHD); it was recently approved in the USA.

In Britain, obesity in children is worrying health experts, who have called for a ban on the advertising of snacks on TV. In the States, epidemic levels of childhood obesity have prompted the country's leading professional heart association to issue its first-ever guidelines for preventing heart disease in children.

Finally, a study by British researchers seems to be showing that biology, not nurture, gives girls their feminine traits and boys their masculinity, or not – as the case may be...

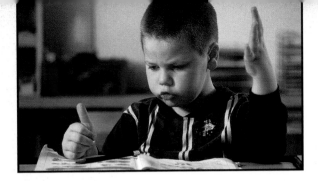

## Drug development
# Nonstimulant ADHD drug excites parents

Few parents want people to know that their children take methylphenidate (Ritalin), the most commonly prescribed drug for one of the most commonly diagnosed behavioural disorders in children – attention deficit hyperactivity disorder, or ADHD.

That's because the stimulant, classified as a Class B controlled substance, has been given some bad press in recent years: reports about the large numbers of children taking the medication, concern about possible long-term effects, and stories of adolescents selling their medications to others who want the speed-like 'high' that they could provide. But for 30 years, parents haven't had a choice. Stimulants – Ritalin and amphetamines such as Dexedrine – were the only drugs available for the treatment of ADHD.

In the USA that changed in December 2002, when the government approved the nonstimulant drug atomoxetine (Strattera). The manufacturer, Eli Lilly, hopes that the drug will be licensed in Europe very soon. Like their American counterparts, doctors here would no doubt be delighted to have another option available in the treatment of ADHD.

**How it works** Researchers don't know exactly how Strattera improves ADHD symptoms but they theorize that it prevents certain receptors in the brain from soaking up adrenaline, which is believed to play a role in ADHD. Stimulant medications also work on adrenaline receptors, as well as on receptors for another brain chemical, dopamine.

While it is not yet known if the new drug works better than stimulants, it does offer advantages. 'It doesn't have the stigma of the stimulants,' says Dr Daniel Coury, professor of clinical paediatrics

and director of behavioural-developmental paediatrics at Columbus Children's Hospital in Ohio. 'Often we see kids whose parents say: "Do anything, but please don't put him on Ritalin."'

Strattera is also easier to prescribe than Ritalin because it isn't a controlled substance. With stimulant drugs, patients have to see their doctors every month for a new prescription. Doctors can write prescriptions for Strattera for months at a time. There's also no opportunity for abuse with Strattera, says Dr Coury, who led some of the clinical trials on the drug. This makes it particularly useful for adolescents who may be experimenting with drugs, or for those who live with a family member who has a substance abuse problem.

Another advantage is that one dose is effective for 24 hours. Even long-acting forms of methylphenidate and amphetamine work for only 8 to 12 hours.

**Side effects** Strattera can cause nausea, weight loss and dizziness, all of which usually disappear after a couple of months of taking the medication.

Alternative answers

# Biofeedback improves focus

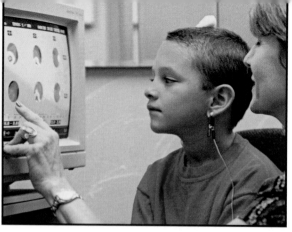

By measuring brainwave patterns, EEG biofeedback helps kids use their brains in ways associated with sustained attention and focus.

Could a group of children suffering from ADHD benefit from biofeedback? One psychologist in New York State decided to experiment and paid some of the children to undergo the therapy.

The results of the study were published in the December 2002 issue of *Applied Psychophysiology and Biofeedback*. Psychologist Dr Vince Monastra, Ph.D. found that while a year's worth of counselling and medication relieved some ADHD symptoms among a group of children, only those receiving biofeedback therapy managed to maintain those gains after coming off the medication.

**How it works** Dr Monastra, clinical director of the FPI Attention Disorders Clinic in Endicott, New York, studied 100 children between the ages of 6 and 19 who had ADHD. They were all treated identically in terms of medication, counselling, and even training for their parents. But half also had weekly EEG biofeedback sessions in which they learned to modify their brain activity.

With leads placed on their heads to measure the electrical activity of their brains, the kids spent a half-hour per week in front of a computer using only their brainwaves to 'play' a video game, then spent another half-hour doing homework.

When they 'turned on' the front part of the brain, which is responsible for sustaining attention, focus, concentration and problem-solving, they were rewarded either with points that later entitled them to money or with a move in their game on the video screen. When the study ended, Dr Monastra took all 100 children off their medication for a week, then retested them. Those who had not participated in the biofeedback training had all relapsed, with no sustained improvement as gauged by either observational or computerized tests. Those who did receive the training continued to show enough improvement to reduce their medication by at least half and 40 per cent were able to stop taking it.

Dr Monastra is adamant that biofeedback is not a substitute for medication. It may, however, prove an important adjunct and, in some instances, may bring on the kind of permanent changes in the brain that may eventually enable some children (and adults) to forgo some or all of their medication.

**Availability** Biofeedback is not widely available in the UK, although it is starting to be used by some psychologists. The Biofeedback Foundation of Europe has undertaken research into the use of biofeedback in ADHD.

---

RESEARCH ROUND-UP

### Study absolves ADHD medications

Thanks to sophisticated imaging techniques such as PET scanning and functional MRIs, researchers know that ADHD involves physical changes in the brain. In people with ADHD, certain areas of the brain appear smaller or structurally abnormal when compared to the brains of people without the condition. This has led to speculation that the drugs commonly prescribed for ADHD, methylphenidate (Ritalin) and amphetamine (Dexedrine), may be

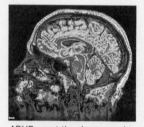

*ADHD – not the drugs used to treat it – changes the brain.*

responsible. However, a 10-year study by the US National Institute of Mental Health, reported in the *Journal of the American Medical Association* in October 2002, found that while the brains of children and adolescents with ADHD are 3 to 4 per cent smaller than those of children who don't have the disorder, medication is not the cause. In fact, researchers suggest that the medication may actually help the brain to mature.

## Key discovery
# Is autism on the increase?

For years the British public has worried that autism rates are on the rise, prompting a national health crisis as many parents boycotted the MMR vaccine fearing a link with the troubling disorder. Though convincing studies have begun to dispel this specific concern, there is little doubt that diagnosed cases of autism have risen dramatically in the past 25 years.

The National Autistic Society estimates that at least half a million children are suffering from autism or related disorders. But what is perhaps most disturbing is the apparent rate of increase in incidence of the disorder. According to a noted autism epidemiologist – Professor Eric Fombonne – formerly of the Institute of Psychiatry in London but now working at Montreal's McGill University, the average increase in autism has been a massive 1300 per cent over the past 25 years, or on average, a doubling of the incidence of the prevalence of autism every two years between 1976 and 2001.

But some feel these figures may be an exaggeration of the real situation. Keith Lovett of Autism Independent, formerly the Society for the Autistically Handicapped, agrees that cases of classical autism have risen but not as dramatically as some statistics suggest. 'In 25 years, they have risen from around 4 per 10,000 to 6-7 in 10,000 now,' he says.

He points out that what is now included are disorders that are related to autism but in some cases ill-defined. The so-called spectrum covers Asperger's syndrome, for instance, which has a name but no established diagnosis.

'There has been a huge groundswell of Asperger's syndrome – sometimes just because parents want a label for their child's disorder – and a lot

of misdiagnosis. Hopefully, some time in the future, genetic studies will reveal what it really is. Meanwhile, we have diagnoses made by clinicians, but they are not clinical diagnoses; they are observations of different types of behaviour by different people.'

The rise in autism is not limited to Britain. In the USA researchers recently published a study showing that the autism rates in five counties around Atlanta were 10 times higher in 1996 than those found in a study conducted in the 1980s.

The question on everyone's lips is 'Why?' Several theories have been put forward. Suspects include a broadening of the definition of the disorder in the mid-1990s and increased public awareness, which could lead to more children being diagnosed.

While the MMR vaccine is now less suspect following studies showing that autism increased even when the vaccination rate remained a constant, no-one is quite sure. The reasons behind autism remain frustratingly illusive and better diagnostic criteria and more research is desperately required.

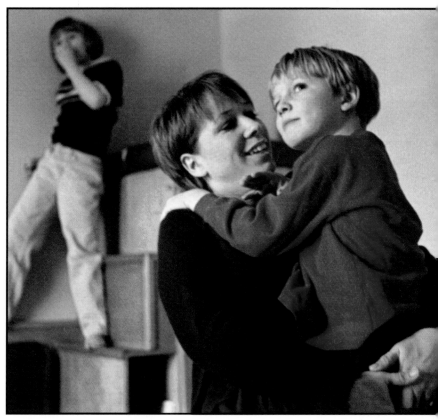

Bobbie Gallagher, above, contacted federal authorities after she learned that both her children, and numerous others in her New Jersey township, were autistic. The apparent and unexplained rise in the disorder is being studied by scientists across the globe.

Key discovery

# Spare the rod, improve the parent

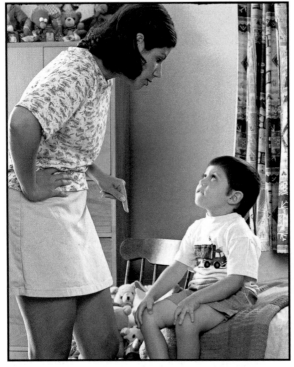

Not sure how to discipline your child? Programmes that teach parents to manage children result in far fewer behaviour problems.

You need a licence to cut hair and drive a car. But no instruction is required for the most difficult job of all: raising children. Maybe it should be. A study in the December 2002 issue of *Archives of Disease in Childhood* found that parents who undergo 20 hours of specialized training cope better with their children, improving their children's behaviour.

Although numerous studies have shown that training can improve parenting skills for at-risk parents and those with children already identified as having behavioural problems, this was one of the first to evaluate the effect on parents who weren't significantly concerned about their kids' behaviour.

The parents, whose children ranged in age from three to 10, were chosen from one general practice and asked to complete a questionnaire. Researchers selected 116 parents who, based on the answers to the questionnaire, had the greatest disciplinary problems with their children.

'They were the sort of problems all parents have and express,' says study author Dr Sarah Stewart-Brown Ph.D. B.M. BCh, professor of public health at Warwick University in Coventry. 'There were times they didn't feel in control, they didn't know how to handle certain problems, their children were throwing temper tantrums.' In the UK, 60 per cent of children under one and 90 per cent of those under four are spanked, she says. 'Most parents aren't happy about that. They say they lose their temper and would rather have other strategies, but they don't know what else to do. These positive discipline strategies are good to learn.'

**How it works** Half the parents received weekly two-hour group counselling sessions for 10 weeks, and half did not. The sessions followed the Webster-Stratton parenting programme, which teaches parents how to manage their children's behaviour with positive reinforcement, setting limits, non-physical discipline alternatives and effective communication skills, among other strategies. Six months after the sessions, researchers retested both sets of parents and found that there were far fewer behaviour problems reported by the group that received the training than by the control group.

Interestingly, in a follow-up a year after the training, the difference between the two groups had diminished – not because parents in the counselling group reported more problems with their children but because those in the control group, some of whom had gone on their own to get counselling, reported fewer problems with *their* children. Filling out the questionnaire and talking to the researchers, some parents said, had made them realize that they needed some help with their kids.

**What it means** Programmes using the Webster-Stratton approach are offered throughout the UK and in other countries. The fact that a 10-week programme made such a difference in a 'typical' group of parents means that 'there are things that parents can do that really make a difference to their children's health and well being, and to their own family life,' says Dr Stewart-Brown. 'The vast majority of parents who go through the training say: "Why didn't someone tell me this a long time ago?"'

Such is its success that the approach has now been listed as a useful resource on a government web site to reduce crime among persistent young offenders.

## Key discovery
# Helping kids to survive divorce

Divorce is painful but parents also worry about its effect on children. The results of a long-term US study show that a short intervention programme to improve communication skills and support healthy parenting can make a significant difference in children's behaviour and overall mental well-being.

The authors of the study, published in the *Journal of the American Medical Association* in October 2002, spent six years tracking 218 families in the midst of divorce. At the start, the children were between 9 and 12 years old, all lived primarily with their mothers, and none were receiving treatment for psychological problems. The families were then randomly assigned to either an intervention programme for the mothers, a programme for both mothers and children, or a control group that was simply given three books about adjusting to divorce.

The programmes focused on helping the mothers increase the positive quality of their relationships with their children, using more effective discipline, increasing the fathers' access to the children, and reducing conflict between the parents. The mothers were taught how to provide 'sensitive parenting,' which included:

- Spending more positive time with their children on a regular basis.
- Listening to their concerns and worries.
- Noticing their good behaviour.
- Providing clear, consistent discipline.

Families were interviewed immediately after completing the programme, three months later, six months later, and six years later.

**The results** After six years, the researchers found that both the mother-only programme and the mother-plus-child programme had positive long-term effects. Teenagers who had entered the programme with significant behaviour problems and whose mothers had participated in the mother-only programme were less aggressive; used less marijuana, alcohol and other drugs; and had fewer symptoms of mental disorders than those in the control group. Teens in the mother-plus-child programme were also less aggressive, were 50 per cent less likely to be diagnosed with a mental

disorder than those in the control group, and reported having fewer sexual partners. The study found that children who had been having the most problems when they entered the programme benefited the most.

**What it means** Not all children have adjustment problems after divorce. 'No child will happily accept a divorce, but most adjust fine with time and some sensitive parenting,' says study author Sharlene Wolchik Ph.D., a clinical psychologist at Arizona State University – a finding supported by studies in Finland and Australia. But for the 20 to 30 per cent who show more serious problems, 'these findings provide strong evidence that the problems children experience after parental divorce are preventable'.

The bottom line: 'Keep the focus on the children, not the spouse you're divorcing. In the long run, that will be the most important factor in how your children turn out,' says Dr Wolchik.

## ALSO in the NEWS

### Can pets reduce allergies?

In one of the best designed studies ever conducted on the issue, US researchers have found that owning dogs and cats during a child's early years may actually reduce the overall risk of allergies.

Michigan researchers tracked 835 children from birth, checking them once a year until they were 7, (when 474 of the children remained in the study). Using blood and skin tests, they tested for reactions to a range of common allergens, then compared the results with information on whether there was a household pet and how long it had lived there. They found that children who had been exposed to two or more cats or dogs in their first year of life had half the rate of allergies of those who had less or no exposure.

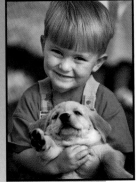

'The study shows that what a child is exposed to in early life is very important in terms of influencing whether they develop allergies and asthma later in childhood,' said a spokesman for the National Asthma Campaign.

# ALSO in the NEWS

## Fighting children's diarrhoea

Outbreaks of a common waterborne parasite caused a spate of sickness and closed swimming pools from Bristol to Glasgow in the summer and autumn of 2003. The parasite – cryptosporidium – a distant relative of the malaria parasite, is transmitted through contaminated water and food. Infection can cause diarrhoea and vomiting and is particularly dangerous for those with weakened immunity. There is, as yet, no effective treatment in the UK. In the USA, where the parasite was largely responsible for a near doubling of outbreaks of waterborne illnesses from 1997 and 2000, a newly approved drug may offer the first effective treatment. Called nitazoxinide (Alinia), the liquid medication can be used for children aged 1 to 11. Nitazoxinide is an antihelminthic drug (meaning it fights worm infestation) that has been available for several years in developing countries. A licensing application is expected this year in Europe but the drug is unlikely to be approved in Britain before 2005.

## Don't blame the obstetrician

In the USA, obstetricians have been among the hardest hit in an ongoing malpractice insurance crisis; some consultants face annual premiums of more than $100,000 (£60,000). One reason is the long-held belief that one of the more common birth defects, cerebral palsy, stems from problems during labour and delivery, which are often blamed on the doctor.

Now, a landmark scientific report published by the American College of Obstetricians and Gynaecologists and the American Academy of Pediatrics reveals that nearly all brain damage in newborns occurs as a result of developmental or metabolic abnormalities, auto-immune and blood defects, infection, trauma, or combinations of these factors during conception or pregnancy, not during labour or delivery. The findings could open new avenues of research into the causes of these conditions, potentially leading to earlier interventions.

The report should please UK obstetricians who also face a high risk of litigation and insurance premiums that are weighted but not nearly as high as in the USA.

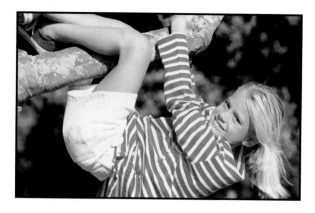

## Key discovery
# Tomboys are born, not made

Give a little boy a doll, and the chances are he'll beat something with it. Give a little girl a tool belt, and see if she doesn't decorate it with sequins and pink felt tip. Anyone who has tried to raise a child in a gender-neutral environment can tell you: children seem programmed to behave in certain gender-specific ways. There are exceptions, of course, such as the tomboyish girl who'd rather climb a tree than dress a Barbie. But are the exceptions the result of upbringing or biology? A surprising new study points to biology.

British researchers, who published the results of their study in the journal *Child Development* in November 2002, evaluated data on 679 children and their mothers. They took blood samples during the women's pregnancy. Then, when the children were 3½ years old, they gave the primary caregivers a survey designed to assess certain gender-specific behaviours in the children, such as which toys, games, and other activities they preferred. It turns out that high testosterone levels in mothers during pregnancy corresponded with high masculinity scores in preschool girls.

The correlation remained even after taking into account such variables as the presence of older siblings and/or a male adult in the home and parental adherence to traditional sex roles. But the researchers didn't find any relationship between testosterone levels and boys' gender-role behaviour.

The reason for that discrepancy, they suggest, is that boys are not only exposed to more prenatal testosterone, they are also discouraged more strongly from engaging in 'girlish' activities than girls are dissuaded from 'acting like boys'.

## Diagnostic advance
# Thermometer shape proves a success

Getting children to keep a thermometer under their tongue until it beeps is about as easy as getting them to eat up their greens. Parents thought they had the problem beaten with the introduction of the infrared thermometer, a device you put in your child's ear for a second and click – until an article published in the August 2002 issue of *The Lancet* found that such devices don't give very accurate readings.

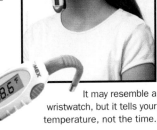

It may resemble a wristwatch, but it tells your temperature, not the time.

Then, in February 2003, a new thermometer from Timex was launched in the USA, providing fresh hope of getting an accurate temperature reading from even the squirmiest four year-old. The AccuCurve 30-Second Digital Thermometer sits neatly under the tongue and one version even talks to you: 'Your current temperature is…'

The plastic thermometer is shaped like a hook. The curved end, which contains the temperature-sensing tip, rests comfortably in the mouth. As advertised, it provides a temperature reading in about 30 seconds and comes in a standard size for older children and adults and small for little ones.

'It's one of those ideas you look at and think, "Why didn't someone come up with this before?"' says Stephen Fanning, a family doctor in Greenville, Rhode Island. Eighteen years of treating young children has taught him all about the difficulties of temperature taking and how hard it is to keep a conventional thermometer under a child's tongue.

Why? 'That's the million-dollar question,' he says. 'Even adults have a hard time keeping them under their tongues and keeping their mouths closed. It's just a fact of life.'

However, Timex UK have no immediate plans to launch the new thermometer here.

---

**BEHIND THE BREAKTHROUGHS**

### Three mums rethink the thermometer

The Rhode Island-based Lindon Group, which designs medical devices, has just three employees: Mindy Penney, Sherry Lussier, and Dalita Tomellini. Between them, they have eight children ranging in age from one to nine, and they know first-hand the challenges of temperature-taking. So, when asked to redesign the traditional thermometer, they turned to the experts: 20 neighbourhood mums, who said they were frustrated with trying to get their youngsters to keep thermometers in their mouths long enough to get accurate readings.

The Lindon executives returned to their corporate offices (in the Penney basement) and brainstormed. One of them (no one recalls who) put her finger in her mouth and curved it down along her chin.

'We should do it like this,' she said. So they moulded aluminium foil into the appropriate shape and coopted their children, husbands, and friends for product testing, finding that regardless of the size or shape of the tester's mouth, the curved shape fitted the 'hot spot' for everyone. *Voilà*! The AccuCurve was born.

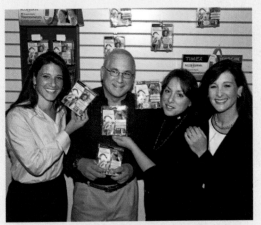

The inventors (from left, Mindy Penney, Dalita Tomellini and Sherry Lussier with Jeff Jacober, chairman of the manufacturers, Medport) used good sense as their guide.

### Key discovery

# Cycle helmets are catching on

More and more children (and also adults) are wearing cycling helmets according to research unveiled by the Department for Transport in June 2003. Between 1994 and 2002, the use of helmets rose from 16 per cent to 25 per cent among the cycling population though teenage boys continued to resist the trend; their rate of helmet use appears to be around 12 per cent.

Ministers are encouraged by the general trend although cycling fatalities remain unacceptably high. In Britain, every week a child under sixteen dies as a result of head injuries suffered in a cycle accident. In 2001 nearly 3,000 cyclists aged between 12 and 16 were killed or injured on the roads. Boy cyclists, who are only half as likely as girls to wear a cycle helmet, are five times more likely to have serious accidents.

The road safety department has targeted teenage boys with a hard-hitting advertising campaign and launched a web site – www.cyclesense.net. The site, which features an X-rayed skull, spells out the helmet message, explains how to carry out a 10-second bike check and offers other basic safety tips.

'It's great news that cycle helmets are catching on but disappointing that teenage boys do not appear to be getting the message,' commented road safety minister, David Jamieson. 'We want to encourage more children to cycle but to do so in a safer manner. Cycle helmets can be effective at reducing the severity of injuries to the head in the event of an accident, and we encourage all cyclists to wear one. I hope that by making cycling safer, more people will take to their bikes.'

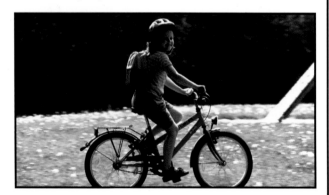

Girls are twice as likely to wear a protective helmet as boys, who are five times more likely to be involved in serious cycling accidents.

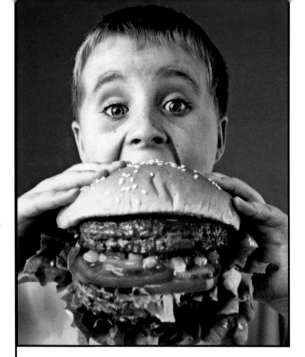

### Progress in prevention

# Preventing heart disease in children

Take hours in front of the TV or playing video games, add snack foods, chips and sugary soft drinks and you have the recipe for what is becoming an epidemic of weight problems in children today. Recent UK research has shown that as many as a fifth of 7 to 11 year olds are overweight and more than a tenth are obese.

Most worryingly, a study of more than 2,500 infants revealed that obesity rates in pre-school children rose by 80 per cent over a single decade.

The time has come to protect children from food advertising, says Dr Geof Rayner, chair of the UK Public Health Association, who presented a report in June 2003 to the Health Select Committee.

'Smoking is still the leading preventable cause of death in this country. That is why advertising aimed at children has been banned for many years. But there is no health protection for our children from the advertising of high-salt, high-fat snack foods or sugary fizzy drinks,' Dr Rayner told the committee.

Professor Sian Griffiths, president of the Faculty of Public Health, agrees and is calling for a joint effort from doctors, teachers, nurses and community workers, as well as parents to combat obesity. 'All parents worry about children smoking but we know that they can always give up. Once obese your chances of developing diabetes are extremely high and the effects are likely to be irreversible. The government should therefore investigate ways of protecting children's health and promoting more physically active lifestyles.'

**Many US teenagers already have arteries clogged so badly they could suffer heart attacks.**

That extra weight can also bring heart disease, according to researchers in the USA, which faces an even greater obesity problem. One US study found that the arteries of many teenagers are already clogged so badly that they could trigger heart attacks and that high blood pressure in children, once considered rare, is now increasingly common. Other studies find that the warning signs of heart disease – including high blood pressure and streaks of fatty plaque on arteries – can be seen in children as young as two. This and other research prompted the American Heart Association (AHA) in March 2003 to issue its first-ever guidelines for preventing cardiovascular disease in children. The guidelines urge doctors to intervene in childhood obesity and in the habits that can lead to it. They also recommend that doctors be 'vigilant for the subtle signs indicating the development of

Children love pizza, but this gooey food favourite – especially the pepperoni version – is loaded with saturated fat, the kind that contributes to clogged arteries in children.

insulin resistance, glucose intolerance, and Type 2 diabetes', which are all increasing in the country's children. The AHA suggests that doctors should measure children's blood pressure at age three and cholesterol levels at five. The American Academy of Pediatrics recommends cholesterol tests for children aged two and older if their parents or grandparents had heart disease before age 55 or if their parents have high cholesterol levels.

## AN EARLY START ON CHOLESTEROL DRUGS?

Is it possible that a child should be prescribed cholesterol lowering drugs? In the USA where up to one-third of children, from the age of two right to teenage years, have high cholesterol, the answer appears to be yes, though it is highly unlikely that specialists in Britain would agree.

The USA's National Cholesterol Education Program now recommends cholesterol-lowering drugs for children over age 10 whose LDL (that's the 'bad' cholesterol) remains high even after they have reformed their diets. However, statins, the most common class of such drugs, are not yet approved for use in children and few large studies have been conducted to determine their effects in children.

That may change as a study published in an October 2002 issue of 'Circulation', the journal of the American Heart Association, found that the cholesterol-lowering drug simvastatin (Zocor) significantly reduced cholesterol levels in children with an inherited form of high cholesterol. The study, which looked at 173 children between the ages of nine and 18, also found that even after 48 weeks on the drug, there was no effect on growth or onset of puberty in the target group.

In Britain, one inherited form of high cholesterol — familial hypercholesterolaemia (FH) — affects 1 in 500 people or around 110,000 people nationwide. Testing for FH is recommended after the age of two. Dietary therapy, rather than medication, is the cornerstone of treatment for children and adults.

Children may also be treated with a so-called resin, a drug which binds with excess cholesterol as it passes through the gut and is then excreted. In Britain, statin drug therapy is not recommended until after puberty, and then only if there is a particular risk of coronary heart disease in the family.

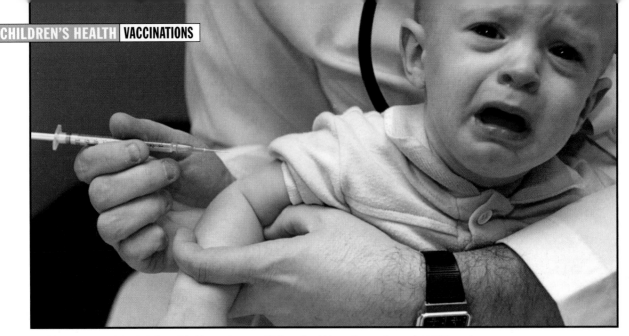

Health experts say it is vital that all babies and young children should have the controversial MMR vaccine.

## Progress in prevention
# MMR catch-up campaign urged

The UK's Health Protection Agency has appealed to the government to consider measures to reverse the dramatic decline in uptake for the mumps, measles and rubella vaccine (MMR). The agency fears that the low uptake which has dropped from 95 per cent to below 80 per cent, is putting youngsters at severe risk of measles and mumps, and has called for an MMR catch-up campaign.

Before the end of 2003, the number of reported measles cases was reported to be up by about 300 per cent and reported mumps cases were also rising. In Sunderland, more than 100 cases of mumps had been reported by September, compared with 14 for the whole of 2002. As a result, teenagers have been reminded that Department of Health guidelines recommend two doses of the MMR vaccine between the ages of 13 and 20 years.

According to the guidelines babies should first have the MMR vaccine at around 13 months, with a second dose between the ages of three and five. However, research suggesting a possible link between the vaccine and the increased incidence of autism, has caused many parents to boycott the vaccine or to try to find practitioners who could give it in single doses rather than in combination.

**RESEARCH ROUND-UP**

### Mother's milk – a baby's painkiller
When you next take your baby in for vaccinations, try feeding him or her while the needle goes in. A study published in the *British Medical Journal* in January 2003 suggests it may ease the pain.

Researchers evaluated 180 newborns during routine heel pricks. They split the babies into four groups: some were breastfed, some were held in their mothers' arms, some received a sugar solution on a soother and some received sterile water. Researchers evaluated the babies' pain based on facial expressions, movement of their arms and legs, the cries they made, their heart rates and the amount of oxygen in their blood (when you're in a lot of pain, your breathing is shallow, so you take in less oxygen). They found no difference between the babies who were held in their mothers' arms and those who received sterile water, but of the babies who were breastfed, all had scores reflecting minimal or no pain, similar to the results of those who sucked on a soother with a sweet solution on it.

Meanwhile, that too brought problems last year, when two private clinics administering single vaccines were accused of exposing thousands of children to the risk of measles, mumps and rubella by givingvaccines that were prepared in advance, against manufacturers' guidelines .

Progress in prevention

# Could vaccine for chickenpox save lives?

Every year hundreds of thousands of children in Canada and the United States are vaccinated against chickenpox – a programme that has not been adopted here. In April 2003, a leading proponent of the vaccine, Anne Gershon, professor of paediatrics at Columbia University in New York, told the Society for General Microbiology's spring meeting in Edinburgh that the US vaccination programme saves hundreds of lives and 'appears to significantly cut outbreaks of the disease'.

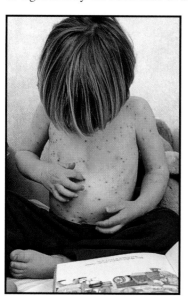

The UK's Department of Health, however, has said that there is not yet enough evidence to merit a mass programme of immunization against chicken-pox in the UK. There has also been a study in the UK that suggests vaccinating children against chickenpox may put adults at risk as being exposed to the childhood disease appears to protect adults from later developing shingles.

Questioned on this, Dr Gershon pointed out that chickenpox was a more potentially fatal disease than shingles: 'Fatalities from shingles are rare.'

Meanwhile, in the USA, children may soon be getting a double dose of the vaccine. It appears that those who receive a single dose may remain susceptible to the virus. A study published in a December 2002 issue of the *New England Journal of Medicine* found that the varicella vaccine protected children against mild and uncomplicated forms of chickenpox, the most common forms, less than half the time. It performed better against moderate and severe forms of the disease, providing protection 86 per cent of the time.

Dr Gershon wrote in an accompanying editorial that the study was a warning signal to doctors. 'The time for exploring the possibility of routinely administering two doses of varicella vaccine to children seems to have arrived,' she said.

## ALSO in the NEWS

### Babies take cues from TV

If you thought you would not have to worry about unsuitable television content until your infant could talk, think again. New research finds that your baby really does watch TV.

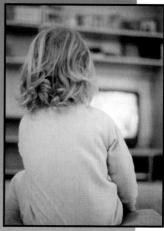

At Tufts University, Boston in the USA, psychology professor Donna Mumme Ph.D. and colleagues already knew that infants watch the emotional reactions of other people and take cues from them. That's why if you're upset, your baby may become upset. But in this study, published in the January/February 2003 issue of *Child Development*, the researchers learned that infants as young as one year old can also pick up such cues from television characters.

First, babies watched a video in which an actress looked at and responded to an object (a red spiral letter holder, a bumpy blue ball, or a yellow garden hose attachment). Then researchers gave identical items to the babies. They found that the babies reacted the same way the actress had. For instance, after watching the actress respond negatively to an object, the babies avoided that object and played with another one instead. 'This means that adults might want to think twice before they speak in a harsh or surprising tone or let an infant see television programmes meant for an older person,' says Dr Mumme.

# WELLNESS

## THE BIG NEWS THIS YEAR WAS ABOUT THE FOOD ON OUR PLATES

We learned that certain types of fish aren't quite as healthy as we thought, thanks to a modern-day problem: mercury contamination. New research reveals high levels of mercury in swordfish, marlin and even, to a lesser extent, tuna, which could damage an unborn child.

Meanwhile, in other nutrition news, one study vindicated the Atkins diet by finding that the low-carbohydrate, high-fat regimen actually lowers cholesterol – although other studies report long-term detrimental effects such as kidney damage. And beer drinkers can rejoice: it turns out that all types of alcohol are as good as wine at guarding against heart disease.

If a sweet tooth is your Achilles' heel, take heed: the World Health Organization issued a strong statement against sugar, calling on everyone to drastically limit their consumption of the sweet stuff to just 10 per cent of daily calorie intake.

## Progress in prevention

# Beer drinkers have their day

Britain's many thousands of beer drinkers will be raising their glasses to a new US study. The research into the effects of alcohol on the heart appears to show that beer and other alcoholic drinks – not just red wine – are beneficial.

Carried out by Dr Mukamal, a junior house doctor at Beth Israel Deaconess Medical Center in Boston, the study was the largest to date on alcohol and heart disease. Researchers analysed data from more than 38,000 men aged between 40 and 75, looking at each one's consumption of beer, red wine, white wine, and spirits by amount and frequency over 12 years. The results, which were published in the January 2003 issue of the *New England Journal of Medicine*, showed that men who consumed moderate amounts of alcohol three or more times a week had a much lower risk of heart disease than those who drank less often. Those with the lowest risk drank five to seven days a week. Moreover, despite the widespread belief that red wine

# TOP TRENDS

## EXERCISERS GET ON THE BALL

Power yoga was the exercise of choice in the late 90s. Pilates became the rage of the early millennium. The new trend is balance training using large, air-filled fitness balls (sometimes called Swiss balls). Exercisers sit on the balls as they perform traditional strength-training moves such as abdominal crunches and bicep curls. Research at the University of Waterloo in Ontario, Canada, shows that the instability of the balls causes people to use more muscles in order to stay balanced than they'd use without the ball.

## ACTION AGAINST DRUG ERRORS

An alarming number of drug errors are occurring in hospitals, according to a *British Medical Journal* report published in March 2003. The report suggests that mistakes are made in about half of all intravenous drug doses, about a third of which are potentially harmful. As a result, a trial scheme has been introduced in six NHS hospital trusts to change the way drugs are administered. This will involve improvements in medicine labelling, a reduction in the number of different infusion devices and special training for medical staff on using equipment, as well as an overhaul in the procedures for reporting errors.

This is by no means a problem unique to the UK. In the US, the increasing number of drug errors has led to the introduction of barcodes on drugs. Before dispensing medication, a nurse scans the code on the drug bottle and one on the patient's bracelet to be sure they match. If they don't, an alarm beeps.

## SMOKERS UNDER PRESSURE TO QUIT

From January 2003, tobacco products sold in the UK have carried stark health warnings, covering 30 per cent of the front and 40 per cent of the back of cigarette packets. And it seems to be working: during the first four months of this year, the NHS Smoking Helpline received calls from over 10,000 people wanting to quit as a result of having read the warnings, an increase in call levels of 12 per cent. Coupled with the ban on tobacco advertising in the UK, which took effect in February 2003, increasing restrictions on smoking in public places and the Cancer Research UK campaign against so-called 'light' cigarettes, smokers are finding themselves under mounting pressure to extinguish their cigarettes permanently.

## FAST FOOD JOINT LIGHTENS UP MENU

McDonald's have introduced a range of salads to their menu, hoping to lure health-conscious consumers. These light options, introduced during the summer in 2003, include Pasta and Chicken Salad and Feta Cheese and Pasta salad, and contain less than 400 calories and 5 per cent fat. Other healthy additions are a Fruit Bag, which can be bought as a Happy Meal option, and Robinson's Fruit Shoot, a no-added-sugar drink.

In the USA, McDonald's have been criticized for some of their new salads that are said to be higher in calories, fat and sodium than a Big Mac. You can check the nutritional content of all your favourite burgers and salads yourself by using the calorie-counters provided on the web sites of McDonald's, Burger King and Kentucky Fried Chicken.

is better for your heart than other types of alcohol, the study found that all types lowered heart disease risk similarly.

**How it works** Red wine has long been thought to offer protection against heart disease because it contains antioxidant plant substances called flavonoids. But while flavonoids may be good for your health in other ways, they don't seem to offer additional protection against heart disease, says Dr Mukamal. Some other component of alcohol seems to do the trick, possibly by raising levels of 'good' (HDL) cholesterol and reducing the risk of potentially dangerous clots. All types of alcohol are good for your heart,' says Dr Mukamal. 'Red wine is probably still more beneficial than other types of alcohol for other diseases, but for heart disease, it looks like it's the alcohol per se, and in fact the frequency with which people drink alcohol, that make the most difference,' he says.

Iain R. Loe from the Campaign for Real Ale (CAMRA) welcomes the findings: 'CAMRA does believe that beer in moderation is generally good for you, at least as good as red wine … Vitamins and antioxidants in beer have beneficial effects on health; hops, unique to beer, have the potential to protect against some forms of cancer and there is strong evidence that people who are moderate drinkers of beer have a substantially reduced risk of coronary heart disease.'

Dr Mukamal warns that this doesn't mean you can drink as much as you like. You need only consume one alcoholic drink (half a pint of beer, a 125ml glass of wine, or a standard 25ml measure of spirits) most days of the week to see an effect. Alison Shaw from the British Heart Foundation (BHF) agrees: 'In the short term, the good news is we can all enjoy the odd drink. However, as the researchers recognize, too much drink can have an adverse effect on health.' According to the BHF, the best way to reduce heart disease is to stop smoking, exercise and cut back on fat.

## Key discovery
# Low oestrogen linked to heart attack risk

Women who haven't yet gone through the menopause usually benefit from natural protection against heart attacks because of their high levels of oestrogen. But if they have oestrogen levels that are below the average – possibly due to stress or depression – their risk could actually be higher than normal.

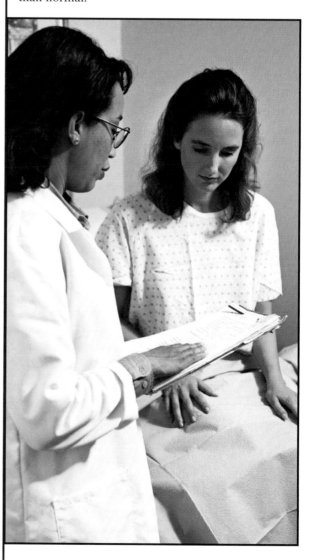

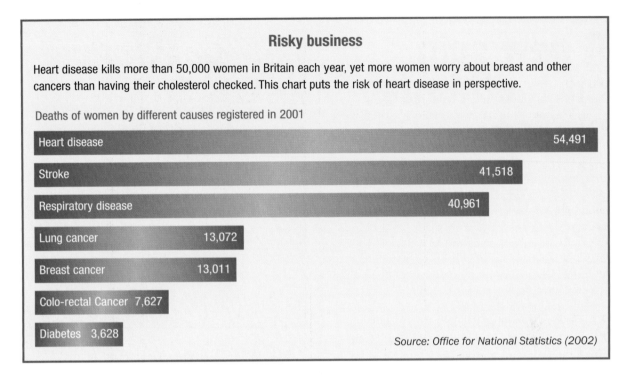

**Risky business**

Heart disease kills more than 50,000 women in Britain each year, yet more women worry about breast and other cancers than having their cholesterol checked. This chart puts the risk of heart disease in perspective.

Deaths of women by different causes registered in 2001

|  |  |
|---|---|
| Heart disease | 54,491 |
| Stroke | 41,518 |
| Respiratory disease | 40,961 |
| Lung cancer | 13,072 |
| Breast cancer | 13,011 |
| Colo-rectal Cancer | 7,627 |
| Diabetes | 3,628 |

*Source: Office for National Statistics (2002)*

In a study published in the February 2003 issue of the *Journal of the American College of Cardiology*, researchers tested oestrogen levels and heart disease prevalence in 95 premenopausal women as part of a much larger study about women and heart disease. They found that women in their forties with chronically low oestrogen levels were more likely to have advanced heart disease than women with normal levels. They also found that women who were taking prescription anti-anxiety or antidepressant medication were more likely to be low in oestrogen, suggesting that emotional problems may lower oestrogen levels and contribute to heart disease.

Although researchers aren't sure exactly how emotional stress factors into the low oestrogen equation, they know from animal studies that emotional and environmental stress can lower oestrogen levels and lead to disrupted menstrual cycles, even stopping ovulation.

**Oestrogen and the menstrual cycle** These findings would appear to confirm an earlier UK study, carried out by a team at St Thomas' hospital in London and published in July 2000 in the journal

*Heart*, which found that women with heart disease suffer worse symptoms during and immediately after their period, when oestrogen levels are at their lowest. The study examined nine premenopausal women with arterial disease and symptoms of angina while exercising on a treadmill at the same time every day over a period of four weeks. They found that the women were most likely to suffer from angina – a pain associated with heart disease – in the week during and after their period.

A British Heart Foundation spokeswoman said that the study raised some interesting questions about the effects of the sex hormones on the heart: 'We understand that oestrogens may have a protective effect on the heart in premenopausal women so it does seem logical that when hormone levels are low this protection may diminish temporarily.' She emphasized, however, that further research is needed to prove this theory conclusively.

**Know your risk** Researchers are a long way from recommending oestrogen screening for premenopausal women, and even further from recommending supplemental oestrogen. However, they do advise all women to talk to their doctors about their heart disease risk factors. If you're premenopausal and don't menstruate regularly, you would be well advised to consult a doctor to find out why.

Factors that lower oestrogen levels – including menopause and possibly stress or depression – may contribute to heart disease. Talk to your doctor about how to lower your risk.

## Progress in prevention
# A new spin on toothbrush choice

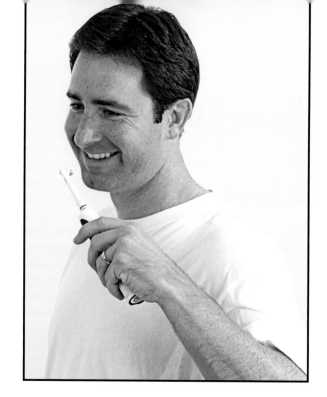

Picking out a toothbrush these days isn't an easy task. Should you go with a big head or a small one, soft bristles or hard, manual or electric? Even among powered brushes, there's more selection than any consumer knows how to deal with, with some offering side-to-side brushing action, others a vibrating action, and still others a circular motion. It's enough to make your head spin.

But recent research could help you to narrow down the selection. The results were released in January 2003 by the Cochrane Collaboration, an international nonprofit organization that reviews existing studies in order to help health consumers make better decisions. They found that electric toothbrushes that provide 'rotation oscillation' – in which the toothbrush spins in one direction and then reverses – removed more plaque and were more effective in preventing gum disease than manual and other types of electric toothbrushes. 'Other powered

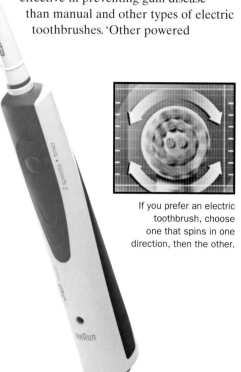

If you prefer an electric toothbrush, choose one that spins in one direction, then the other.

brushes were as good as manual brushes. Only rotation oscillation brushes were better,' says Dr William Shaw Ph.D., coordinator of the study and professor of orthodontics at the University of Manchester.

Types of rotation oscillation brushes include numerous Braun Oral B models and the Crest SpinBrush. Use of such brushes resulted in a 7 per cent reduction in plaque and a 17 per cent reduction in gum disease compared with manual brushing and outperformed other powered brushes such as Interplak and Philips Sonicare as well.

**Don't rush for a new brush** One drawback of the study is that it compared existing studies – many of them carried out by the manufacturers of the toothbrushes that were evaluated. Even the researchers who conducted the review concede that the studies were not as well designed as they would have liked. 'Despite this being a multibillion-dollar industry, no single trial was of sufficient duration to allow the long-term value of powered toothbrushes to be assessed,' says Dr Shaw.

In fact, it may be the toothpaste and not the brush that makes the most difference in whether or not you develop cavities or gum disease. Past research shows that fluoride is most effective in helping to prevent cavities. So use a fluoride toothpaste, advises Dr Shaw, and brush well. 'The most important tip in brushing is that each time you do it, it should not be for less than 2 minutes.'

Key discovery

# Mobile phones not so mobile after all

Since December 2003, motorists in the UK caught using a hand-held mobile phone while driving have faced a fine of up to £1,000. The legislation was welcomed by safety campaigners but many still believe that this is not enough and would like to see hands-free phones included in the ban.

A study on the effects of mobile phone use on driving behaviour carried out by Dr Frank Drews, assistant professor of psychology at the University of Utah in Salt Lake City, would appear to confirm these fears. According to Dr Drews' research, published in the March 2003 issue of the *Journal of Experimental Psychology,* even people who use hands-free mobile phones exhibit impaired reaction times and poorer driving behaviour.

For the study, 110 people were asked to drive inside a driver training simulator while talking on a hands-free mobile phone or to a passenger. When the participants conversed on the mobile phone, they braked more slowly in response to traffic; some of them even drove into the back of the simulated cars ahead.

**How it works** It seems counterintuitive that you can drive effectively while talking to a passenger but not while talking on a hands-free phone. That's why Dr Drews and his colleagues are now studying precisely why mobile phone users get into accidents. Their preliminary data suggests that passengers converse with drivers differently than with people on the other end of a mobile phone conversation.

'Car passengers modulate their conversation depending on traffic density,' says Dr Drews. 'When a driver approaches a traffic jam, the passenger actually slows down or stops talking completely.' On the other hand, a person speaking to a driver on a mobile phone has no idea about traffic density and continues to talk and question the driver in all driving conditions.

Dr Drews is sceptical that any new mobile phone technology could make talking while driving safer and Kevin Clinton, head of road safety at the Royal Society for the Prevention of Accidents in the UK (Rospa), agrees, 'The main problem is that drivers are mentally distracted and switch off from what is happening around them, so it doesn't matter what sort of phone it is.'

The suggestion of banning hands-free mobiles in the UK has encountered much resistance, however, so safety campaigners are likely to have an uphill struggle in their calls for further legislation against mobile phones. In the meantime, Rospa advise that you should limit your use of the mobile phone in the car to emergency calls and only then when the car is stationary.

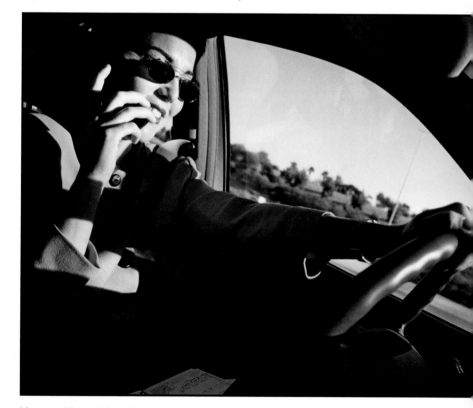

It's an accident waiting to happen: new research shows that using a mobile phone while driving causes delayed reactions and bad driving.

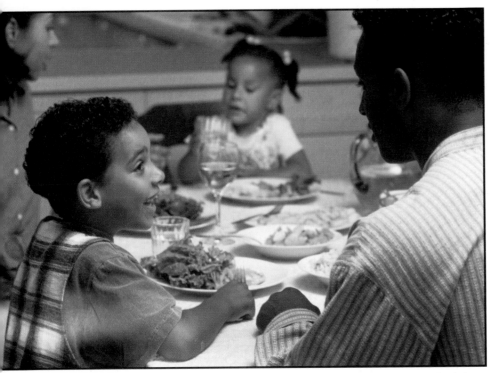

Set the table and gather around. Research shows that routines such as eating dinner together help families thrive, both emotionally and physically.

## Key discovery
# Family dinner a big helping of therapy

Professor Barbara Fiese Ph.D. has made dinnertime a priority for her family ever since her son was a toddler. She held firm to the routine even during his secondary school years, when extracurricular activities often made it hard for the family to find a common eating time.

She did so in part because of a growing body of research linking family routines such as eating dinner together to the physical and emotional well-being of families. Dr Fiese and her colleagues at Syracuse University in New York, where she is professor and head of psychology, recently examined 50 years' worth of studies on routines and rituals. Overall, families who practised routines such as eating dinner together reported better children's health and academic achievement and stronger marital and family relationships. They also found that children in these families experienced shorter bouts of respiratory infections, and that predictable bedtime routines helped youngsters to fall asleep sooner and wake less frequently during the night.

**A security blanket** Routines, such as reading your child a story at bedtime every night, and rituals, such as birthdays and festive celebrations, may boost family health by creating a sense of security and making family members feel that they're part of a special group. Such routines can be especially important during tough times. 'We know that all families go through transitions and changes, and it's during these transitions that individuals are the most vulnerable in terms of their physical or mental health,' says Dr Fiese. 'The studies that have been done during these transitions, such as becoming a parent for the first time or going through a divorce, show that the predictability of these routines tends to provide a buffer. In the case of divorced families, it provides parents and particularly kids with a feeling that some things in life are going to stay the same.'

**Keep it simple** You may already have established routines and not even be aware of them. They can be as simple as a comment you make every night to your spouse or children, or how you greet your spouse or children when they arrive home.

As for dinner, don't stress yourself by trying to enforce a long, elaborate family dinner every day. 'Most of the mealtimes [in the studies] lasted only 20 minutes and took place about four days a week,' says Dr Fiese. 'We're not talking about long, drawn-out, hour-and-a-half meals.'

## Progress in prevention
# Thwarting hospital-acquired infections

Hospitals are rife with infection and it's not exactly surprising, considering how many germs sick people bring into hospital with them. One bug that poses a serious threat is the dreaded *Staphylococcus aureus* bacterium. Poor sanitation allows this bug to linger on hospital equipment and work surfaces for weeks, where it can quickly spread from one patient to another.

Antibiotics can't always help when you've been infected either. Once routed by penicillin, the superbug has rapidly evolved to resist every new antibiotic drug, including methicillin, one of the most powerful drugs introduced in recent years. The new variant methicillin resistant staphylococcus aureus (commonly known as MRSA) is a major concern in hospitals around the world and particularly in the UK, which has the highest rates of MRSA in Europe, according to research findings by the European Antimicrobial Resistance Surveillance System (EARSS) in 2002.

Reports from the National Audit office in 2002 show that around 100,000 patients are infected with MRSA in NHS hospitals every year. And, of even greater concern, these infections account for up to 5,000 deaths a year. The elderly and people with compromised immune systems – such as patients in intensive care units – are especially susceptible.

The spiralling number of MRSA infections may be due in part to poor hygiene in hospitals. Peter Wilson, consultant microbiologist at University College Hospital, London, believes that, if hospital staff washed their hands after every contact with a patient, the number of infections would be cut by a third. The sterilization of equipment after every use would also help to prevent infection spreading. Another contributing factor is believed to be antibiotics themselves. The overprescription and misuse of antibiotics – for example, the prescription of antibiotics for non-bacterial complaints such as coughs and colds – is thought to have promoted the evolution of drug-resistant strains.

Research published in the January 2003 issue of *Archives of Internal Medicine* shows that hospitals could gain the upper hand by screening incoming patients for drug-resistant infections and then isolating those who test positive to prevent the spread of infection. The US researchers tracked drug-resistant infections at 14 intensive care units for six months. They screened all 2,347 patients entering the ICU, identified 96 who carried the infections, and took steps to isolate them. Those steps helped to prevent the spread of the diseases to other patients. Screening guidelines are being drafted for hospitals in the US but there are currently no plans to introduce these measures in the UK.

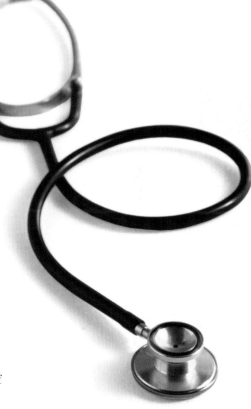

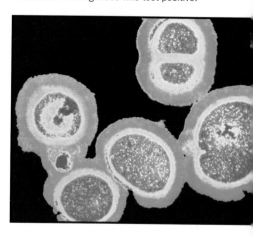

The bacteria can ride on instruments like this, passing from one patient to another. A US study advocates screening patients for MRSA and isolating those who test positive.

# ALSO in the NEWS

## Warning over high vitamin doses

According to the Food Standards Agency (FSA), people taking large doses of certain vitamins and minerals risk seriously damaging their health. A review of 31 vitamins and minerals published by the FSA in May 2003 found that high doses of beta-carotene, zinc, manganese, nicotinic acid and phosphorus taken over a long period can have irreversible effects on health. The FSA also reiterated warnings that high doses of vitamin C (above 1,000mg a day), calcium (above 1,500mg a day) and iron (above 17mg a day) could cause abdominal pain and diarrhoea, although symptoms disappear once people stop taking them. The FSA have even called for a ban on chromium picolinate amid fears that it may cause cancer.

The doses found in the majority of multivitamin supplements are well within safe limits but consumers buying supplements individually may occasionally find themselves exceeding the recommended dose. For example, most beta-carotene supplements contain as much as 20mg – well over the recommended daily dose of 7mg.

## Cruise ships clean up their act

Epidemics of stomach flu swept through cruise ships in the winter of 2002, causing 23 outbreaks on 19 ships and grounding the Disney Magic and the Holland America Amsterdam. In October 2003, more than 430 passengers onboard the British cruise ship Aurora in the Mediterranean were infected with the norovirus stomach bug. The bug is the most common cause of infectious gastroenteritis in the UK and is often found on cruise ships and in hospitals and schools. Norovirus, also known as Norwalk-like virus, is usually caused by inadequate sanitation. Although outbreaks on cruises are still common, a report released by the Vessel Sanitation Program, the National Center for Environmental Health, and the Centers for Disease Control in the USA found that stomach flu rates onboard cruises dropped in the 1990s as a result of mandatory hygiene inspections. You can see the ship inspection scores at http://www2.cdc.gov/nceh/vsp/vspmain.asp.

In the meantime, there is mounting pressure on drug companies to come up with new antibiotics to conquer the continually evolving strains of MRSA. In early 2003, Scottish researchers at AquaPharm Bio-Discovery in Edinburgh discovered bacteria in rock pools that may promise a potent new cure for MRSA. David Livermore, director of antibiotic resistance at the Public Health Laboratory Service, believes the development of new drugs such as these is key in the struggle against MRSA: 'However we use antibiotics and however good we are at stopping the spread of infection, I honestly don't believe we can beat evolution.'

## THE LONG AND THE SHORT OF ANTIBIOTICS

The next time you get a prescription for antibiotics, you may find so few pills – just enough to last a day or two – that you may wonder where the rest went. The chances are, however, that it's not a mistake.

A report by the Standing Medical Advisory Committee (SMAC) in 1998 recommended a reduction in the prescription of antibiotics to help stem the growth of antibiotic-resistant bacteria. This has resulted in higher doses of antibiotics being used for shorter periods of time. For example, urinary tract infections are now treated for 3 days rather than 7, and sinus infections for 7 days instead of 10. Childhood ear infections can be treated in 1 to 3 days. For certain conditions, such as simple coughs, colds and viral sore throats, doctors were advised to avoid prescribing antibiotics altogether, where possible. As a result of this policy, GP prescriptions of antibiotics have fallen by around 20 per cent.

Higher doses kill more bacteria and do it faster, making it easier for the immune system to take over and destroy any stragglers, some of which may be naturally drug resistant. If allowed to linger, these bugs could multiply into an entire drug-resistant colony, contributing to a growing problem. Certain bacteria strains – particularly sexually transmitted bacteria and those that cause urinary tract infections – are now completely resistant to nearly all available drug treatments.

Always finish the prescribed course of antibiotics, even if you start to feel better before you've taken all the pills, since a few germs may still linger.

Progress in prevention

# Saturated fat link to diabetes

You may already know that saturated fat is bad for your heart. But here's something that you probably didn't know: it may also be bad for your blood sugar levels. Intriguing new findings, published in the April 2003 issue of the US *Journal of Biological Chemistry*, explain why – and present the tantalizing prospect of a brand new way to treat, and perhaps prevent, diabetes.

People with Type 2 diabetes are resistant to the hormone insulin. Insulin normally helps blood sugar enter cells, including muscle cells, which use it for energy. When the body doesn't respond to insulin as it should, blood sugar is 'locked out' of the cell and accumulates in the bloodstream. High blood sugar levels wreak havoc throughout the body and can contribute to serious health problems, including kidney failure and blindness.

Previous research has shown that eating too much saturated fat is linked to insulin resistance. In fact, scientists have known for some time that the accumulation of fat inside muscle tissue – much like the marbling you see on a piece of prime steak – seems to contribute to the condition. But no one was sure why, until now. The culprit, as it turns out, is a chemical called ceramide, a by-product of the breakdown of saturated fat.

**How it works** When people with diabetes eat foods that are high in saturated fats, their bodies convert too much of the fat into ceramide. Ceramide then accumulates inside the muscles, inhibiting the entry of blood sugar. The implications are significant. According to the researchers, 'These findings suggest that medication aimed to prevent ceramide accumulation in the body tissue might lessen or even prevent insulin resistance and lead to breakthroughs in the treatment of Type 2 diabetes.' In their laboratory study, the researchers used drugs to block the conversion of the fats into ceramide – and this prevented insulin resistance.

Debbie Hammond from Diabetes UK agrees with the study's findings: 'All types of fat, if eaten in excess, can cause a person to gain weight. It is known that obesity is a risk factor for developing Type 2 diabetes and this may be significant in the recently published research from the USA.'

There's also another reason to go easy on saturated fat: some research shows that an accumulation of ceramide may destroy insulin-producing beta cells in the pancreas.

According to Scott Summers Ph.D., assistant professor of biochemistry and molecular biology at Colorado State University in Fort Collins, exercise is an important preventative measure: 'We know that exercise improves insulin's ability to shuttle sugar into cells while simultaneously lowering ceramide levels.'

**Availability** Before drugs can be developed to block the conversion of saturated fat to ceramide, further studies need to be done. Current drugs that block ceramide have been linked to cancer, so new drugs must be developed before human trials can be carried out. In the meantime, Diabetes UK encourages people to eat a diet low in saturated fat, salt and sugar and high in fruit and vegetables.

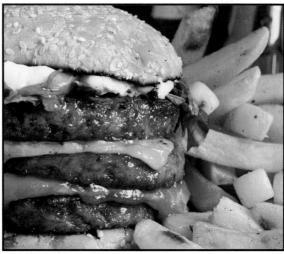

A juicy burger could do more than pack on the pounds; it could also raise your risk of developing diabetes.

## Key discovery
# Fish – could it ever be a danger to your health?

Fish has long been promoted as the ideal heart-healthy food but is this still the case? Research published in April 2003 in the USA revealed dangerously high levels of mercury in those who eat a lot of fish, particularly large predatory fish such as swordfish and shark.

Run by Dr H. Hightower, a junior house doctor in San Francisco, the study showed a startling 89 per cent of the 113 fish-eating people who were tested for mercury contamination had higher than recommended levels and were even suffering from toxic symptoms such as hair loss and fatigue.

However, recent research findings published in the journal *Science* in August 2003 claim that warnings over mercury contamination in fish are overestimated. Researchers at the University of Saskatchewan in Canada believe that mercury may be stored in a less harmful form in the body of fish. But UK experts have cautioned that further research is needed.

**The story in the UK** Although levels of mercury were found to be high in fish in the USA, this is not the case everywhere in the world. A report released by the Food Standards Agency (FSA) in 2002 revealed that mercury levels in most fish in the UK were within the safety limits set out in World Health Organization guidelines.

### Nutritional differences between types of seafood

|  | white fish | oily fish | shellfish |
|---|---|---|---|
| energy | 80 kcals | 180kcals | 76kcals |
| protein | 18.3g | 20.2g | 17.6g |
| fat* | 0.7g | 11.0g | 0.6g |
| polyunsaturates | 0.3g | 3.1g | 0.1g |
| monounsaturates | 0.1g | 4.4g | 0.2g |
| saturates | 0.1g | 1.9g | 0.1g |
| carbohydrate | 0.0g | 0.0g | 0.0g |
| fibre | 0.0g | 0.0g | 0.0g |
| sodium | 60.0mg | 45.0mg | 190mg |

(typical values per 100g/3½oz raw edible fish)

*The total fat figure includes fatty compounds and other fatty acids in addition to mono and polyunsaturates.

The FSA surveyed 336 fresh, frozen and processed sea fish and shellfish for mercury content, including trout, salmon, tuna, halibut, seabass, lobster, mussels and prawns. But only shark, swordfish and marlin were found to contain relatively high levels of mercury – and those levels are only harmful to foetuses or breastfed babies and young children. Fresh and canned tuna contained levels that could damage the nervous system of an unborn child or breastfed baby if they are consumed too frequently. But for most adults and children, reasonable consumption of tuna – not more than a couple of sandwiches a day – is perfectly safe and healthy.

As a result of these findings, the FSA advised pregnant and breastfeeding women, and those planning babies, to avoid eating shark, swordfish and marlin and restrict their consumption of tuna to no more than one portion of fresh tuna or two medium-sized cans a week. 'It is unlikely that many pregnant or breastfeeding women eat more than the recommended amounts of these fish every week. But for any that currently do, it would be a sensible precaution to change their diets slightly,' said Andrew Wadge, acting food safety director of the

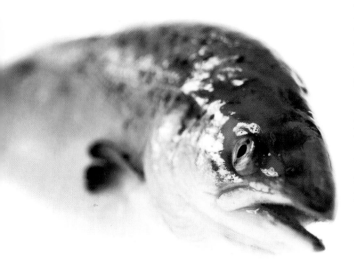

FSA. Children under 16 were also cautioned against eating shark, swordfish and marlin and, as a precaution, other adults were advised to eat no more than one portion of these fish a week. No restrictions are recommended for the consumption of tuna, however.

**Mercury on your plate?** Fish become tainted with mercury in polluted waterways. Industrial power plants, waste facilities, and incinerators release mercury into the air. It eventually rains into lakes and streams, where bacteria absorb it and convert it into methylmercury, an absorbable neurotoxin. Small fish then eat the bacteria, and larger fish eat the small fish. Neither fish nor humans can eliminate mercury easily once they ingest it, so mercury becomes increasingly concentrated as it travels up the food chain.

**What should you do?** Despite the concerns in the USA, where heavy metal pollution is much more widespread, the FSA actively encourage the consumption of fish because of its health benefits. Species that live in cold water contain important omega-3 fatty acids. Omega-3s can not only reduce heart disease risk but also help lift depression, ease joint pain related to inflammation, and possibly even promote weight loss. They are also important for a baby's brain development and can help prevent postnatal depression in women. Fish such as salmon and rainbow trout are packed with healthy Omega-3 acids and can be safely eaten by pregnant and breastfeeding women.

The FSA's general guidelines on fish consumption suggest eating two portions of fish a week, one of which should be oily, as part of a balanced and varied diet. 'Fish is an important part of our diet,' says Diane Bedford, senior toxicologist at the FSA, 'It's an excellent source of protein and other nutrients. People should continue to eat at least two portions of fish a week.'

On average, UK consumers eat three-quarters of a portion of white fish and only one-quarter of a portion of oily fish a week so the advice is to eat more fish, not less.

## How mercury gets to your dinner table

Man-made pollution has increased the amount of mercury in certain fish to levels that may be harmful for an unborn child.

Coal-fired industrial power plants release mercury into the atmosphere.

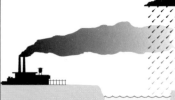

The mercury can travel hundreds of miles before falling as rain into lakes and streams.

Consumed by micro-organisms, mercury moves up the food chain and towards the ocean.

Large fish at the top of the marine food chain accumulate levels of mercury that can cause damage to the nervous system of an unborn child if eaten regularly by a pregnant woman.

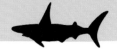
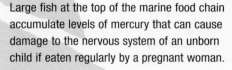

**Large predatory fish** At the top of the food chain, swordfish, shark and marlin have mercury levels higher than 1.0mg of mercury per kilogram of fish – the EU limit for larger predatory species of fish. The FSA advises that pregnant women, infants and children under 16 avoid eating these types of fish.

**Smaller saltwater fish** Mercury levels in all fish in this group were in line with EU regulations except fresh tuna and, to a slightly lesser extent, canned tuna. The FSA recommends that pregnant women consume no more than one portion of fresh tuna and two portions of canned tuna a week.

**Shellfish and freshwater fish** Mercury levels in all fish in this group – which includes crab, prawns and salmon – were found to be well under the EU limit of 0.5mg of mercury per kilogram of fish.

Progress in prevention

# Sugar's reputation sours

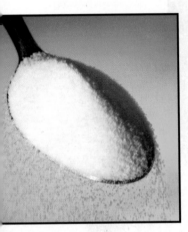

During the 1990s, health experts told us that fat was the arch enemy of good health. Now, another villain has taken its place: sugar.

Not only does sugar contribute to tooth decay, it has also been implicated as one of the main causes of high blood pressure, heart disease, obesity and syndrome X – a cluster of symptoms that include high blood pressure, high triglycerides (an artery-clogging type of fat in the blood) and low levels of heart-healthy HDL cholesterol.

In response to a growing body of research detailing sugar's bad effects on the body, the World Health Organization (WHO) and the Food and Agriculture Organization (FAO) – the United Nations agencies in charge of health and nutrition – recommended in March 2003 that we restrict our sugar consumption to just 10 per cent of daily calories. For most people, that's the amount of sugar in a single can of cola. That suggested limit, which matches the British Nutrition Foundation's own recommendations, received applause from health experts. In the average British diet sugar accounts for 40 per cent of the total carbohydrate intake.

'It's about time somebody took a stand against the sugar industry – eating too much sugar is the dietary equivalent of standing in oncoming traffic,' says Susan Kleiner R.D. Ph.D., author of *High Performance Nutrition*.

**What's wrong with sugar?** Most of the problems stem from its effects on blood sugar (glucose) levels. The body digests sugar – particularly white table sugar or the type listed on food labels as high-fructose syrup – very quickly, dramatically raising blood sugar levels. Your pancreas responds by overproducing insulin, the hormone that is needed to shuttle glucose into cells. But too much insulin, however, will lower blood sugar too quickly. An hour after you have eaten a bar of chocolate, for example, your blood sugar levels are lower than before you ate, and you feel tired and hungry. So you eat again, even though you don't need the calories. Over time, this habit piles on the pounds. Chronic blood sugar problems can lead to many health problems, such as yeast and fungal infections, low immunity and also Type 2 diabetes.

**What should you do?** Some sugars – such as fructose in fruit, lactose in milk, and maltosein in pulses – exist in wholesome plant foods along with important vitamins, minerals and other nutrients that help keep you healthy. You don't have to cut back on those types of sugar. High-fructose syrup and white (refined) table sugar, on the other hand, contain nothing but empty calories, and those are the forms you should restrict to less than 10 per cent of your total calories.

To get your sugar consumption under control, read product labels. Choose packaged foods that contain fewer than 2g of sugar (it's listed on the food label under 'carbohydrates') per 100 calories. You should aim for fewer than 40g of sugar a day, advises Marie Spano M.S. R.D., a health scientist at the US Centers for Disease Control and Prevention.

'And cut out sugary drinks – they're the greatest contributor to sugar intake," Dr Kleiner says.

Is it all right to get the sweetness you crave from a sugar substitute? In moderation, yes, says Spano. 'But "sugar-free" does not mean a food is healthy or even low-calorie,' she notes. She also cautions against the sugar alcohols (such as sorbitol and mannitol) that are contained in many sugar-free sweets, chewing gum and desserts. Many people don't tolerate sugar alcohols very well and experience bloating, cramps, and diarrhoea as a result of eating them.

Key discovery

# Scandal escalates over tainted chicken

A shock report by *The Guardian* and BBC1's 'Panorama' programme in May 2003 revealed that vast quantities of chicken imported into the UK have been injected with beef and pork proteins and water and this elaborate practice has continued for more than a decade.

An undercover investigation televised on BBC1's Panorama showed Dutch manufacturers employing sophisticated techniques to adulterate poultry, most of which is destined for the UK market. It even showed them manipulating beef and pork DNA so that the proteins remain undetected in safety authorities' tests.

The UK's food watchdog, the Food Standards Agency (FSA) was first warned of this practice in 2000 and its own tests identified the presence of pork proteins in poultry in December 2001. In a follow-up investigation, Hull Trading Standards officials examined 25 chicken samples taken from processing plants in Belgium and Holland, including one plant in the UK. They found 15 of the samples contained less chicken than the claims made on their labels. Twelve samples contained pork or beef protein and 11 of these were wrongly labelled as 'Halal'. Also, 18 of the 25 samples were inaccurately described as chicken breast or fillet. Chicken pieces were also found to contain added water accounting for up to 55 per cent of the product's total weight.

**Customer rip-off**
Hydrolyzed proteins – proteins extracted from parts such as the skin, hide and bone of animals – are injected into chicken by processors because this enables the product to retain more water, which in turn helps to bulk up the portions. Meat processors are legally permitted to add water to meat to

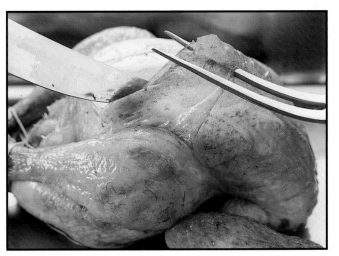

compensate for the liquid that is lost when the meat is cooked although the added proteins actually prevent the water from escaping. Adding water also dilutes the salt and thereby enables the processors to exploit an EU tax loophole on the importation of salted meats.

**A legal practice** There is currently no law against the practice of adding beef and pork proteins and water, although processors are legally bound to declare it on the packaging. Surveys run by the FSA, however, found that in a large number of cases labels are misleading and inaccurate and, as a result, the agency have called for EU legislation to crack down on labelling. They say labels should contain wording such as 'chicken product with beef' or 'chicken product with pork'.

This is particularly an issue for the Muslim community, whose religion forbids them to eat pork, and for Hindus who do not eat beef. FSA tests found pork protein in half of chicken products marked 'Halal', which denotes that the food is suitable for Muslims.

**Call for new legislation** The FSA has called on the European Commission to introduce a 15 per cent limit on the amount of water allowed in processed chicken as well as a separate ban on adding non-chicken proteins to poultry products. Sir John Krebs, chairman of the FSA, remarked on the practice: 'It may be legal but it doesn't make it acceptable. The only reason to add proteins is to pump up the water to high levels and that's a recipe for ripping customers off. That is why we think that the amount of water that can be added to chicken should be limited and the use of non-chicken proteins banned.'

**117**

# ALSO in the NEWS

## New weight-loss secret: get a skinny doctor

If you want more motivation to lose weight, chose a lean GP. A January 2003 study of 226 patients at five US surgeries found that patients who saw slimmer doctors felt more confident about the weight and fitness counselling they received than those who visited obese doctors.

'It takes a good example to motivate people to accept a change in behaviour,' says Dr Larrian Gillespie, author of *The Menopause Diet*, *The Goddess Diet*, and *The Gladiator Diet*. A GP who is overweight, smokes, and otherwise displays behaviour known to incur poor health does not provide a good example, she says.

## Stubborn wound? Give it oxygen

When rally driver Colin McRae fractured his cheekbone in a crash in February 2003, he underwent pressurized oxygen treatment to speed his recovery. Known as hyperbaric treatment, this therapy was first developed to help divers who had the 'bends', but has since been used for many other medical conditions. According to Dr Stephen Watt from the Aberdeen Royal Infirmary, 100 per cent oxygen can help to reduce inflammation in damaged tissues, such as those caused by open wounds, burns and frostbite, thereby speeding the healing process.

In the past, doctors placed you in a pressurized chamber filled with 100 per cent pure oxygen – a cumbersome treatment, to say the least. But a January 2003 study by Dr Gayle Gordillo, a plastic surgeon and assistant professor at the Ohio State University College of Medicine and Public Health in Columbus, shows that simply placing a bag filled with oxygen on top of a wound can equally speed healing time. This study paves the way for widespread use of bagged oxygen rather than traditional oxygen chambers for patients whose wounds heal more slowly due to age, diabetes, cancer, or other ailments. 'We hope the results of our study will make oxygen therapy accessible to more patients, especially those suffering from chronic wounds,' Dr Gordillo says.

## Key discovery

# Can research vindicate high-protein diets?

The popularity of high-protein diets, such as the famous Atkins diet, has soared in the UK over the past year. More and more people are being seduced by the promise of fast weight loss on a diet of fatty foods and celebrity devotees of the Atkins diet, such as Geri Halliwell and Jennifer Anniston, have made it the fashionable way to lose weight. But the diet has also sparked much controversy in the world of medicine. Although one study published at the end of 2002 appeared to vindicate the diet, it has since come under fire once again after more recent research suggests it may lead to kidney problems and bone loss.

In November 2002, the results of a study on the Atkins diet, conducted by Dr Eric Westman, associate professor of medicine at Duke University in Durham, North Carolina, were presented at the annual meeting of the American Heart Association. These results were astounding: they found that instead of raising cholesterol levels – as many doctors and even the researchers conducting the study had expected – the Atkins diet actually lowers them.

Dr Westman's study followed 60 people on the low-carbohydrate Atkins diet as well as 60 people who went on a low-fat diet for six months. After six months, those on the Atkins diet had all lost weight and the diet hadn't increased their cholesterol. In fact, their 'bad' LDL cholesterol actually dropped by 10 points and their 'good' HDL cholesterol increased by 10 points. (Those on the low-fat diet experienced a very similar reduction in total cholesterol, but some of it came from a drop in healthy HDL cholesterol.)

**How it works** Dr Robert C. Atkins, who died in April 2003, developed the Atkins diet in the 1970s. Precisely how it reduces blood cholesterol levels is not well understood. Dr Atkins' theory was that the body doesn't metabolize fat and carbohydrate well at the same time. When you cut carbohydrate out of your diet, your body starts to burn the fat that you eat to create energy, rather than storing it. This means that there's less excess fat floating around in your bloodstream and therefore less need for cholesterol to transport it to your fat cells.

**The downside** Critics of such high-protein diets say that Dr Westman's study, and others like it, do not provide conclusive evidence. The study lasted only six months – not long enough to gauge the true health impact of the diets. And because the study subjects were still losing weight, the weight loss in itself could have affected their cholesterol levels favourably. Dr Westman admits this himself and also cautions that one in 60 people may find their cholesterol levels increase when following a low carbohydrate diet. Such people may have a genetic disposition to a rise in cholesterol with such a diet.

There is also a growing mass of medical research highlighting the detrimental effects of high-protein, low-carbohydrate diets. A US study carried out by the Brigham and Women's Hospital and Harvard School of Public Health in Boston in early 2003 found that high-protein diets can accelerate kidney disease in those with mild kidney problems. Elizabeth Ward, founder and president of the British Kidney Patient Association comments: 'If you have healthy kidneys, you can't eat enough protein to damage your kidneys. But there are a number of kidney diseases, which do not produce symptoms until much later on in the illness.' She advises any-one thinking of trying one of these diets to go to their GP for a urine test first.

Research carried out by Dr Shalini Reddy from the University of Chicago in 2002 found that high-protein diets can also increase the risk of kidney stones and, in the long term, may affect the body's ability to absorb calcium, leaving people vulnerable to bone damage.

Amanda Wynne from the British Dietetic Association does not recommend these diets: 'The Atkins diet is unhealthy because it focuses very much on fat and protein, and cuts out your healthy wholegrain foods. You are also not having a lot of fruit and vegetables, and those are foods that are important for your health.'

**Should you try it?** More research is needed to evaluate the long-term health impact of high-protein diets before they will be approved by doctors and dieticians. In the meantime, if you decide to try a high-protein diet, you should inform your doctor.

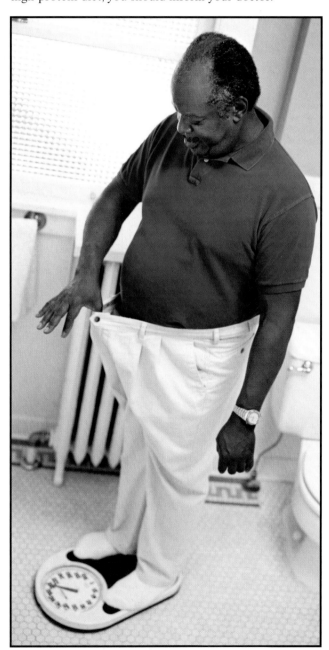

The debate rages on: new studies have found that the Atkins diet could actually lower your cholesterol levels but it may also lead to kidney problems and bone wastage.

Key discovery
# Diet trials – see how they measure up

The diet industry makes millions of pounds from the sales of books, magazines and dietary supplements but there is little hard evidence to back up the claims made by diet companies. How do you know which diet works best? Which is the easiest to stick to? And which is best suited to your lifestyle?

In March 2003 BBC 1 ran a three-week series called 'Diet Trials', which set out to find the most effective diet plan. Led by the University of Surrey in association with other leading academic centres, the study examined four of the most popular and best-known weight loss plans: the Slim Fast Plan, Weight 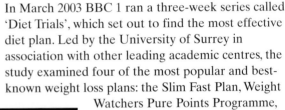 Watchers Pure Points Programme, Rosemary Conley's 'Eat Yourself Slim' Diet & Fitness Plan and Dr Atkins' New Diet Revolution.

The study divided 300 clinically overweight people, aged 21–60 years, into five groups, four of which followed one of the diets and the other 'control' group followed their usual diet, and monitored them over a six-month period. 'We decided that there was only one way to discover the truth – to put some of the most popular (and profitable) diets to the test in a way which was truly scientific and truly independent,' said Gabby Koppel, producer of the 'Diet Trials' series.

**The Slim Fast Plan** This diet involves replacing two of your daily meals with Slim Fast milk shakes, soups, pasta or meal bars, and eating a 600-calorie balanced meal for the remaining meal. In addition, you can eat two to three Slim Fast snacks a day. This provides 1200 to 1400 calories per day – lower than the daily recommended amount, so the dieters lose weight. The Slim Fast products contain vitamins and minerals to ensure a nutritious diet. Dieters are also advised to drink 1.5 to 2 litres of water a day.

**Weight Watchers diet** Based on a points system, this plan does away with complex and confusing calorie counting. Different foods are given a certain number of points

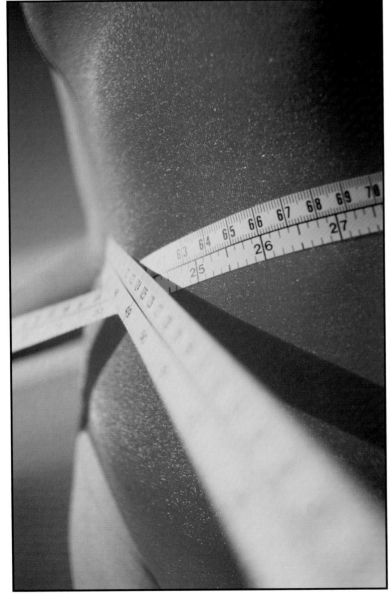

depending on their calorie and saturated fat content. A personal daily points allowance is set for each dieter, based on their weight, age and sex. Dieters are allowed to eat whatever they like as long as they keep within their allowance. Weekly meetings help dieters to track their progress and provide information and advice.

**Rosemary Conley 'Eat Yourself Slim' plan** This plan consists of a low-fat, calorie-controlled eating plan with a strong emphasis on exercise. Dieters are set a daily calorie allowance that is determined by their weight, age and sex. The plan involves regular balanced low-calorie, low-fat meals three times a day and includes one 150-calorie treat a day. Regular exercise is strongly recommended as an important part of the plan and an exercise session is held at each weekly class.

**Dr Atkins, New Diet Revolution** The principle behind this controversial diet is that by restricting the intake of carbohydrates, the body is forced to burn its fat stores thus leading to significant weight loss. Dieters can eat an unlimited amount of protein (meat, fish, eggs and cheese) but must restrict their intake of carbohydrates (pasta, bread, rice, many vegetables, fruit, milk, yoghurt) initially to only 20g each day, although this can increase to 40g after 14 days. Critics argue that the diet can be hazardous to health, leading to kidney problems, bone loss, heart disease and Type 2 diabetes.

**The results** The study revealed considerable variation in weight loss within each diet group. Some achieved substantial losses while a few actually gained weight. There were no significant differences between the diet groups, although all groups lost more weight than the non-dieting group. The results also showed that the men had more success in dieting than the women. 'This is because most of the men tended to have more weight to lose and are also metabolically better at burning fat,' explains Helen Truby from *Lead Scientist*.

It was also found that exercise was a key factor in weight loss. The dieters who exercised had more fat loss and less muscle loss, which made it less likely they would put the weight on again. Although all diets recommend exercise, only the Rosemary Conley plan actually includes it as part of the diet regime.

Finally, those following the Atkins regime did not suffer any harzardous health effects although their intake of nutrients from the diet was inadequate and so they had to take dietary supplements.

## How the different diet plans fared

**The Slim Fast Plan**
**Pros**
- Simple and convenient
- Good short-term way to lose weight
- Diet products contain essential nutrients
- Perfect for busy people
- No group sessions

**Cons**
- Harder to follow at weekends
- Some people reported they missed solid food
- Difficult to stick to diet in the long-term
- Reported decrease in fruit and vegetable intake

**Weight Watchers**
**Pros**
- Easy to fit the diet around a family
- No restrictions on how much and what you can eat
- No exercise involved
- Easy to follow – it had the lowest dropout rate
- Intake of fruit and vegetables increased

**Cons**
- Classes reported to be of variable quality
- Doesn't suit those who dislike group sessions

**The Rosemary Conley Plan**
**Pros**
- Many found this a natural way to eat
- No restrictions on how much you can eat
- Dieters had more fat loss and less muscle loss
- Intake of fruit and vegetables increased

**Cons**
- Doesn't suit those who dislike group sessions
- Unsuitable for those who dislike exercising in public
- Checking labels for fat content is time-consuming

**The Atkins Diet**
**Pros**
- Very rapid initial weight loss, especially in men
- You can eat unlimited amounts of permitted foods
- No need for calorie-counting
- No group sessions
- Side effects found to be overrated by most

**Cons**
- Very restrictive on the foods you can eat
- Potential longer-term health effects
- Diet is deficient in essential vitamins and minerals

# YOUR BODY HEAD TO TOE

In medical science, the wonders never cease. We combed through thousands of studies and reports to produce this collection of important innovations. Learn how the anthrax toxin, and fireflies, are being used to fight cancer. Read about permanently implantable contact lenses and robotic heart surgery, done through pencil-sized holes. Discover the quick, snip-free vasectomy, the cure for warts that you'll find in your hardware store, the patch that calms overactive bladders and much more.

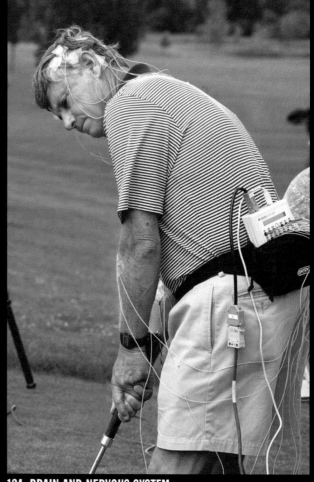

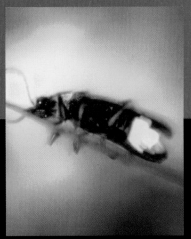

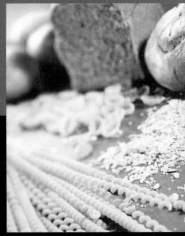

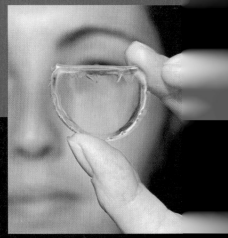

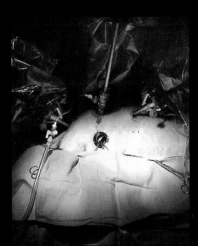

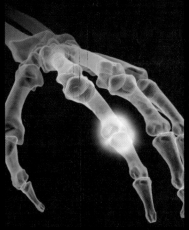

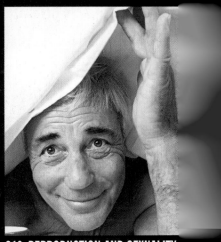

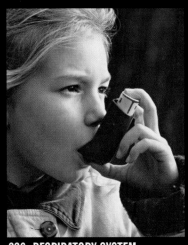

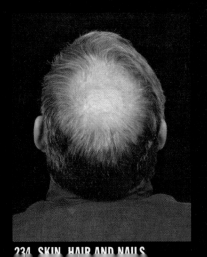

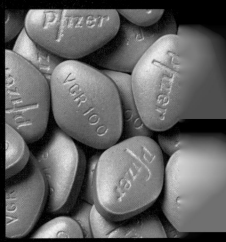

# BRAIN AND NERVOUS SYSTEM

## IF THE SLIGHTEST BUMP, SCRAPE OR CUT MAKES YOU HOWL WITH PAIN, BLAME YOUR GENES

Researchers have identified a genetic blip that helps to determine whether you're a wimp or a stoic. And if you're a woman, the degree of pain you feel depends not only on your genes, it seems, but also on the time of the month.

Elsewhere, a type of brain surgery first used more than a century ago is regaining favour as a treatment for epilepsy, while researchers have concluded that electroshock therapy – in a new benign form – works better than drugs to alleviate severe depression.

One approach that's quite new is a virtual-reality therapy to desensitize people who have a fear of flying. Soon there may be no need to go to an airport or get on a plane to confront your aviation demons.

A different demon, homocysteine (an amino acid), isn't just a heart disease risk anymore; now it's implicated in strokes and Alzheimer's disease. Fortunately, there's a simple way to lower your levels. See page 137 to learn what it is. Finally, there's more reason than ever to have your child tested for levels of lead.

## High-tech help
# Fear of flying – a virtual cure

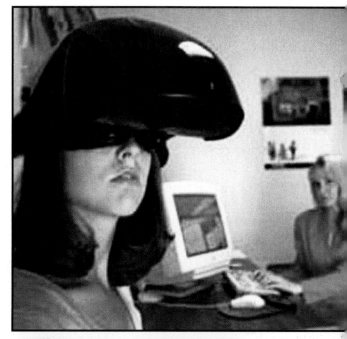

Fear of flying isn't uncommon these days. What with the September 11 terrorist attacks, the would-be shoe bombers, and stepped-up airport security, it's no wonder that, for some of us, having a tooth filled is preferable to flying. About 20 per cent of people, however, have bona fide phobias that make them either extremely anxious or unable to fly at all, even to the point of putting their careers at risk.

For decades, behavioural therapists have known that the best way to treat such anxiety is through a process known as desensitization, in which the phobic person is gradually exposed to the very thing that causes the fear. For instance, individuals who are scared of flying might first visit an airport with the support of a therapist. When feeling comfortable enough, they might sit in the waiting area by the gate, then sit in a stationary plane, and so forth.

In real life, this can be quite time-consuming and expensive, particularly for people who don't live near commercial airports, so therapists have begun taking advantage of a technology more commonly associated with video games. They're using virtual reality, where people are desensitized with computer simulations of airports and aeroplane flights. A study published in the October 2002 issue of the US *Journal of Consulting and Clinical Psychology* found that virtual reality therapy is just as successful as standard exposure therapy in treating fear of flying.

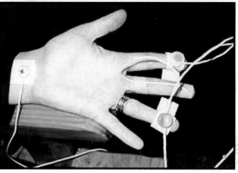

To us it looks like this woman is sitting in an office, but to her eyes and brain, she's sitting in an aeroplane. Sensors track her body's responses.

**How it works** The subject sits in an airline seat wearing a goggle-like device that fits over the head and eyes and transmits extremely realistic images. Researcher Nicholas Maltby Ph.D. of the Anxiety Disorders Center in Hartford, Connecticut, recalls one person who stared straight ahead, gripping the arms of the chair so hard her knuckles turned white. When Dr Maltby suggested that the woman should turn her head and take a look out of the window, she replied, 'No way. We're up too high.'

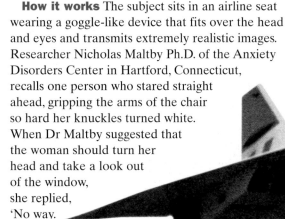

Dr Maltby and his colleagues are now trying to integrate artificial intelligence with the virtual reality device so that sensors could measure anxiety levels (through heart and respiratory rates) to provide feedback. The computer could then adjust the scenario automatically, adding a difficulty factor such as turbulence, for instance, if the subject is able to remain relatively calm during a smooth take-off.

**Availability** This is a new therapy and not widely practised in the UK. For a list of centres abroad where the technology is available, go to www.virtuallybetter.com

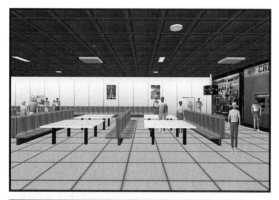

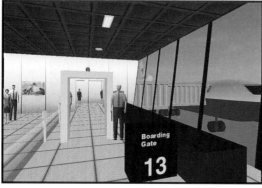

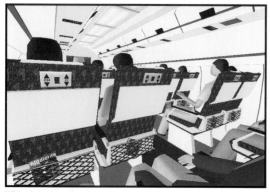

With virtual reality therapy, you can enter the airport, go through security and board a plane without leaving your chair.

# A glowing report for shock therapy

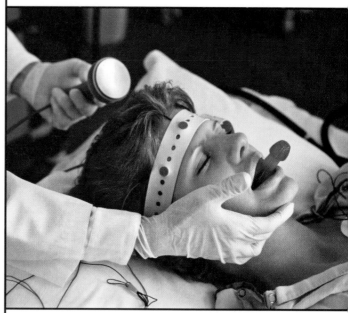

For major depression, electroconvulsive therapy is regaining favour. According to a new study, it works better than drugs.

Despite the dozens of new medications approved to treat severe depression in the past 20 years, a large study has found that the most effective treatment for the often crippling mental condition remains electroconvulsive therapy (ECT), or 'shock therapy'. But instead of being the medieval-like torture depicted in the film classic 'One Flew Over the Cuckoo's Nest', today's shock therapy is a much more civilized procedure. During the treatment, electrodes placed on the patient's head deliver a brief, controlled series of electrical pulses, creating seizures within the brain that last for about a minute.

The study, published in March 2003 in British medical journal *The Lancet*, reviewed 73 trials on the procedure. The results showed not only that ECT was more effective than drugs in treating depression but also that high-dose ECT was better than low dose and that delivering ECT to both sides of the brain (bilateral) was better than delivering it to just one side (unilateral).

## Depression linked to earlier menopause

Many women complain of depression and other mood changes as they move through the menopause, which had led many experts to suggest that dropping oestrogen levels may be to blame. Now, a study published in the January 2003 issue of *Archives of General Psychiatry* adds credence to the idea that low oestrogen and depression are linked.

The study looked at women aged 36 to 45 with and without histories of depression. It followed the women for three years to see how many of them entered so-called perimenopause, when the body's production of reproductive hormones begins to decline.

The researchers, from Harvard's Brigham and Women's Hospital in Boston, found that women who had histories of depression were 20 per cent more likely to experience menopausal symptoms, such as missed periods, changes in menstrual cycles, or hot flushes, earlier than women who hadn't experienced depression before. Women who scored high on a scale of depression during the study were twice as likely to enter perimenopause early; those currently using anti-depressants were three times as likely.

However, what the study does not answer is whether depression lowers oestrogen levels, leading to menopause, or whether low levels of oestrogen result in depression.

## Researchers find depression gene

How do you make a fortune? If you are Salt Lake City-based Myriad Genetics, you discover a gene linked to depression. Pharmaceutical giant Abbott Laboratories, which paid out a million dollars, expects the discovery of the gene, dubbed DEP1, to trigger an entirely new class of drugs to treat depression. Current antidepressants aim to increase the levels of brain chemicals such as serotonin and noradrenaline, but the identification of DEP1 suggests that there may be other chemicals involved – and opens the door to brand new ways to target the disease.

To identify the gene, researchers at Myriad Genetics, which also isolated the two major genes linked to breast cancer, analysed the DNA of more than 400 Utah families who had strong histories of depression. Within three of the 400 families, more than 50 people suffered from depression, all of whom took part in the study.

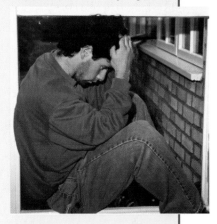

**A controversial treatment** Not all doctors are in favour of using ECT and it has long been viewed with suspicion. The National Institute for Clinical Excellence, an NHS watchdog, has issued guidelines stating that the therapy should be used only as a last resort. NICE says that it should be restricted to people who are severely depressed, catatonic or who have had a prolonged or severe manic episode. It is not appropriate for people with schizophrenia.

There is also the issue of patient consent, with critics arguing that ECT is often used on patients who are unable to give their consent. The NICE guidelines clearly state that informed consent must be obtained wherever possible – this means that patients must fully understand what the treatment entails and should be warned about possible side effects.

On the positive side, ECT offers a solution to severe cases of depression or mania that will not respond to other forms of treatment. It also works quickly. People with the kind of deep, intractable depression that ECT is most commonly used to treat are at high risk of dying from suicide or other medical conditions exacerbated by their depression. They need help fast.

**Today's ECT** People undergoing ECT are put to sleep using general anaesthesia and are carefully monitored during the procedure. The 'shock', when it's given, results in slight twitching. Patients typically have treatments three times a week for six to 12 weeks and begin to improve after the first few sessions. Each treatment takes about a minute.

Still, as with any medical procedure, there are risks as well as benefits. The most common side effects are nausea, headaches and muscle pain that last for a couple of hours after the patient wakes up. More severe but less likely side effects may include memory problems, although many people report that their memory improves. ECT does not help to prevent episodes of depression, as medication can. And it can only be performed in a hospital.

High-tech help
# Mini-brain offers new avenues for drug testing

It sounds like the premise for a horror movie: scientists keep slivers of brain tissue alive for weeks on a 1 inch-square silicon microchip while testing dozens of compounds on it, looking for the next Prozac or Valium. But it's not fiction. A small biotechnology company based in Irvine, California, working in conjunction with researchers at the University of California, is marketing just such a device. The 'Brain on a Chip', as it's known, may one day revolutionize the development of new medications for disorders of the central nervous system, including Alzheimer's disease.

**How it works** The Brain on a Chip consists of a glass chip that contains tens of thousands of inter-connected living brain cells taken from rats or mice. The cells are kept alive in a solution of artificial cerebrospinal fluid, the liquid that surrounds the brain and spinal cord. An array of 64 electrodes on

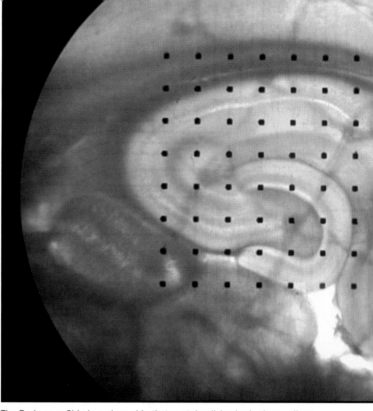

The Brain on a Chip is a glass chip that contains living brain tissue slices. On the chip's surface, 64 tiny electrodes record the activity of the 'mini-brain'.

the chip's surface monitors the electrical activity of the brain tissue just like an electroencephalograph (EEG), which monitors brain waves through the skull. The electrodes then feed the information to a computer. Researchers are using the technology to test chemical compounds for their effect on brain cell activity, a critical step in determining which compounds should undergo further testing.

## ARTIFICIAL
## SPARE PARTS FOR THE BRAIN

While Tensor Bioscience's Brain on a Chip is designed to be primarily a drug development tool, similar technology developed by scientists at the University of Southern California in Los Angeles may one day be able to replace parts of the brain that no longer work. Dubbed 'the world's first brain prosthesis' in a March 2003 issue of New Scientist magazine, the new device is designed to mimic the activities of the hippocampus, the area of the brain responsible for mood, memory, awareness, and consciousness.

It took scientists 10 years to develop the prototype of the artificial hippocampus. Using complex mathematical models, the researchers subjected slices of rat hippocampus to millions of electrical signals, then processed and recorded the slices' responses to those signals before programming them onto a chip, thus creating an artificial hippocampus that acts like a real one. In theory, the chip would be attached to the outside of a human skull and communicate with the brain through electrodes.

The team behind the invention, led by neuroscientist Theodore Berger Ph.D., announced in March 2003 that they were ready to begin testing the chip, first on slices of rat brain, then on live rats and then on monkeys trained to carry out memory tasks, which will – next to humans – be the best indicator of the chip's performance.

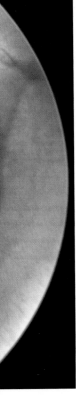

The technology is a major advance from current drug testing, which uses EEGs of the entire brain to see the effects of a drug. This is a crude method, says Miro Pastrnak Ph.D., director of business development for Tensor Biosciences, the company marketing Brain on a Chip. There are various types of circuits in the brain and when scientists research a new drug, they need to examine its effects on a particular circuit. Brain on a Chip enables them to study the EEGs of specific parts of the brain and allows them to 'disturb' an individual circuit to learn more about how the compound affects it. It's akin to following the path of one thread through a sweater rather than examining the sweater as a whole. 'This would be very difficult to do in a whole brain, where many interacting circuits are present,' Dr Pastrnak says.

Early forms of the mini-brain enabled scientists to test just three or four compounds a day, but in the past three years, Tensor has improved the technology to allow testing on up to 16 slices of tissue at once, using 16 interconnected chips. This means researchers can scan 40 to 50 compounds a day. Another benefit: testing brain slices in a petri dish, where the slices exhibit no electrical activity of their own, requires many times the ideal dose of a drug to get an effect. Brain on a Chip enables the recording of natural, rhythmic, electrical brain activity, which previously could be measured only in live animals, says Dr Pastrnak.

Because the brain tissue lives for several weeks, researchers can monitor the effects of drugs such as antidepressants, which don't become fully effective immediately. Other potential uses include screening drugs that target other parts of the body to see if they affect the brain. For instance, a drug meant to treat the heart could be tested on brain tissue to see if it has any negative effects.

Neurophysicist Peter Fromherz of the Max Planck Institute for Biochemistry in Germany, who has developed techniques to grow neurons on silicon, said the chips would be even more useful if they could record the activity of individual neurons. 'The problem is that these electrodes are widely spaced, so you get little information about the neural circuits,' he told *New Scientist* magazine. But he agrees it will be a powerful tool for testing drugs.

# ALSO in the NEWS

## How meditation changes the brain

Scientists have known for some time that when people meditate, their brain waves change, differing from those typical of sleep, dreaming or wakefulness. Now, a study has found that long-time practitioners of transcendental meditation (TM) have brain waves typical of a meditative state even when they're not meditating.

The study's author, Frederick Travis Ph.D., director of the EEG, Consciousness and cognition laboratory at the Maharishi University of Management in Fairfield, Iowa, compared electroencephalograms (EEGs) of the brain wave patterns of 17 people who had been meditating for 24 years with those of people who had meditated for seven years and others who did not meditate at all. The results were published in *Biological Psychology* in November 2002.

The research suggests that people who meditate regularly are able to permanently change the way in which their brain functions. 'In practical terms, this means that you can continue to deal with the day-to-day details, but you never get lost in them because you have this expanded sense of self,' says Dr Travis. More research is needed to understand fully the consequences of these findings.

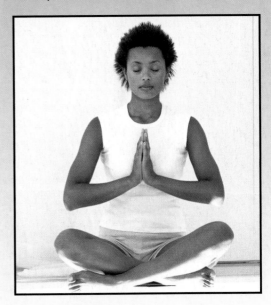

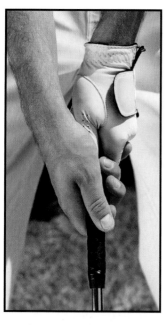

**Key discovery**

# Help for your short game

It's something all golfers dread – the 'yips' – that slight twitch in the hands that makes accurate putting nearly impossible. The yips can curtail a pro golfer's career faster than a 30 handicap and ruin an amateur's weekend fun. Now comes research that suggests that the yips are not all in the mind.

**What the experts found** Researchers from the Mayo Clinic in Rochester, Minnesota, asked 72 good golfers (with an average handicap of 6.7) to complete a survey describing the yips. It was the first time researchers had ever asked golfers to describe the affliction themselves, says lead researcher Aynsley M. Smith Ph.D., who directs sports psychology and sports medicine research at the clinic. Previously, it had been researchers and doctors who had described the disorder.

The results were surprising. More than half of the golfers (55 per cent) described the yips in physical terms, such as 'involuntary jerking of the hands during putting', while just 22 per cent gave more psychological descriptions, such as 'nervousness and a tight feeling in the body prior to and during the putt'. The remainder gave definitions that didn't fit either category.

'We've always known that people with the yips experience a jerk or tremor or freezing made worse by anxiety, but until this study, we didn't see quite as clearly that perhaps there really are two very different groups of golfers who have the yips,' says Dr Smith. One type suffers from a neurological

## WHICH TYPE OF
## YIPS DO YOU HAVE?

Dr Aynsley Smith, who conducted the yips research at the Mayo Clinic in Rochester, Minnesota, says the condition may eventually be categorized into type 1 yips and type 2 yips. Below are some ways golfers describe the yips. Which category do you fall into?

| TYPE 1: DYSTONIA | TYPE 2: PSYCHOLOGICAL |
|---|---|
| Jerky, uncontrollable swing with the putter | Can't start the golf swing |
| Flinching on impact | Adrenaline surges and nervousness sets in at certain times |
| Failure to control the club facet at contact | Inability to consistently make a 3ft (1m) to 4ft (1.3m) putt while putting under pressure |
| Twitch of the hands at a putt | Your mind tells you that you can't make short putts, thus you either push or pull the putt |
| When putting, just before contacting the ball, a sudden spasm causes the player to miss the putt | Nervousness and a tight feeling in the body prior to and during the putt |

problem and the other from extremely high anxiety. That neurological problem is called dystonia, a movement disorder characterized by involuntary muscle contractions (jerks, spasms, tremors) that force certain parts of the body into abnormal, sometimes painful, movements or postures.

**Get a grip – a new one** So what does the new research mean for golfers afflicted with the upsetting disorder?

Well, says Dr Smith, if the findings hold true in future studies, dystonia-affected golfers should make immediate changes in their putting patterns – whether it be a different grip, a different kind of putter, or a different stance – before the yip becomes a habit.

'It's our belief that when you move your hand position or change the grip or start to putt left-handed, you've broken yourself out of this template that had the "hiccup" in it,' says Dr Smith. 'You're firing different motor pathways in the brain.'

To test this theory, she held a putting tournament in July 2003 with 16 self-professed 'yippers'. Half of the participants fell into the dystonia category and half into the psychological category. The golfers were so desperate for help that they paid their own travel and lodging expenses. One man flew all the way to Minnesota from Scotland.

While they putted, researchers monitored their heart rate, stress hormones, grip tension, and even their brain waves in some cases. Dr Smith says she hopes the results, which were due to be published in late 2003, will point to new information about the yips and suggest potential treatments.

'They just want help so badly,' she says.

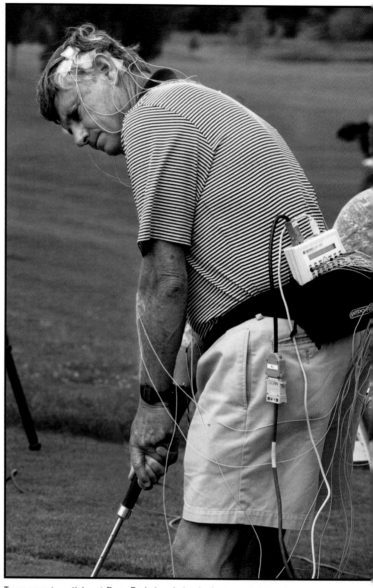

Tournament participant Russ Burkoben is hooked up to monitors that measure his brain waves while he putts. The aim of the study is to get to the bottom of the twitches known as the 'yips'.

# ALSO in the NEWS HRT appears to increase dementia risk

In recent years, tantalizing evidence that oestrogen may protect against or even reverse dementia had fuelled the case in favour of hormone replacement therapy (HRT). But in May 2003, data came in that sharply conflicts with earlier findings. New results from the ongoing US-based Women's Health Initiative found that the most popular hormone combination, Prempro, doubled the risk of dementia in women over 65. The study is the same one that in the summer of 2002 found that Prempro increased women's risk of heart disease, stroke and breast cancer.

Surgical solution

# Surgery gains favour for controlling seizures

Imagine that you have a debilitating illness that leaves you unable to work or lead a normal life. Then imagine that for 18 years, your doctors tried one medication after another before finally recommending the surgery that eventually cured you. By then, however, you had missed out on your youth, your education, and many of life's joys.

That's the reality for the 20 per cent of epileptics whose seizures cannot be controlled by drugs. People with mesial temporal lobe epilepsy (MTLE) commonly fall into this category. Although there is a type of brain surgery that's been in use for more than a century and relieves seizures in 60 to 90 per cent of people for whom drugs don't work, with few risks, it tends to be recommended as a last resort after every medication has been tried.

That could change. In February 2003, the American Academy of Neurology, the American Epilepsy Society, and the American Association of Neurological Surgeons released the first set of

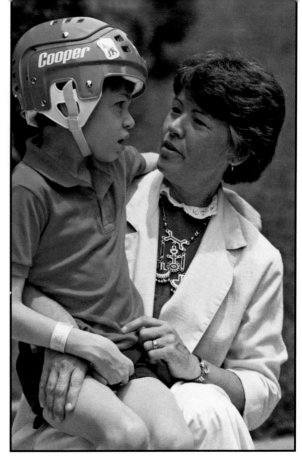

Surgery can help epileptics, whose seizures can't be controlled with drugs, to lead normal lives. The earlier it's done, the less likely it is that recurrent seizures will cause permanent brain damage.

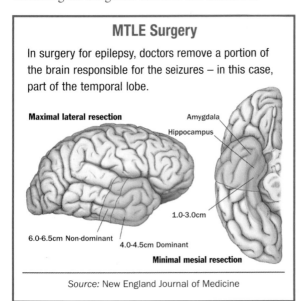

## MTLE Surgery

In surgery for epilepsy, doctors remove a portion of the brain responsible for the seizures – in this case, part of the temporal lobe.

Maximal lateral resection

Amygdala

Hippocampus

1.0-3.0cm

6.0-6.5cm Non-dominant

4.0-4.5cm Dominant

Minimal mesial resection

*Source:* New England Journal of Medicine

guidelines for MTLE surgery, calling on doctors to recommend the surgery for *all* MTLE patients who have disabling seizures and don't respond to anti-epileptic drugs. Although surgery is one of the least used options for treating intractable seizures, the panel found that it's the most effective, says Dr Jerome Engel Ph.D., professor of neurology and neurobiology at the UCLA School of Medicine. Dr Engel headed the committee that developed the parameters, which were published in *Neurology*.

**Support for the surgery** The guidelines rely heavily on one of the best studies ever conducted comparing surgery with drugs. The study, published in the *New England Journal of Medicine* in 2001, followed 40 patients who received drug treatment for a year and 40 who received immediate surgery. One year after the procedure, 64 per cent of those who had the surgery remained seizure-free, while just 8 per cent of those on medication had stopped having seizures. None of the surgical patients died, while one patient on drug therapy did.

The procedure, in which surgeons identify and remove the area of the brain from which the seizures emanate, has been around for more than a century, notes Dr Engel. Ironically, he says, back in the 1960s, when technology was light years behind where it is today, patients were referred for surgery sooner than they are now. 'Doctors tend to drag their feet and keep trying new drugs instead of referring for surgery,' he says, perhaps because there are more drugs available than there once were.

**Spreading the word** There are around 160,000 people with epilepsy in the UK and about half of them have MTLE. Now, the challenge is getting the message across to people with epilepsy and their doctors. The earlier the surgery is done, Dr Engel says, the less likely it is that recurrent seizures will cause permanent brain damage. Because the guidelines don't address when surgery should first be considered, the National Institutes of Health is conducting a large trial to determine if it might be regarded as more effective than medications when only two drugs have failed.

Dr Engel says the therapy could be used to help people who have other forms of epilepsy, enabling them all to lead 'happier, more productive lives with surgical intervention'.

## RESEARCH ROUND-UP

### Gene variation tied to drug rsistance

Researchers have long known that up to a third of people who have epilepsy don't respond to medication, putting them at greater risk of death or other complications from the disease. Now, British researchers from the University College London have identified a gene variation that they suspect may be responsible.

Among the study participants who had drug-resistant epilepsy, the researchers found that about a third had a variation in a gene that results in high levels of a certain protein. That protein seems to put up a kind of wall around cells, which in turn causes the active ingredients in anti-epileptic drugs to 'bounce' against it. Among study subjects who were not drug resistant, just 16 per cent had the gene variation.

Being able to predict which people are likely to be drug resistant could save valuable time in treating them, leading doctors to try other approaches, such as surgery, earlier. The study results were published in an April 2003 issue of the *New England Journal of Medicine*.

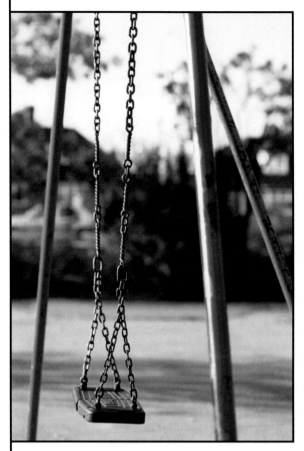

**Key discovery**

# Even 'safe' doses of lead could affect children's IQ

You bought that charming, if run-down, Victorian pile, and now you're sanding and scraping like mad. But if you have children, beware. A major study in the *New England Journal of Medicine* found that even levels of lead in the blood currently considered safe can impair a child's intellectual development. And that old paint you're scraping? It may well contain lead.

Currently the accepted 'safe' level of blood-lead concentration in the UK and US is 10 micrograms per decilitre (mcg/dl), or about 100 parts per billion. But a five-year study has found that even lower concentrations of lead in the blood result in a decline in IQ. In fact, the study found that most of the damage to intellectual ability occurred at concentrations below the 10mcg/dl mark.

**Testing, testing, testing** Currently, children are not routinely tested for lead unless there is a case for suspected poisoning. In the light of this research, the study's lead author, Richard L. Canfield Ph.D., senior research associate in the division of nutritional sciences at Cornell University in Ithaca, New York, reckons parents should request that their children are tested. They should also ask to see the exact test results, he says. Dr Canfield can't say precisely what number

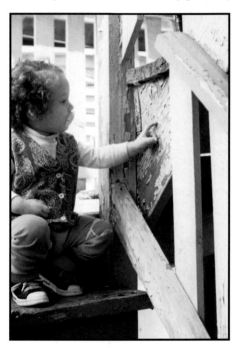

might be considered safe. But he does say: 'If it were my child, and he had a lead level of 5 or greater, I would work very hard to find out where that lead might be coming from.'

Dr Canfield doesn't know why lower levels of lead had a greater effect on IQ than higher levels. An increase from 1mcg/dl to 10mcg/dl resulted in a 7 point drop in IQ, compared with a drop of 2-3 points with an increase in blood lead from 10mcg/dl to 30mcg/dl. One theory is that once lead levels hit 10mcg/dl, a mechanism within the body acts to protect the brain.

**Redefining 'safe'** Dr Gill Lewenden, acting director of public health for North and East Cornwall Primary Care Trust, has studied the effect of lead on children. She says that this is yet more research to suggest 'that there's actually no safe level of lead in the blood'.

Although children's blood-lead concentrations have fallen by more than 80 per cent in the UK over the past 30 years, poorer children tend to be the worst affected. Old housing can contain high levels of lead in the paint. So if you're stripping away that old paint, make sure the kids and their toys are a safe distance away.

## PROTECTING YOUR FAMILY FROM LEAD

Children may be exposed to lead by inhaling lead-paint dust or eating paint flakes, even though such paint was banned in the 1970s. Still, there are many UK homes, particularly older, period houses, that contain some lead-based paint. Houses built before 1970 may also contain lead pipes, which can contaminate the drinking water.

Other sources of either environmental or household lead include car exhaust fumes, lead wicks in candles (now banned), vinyl miniblinds (some contain lead as a stabilizer, and exposure to sunlight and heat makes the plastic deteriorate, forming dust that's high in lead), pottery and other food and drink containers, some home remedies, certain cosmetics, and some fertilizers.

Since lead can build up in the body to toxic levels, it is sensible to avoid exposure from any source. There are steps you can take to make your living environment as lead-free as possible:

- Ask your local health authority about testing paint and dust from your home for lead, especially if you have young children in the house. It is best not to remove the lead yourself. Check the Yellow Pages for a professional technician who is skilled in working with lead paint.

- Wash your child's hands, toys and soothers frequently, especially if lead paint is being stripped from the house. Damp-mop the floors and damp-wipe other surfaces.

- If your house has lead pipes, run the taps for a few minutes first thing in the morning before making up baby milk – to flush out lead in the water that has built up overnight. For drinking water, always use the cold tap – hot water is more likely to contain lead from plumbing.

- Check home remedies and cosmetics (such as kohl eyeliner) for their lead content.

- Take steps to decrease your exposure to lead if you regularly work with lead-based products. For example, always shower and change clothes after finishing tasks.

Key discovery

# The next time it hurts, blame your genes

We all know people who can't tolerate the pain of a paper cut and others who sail through a filling or tooth extraction without any local anaesthetic. Likewise, some women go through childbirth without drugs, while others beg for medication as soon as the first contraction starts.

Are some people simply less brave than others, or is there more to it than that? Researchers at the University of Michigan and the National Institute of Alcohol and Alcoholism in the USA have uncovered a clue to the answer, and it lies in our genes.

**Nature's painkillers** Everyone's brain has receptors that natural painkilling chemicals (encephalins and endorphins) latch on to. Called μ-opioid receptors, they are the same ones to which narcotics such as morphine attach in order to block out pain. Not everyone has the same

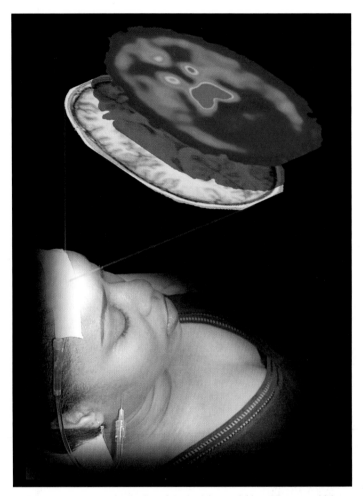

A PET scan shows the distribution of the brain's μ-opioid receptors, to which natural painkillers bind. Warm colours (red) indicate high concentrations and cool colours (blue) are low concentrations. The receptors are activated by the body's response to pain, triggered here by a salt solution infused into the jaw.

## Pain tolerance linked to oestrogen levels

Female hormones may influence pain tolerance, says University of Michigan pain researcher Dr Jon-Kar Zubieta Ph.D. He and his team exposed women to mildly painful stimuli, then used positron emission tomography (PET) scans to examine their brains.

First, they tested women early in their menstrual cycles, when oestrogen levels are at their lowest. They then gave the women oestrogen patches to wear for a week to raise their levels above those normally seen at the end of the monthly cycle. The results showed that the higher the levels of oestrogen, the better the women were at activating their internal anti-pain mechanisms. The lower the oestrogen levels, the

more sensitive women were to the identical type of pain. The researchers presented their findings at the February 2003 meeting of the American Association for the Advancement of Science.

'This makes some evolutionary sense,' says Dr Zubieta. 'During pregnancy [when oestrogen levels are high], you need to be able to withstand pain. At other times, particularly prior to ovulation, women may need to be protected against injury so they can continue having and raising children. The higher pain sensitivity serves as a warning signal that they're in danger.'

That, it seems, is just one more example where Mother Nature is showing that she knows best.

# ALSO in the NEWS

## New hope for cluster headaches

Cluster headaches can be extremely painful. Until now, there have been few ways for patients (mostly men) to find relief. The options can include gulping pure oxygen or taking major pain medication just as the headaches start. But researchers now think that deep brain stimulation – in which a wire implanted in the brain emits small electrical shocks – may be a cure.

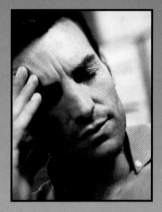

Italian researchers tried the approach with eight people who had suffered severe, disabling headaches for years. They implanted nine elec-trodes in the patients' brains, with a wire running under the skin of the scalp to a small electrical stimulator implanted under the collarbone. After about four weeks, the men's headaches completely disappeared; 26 months after the procedure, three of the eight remained pain-free without any medica-tion, and the remaining five required low doses of medication. None experienced any side effects as a result of the electrical stimulation. The researchers presented the results of their work at a meeting of the American Association of Neurological Surgeons in April 2003.

## Snoring is such a headache

There is perhaps a kind of cruel justice in the discovery that snorers not only give their partners headaches, but suffer from them too. A study published in the April 2003 issue of the US journal *Neurology* found that people who had chronic headaches (at least 15 a month) were more than twice more likely to be snorers than those who had occasional headaches, even considering other factors related to snoring, such as weight and alcohol intake. Researchers don't know yet whether the headaches cause the snoring or the snoring causes the headaches, but they say that finding out could lead to new treatments for both.

number of them, though. And not everyone's natural painkilling system kicks in as readily in response to pain.

To 'watch' the μ-opioid receptors in action, researchers injected minute quantities of saline solution into participants' jaw muscles to simulate a painful condition called temporo-mandibular disorder (TMD). Then they examined the subjects' brains using a positron emission tomography (PET) scan. The scan revealed the μ-opioid receptors and showed when they became activated by the pain.

'We had seen that some subjects had more μ-opioid receptors and some less and that some subjects were more efficient at activating them in response to pain,' says Dr Jon-Kar Zubieta Ph.D., the study's lead researcher. 'But we never knew why.'

**Enzyme answer** To find out, they looked more closely at the brains of their study subjects. Specifically, they looked at the ways in which common variations in an enzyme called catechol-O-methyl transferase (COMT) affected the response to pain. This enzyme is important for 'mopping up' dopamine and noradrenaline, brain chemicals that contribute to pain sensations. The less dopamine and noradrenaline in the brain, the less pain is felt.

The researchers found that people who experienced the greatest pain had weak forms of COMT. Conversely, those with the strongest form of the enzyme were the least affected by pain. The differences in COMT strengths are genetically linked. Dr Zubieta estimates that a quarter of the population have the weaker forms, another quarter have the stronger forms, and half have a mixture, putting them in between pain stoics and pain wimps.

**What it means** The discovery paves the way for a better understanding of why pain medications sometimes have different effects on different people. It may also help explain why some people are more prone to chronic pain or other problems associated with pain, such as depression, says Dr Zubieta. 'Forty per cent of people with chronic pain develop depression,' he notes. 'Why does this happen with some people and not others?

'This is hinting that some people may have more vulnerability to depression or other stress-related conditions.'

Key discovery

# A new culprit in stroke and Alzheimer's

In recent years, a growing body of evidence has thrown suspicion on the naturally occurring amino acid homocysteine as a contributing factor in heart disease, including heart attacks. It appears that it is also a culprit in stroke and Alzheimer's disease.

Homocysteine is formed when the body breaks down protein, especially protein from animal sources. The B vitamins, particularly folate and vitamins $B_6$ and $B_{12}$, break down homocysteine so that cells can use it for energy before disposing of any excess. If this breakdown phase fails to occur – for example, if you don't get enough B vitamins – homocysteine builds up to an unhealthy level, damaging the cells lining the arteries in your heart. It may also make blood cells stickier, encouraging the formation of potentially dangerous blood clots.

A study published in the October 2002 issue of the journal *Stroke* has found that even a moderate elevation in homocysteine levels is associated with a more than fivefold increase in the risk of stroke and almost triple the risk of Alzheimer's disease.

**What the study shows** Researchers from Queens University in Belfast, Ireland, studied 83 people with Alzheimer's disease, 78 with other forms of dementia caused by poor blood flow to the brain (vascular dementia), 64 stroke patients and 71 healthy volunteers. The researchers took into account differences in other risk factors (including diet, smoking, blood pressure and cholesterol levels) and screened for a genetic defect that causes problems with the metabolism of folate. When they looked

RESEARCH ROUND-UP

## Blood pressure drug cuts risk of stroke and heart attack

If you have high blood pressure and are taking the beta-blocker atenolol (Tenormin), you may want to ask your doctor about the benefits of a newer medication, losartan (Cozaar). A large study published in a September 2002 issue of the *Journal of the American Medical Association* found that while both drugs worked equally well at reducing blood pressure, people taking Cozaar had a 46 per cent lower death rate from heart attacks, a 40 per cent lower rate of stroke, and an overall death rate 28 per cent lower than that of people taking Tenormin. They also had a lower incidence of diabetes.

The study evaluated 1,326 people aged 55 to 80 with isolated systolic hypertension, the most common form of high blood pressure, in which the top number (systolic pressure) is too high, but the bottom number (diastolic) is normal. With this form of hypertension, the heart's pumping chambers are also enlarged, because the heart works harder to pump blood out. The study was funded by Merck, which makes Cozaar.

at homocysteine levels, they found that subjects with moderately elevated levels – 13.3mm/l (micromoles per litre) or higher – had a nearly three times greater risk of Alzheimer's than those with lower levels. The subjects' risk of stroke was five and a half times higher, and their risk of vascular dementia was nearly five times greater.

**What it means** Reducing homocysteine levels is pretty simple: just get enough folate, vitamin $B_{12}$, and/or vitamin $B_6$ in your diet (good sources include meats, fortified cereals and breads, potatoes, fish, eggs, bananas, nuts and seeds) or from supplements. If other researchers achieve the same results when the study is repeated, the next step may be to test B vitamin supplements and their ability to reduce the chances of stroke and dementia in people who are at increased risk for them.

Older people may want to talk to their doctors now about supplementing with these vitamins, as studies find that in the USA and possibly here, older people don't get enough folate in their diets to prevent high levels of homocysteine. And with age, the body also absorbs $B_{12}$ less efficiently from food.

# RESEARCHERS ARE BATTLING ON TO FIND NEW CANCER CURES

This year brought further progress. For instance, one of the first trials using gene therapy to treat cancer had spectacular results in several patients with late-stage pancreatic cancer. And a genetically modified version of the infamous anthrax toxin has treated and even eliminated certain cancers in mice. No stone is being left unturned: even the firefly has been tapped as a way to destroy cancer cells.

For women, there's a new – and perfectly painless – imaging technique in development that can actually tell whether a breast cyst is benign or cancerous. And for men, new micro-surgery eliminates suspicious testicular lumps without removing the testes.

Scientists are also making progress in pinpointing the causes of some cancers. They think a common virus may be responsible for some colon cancers, perhaps paving the way for a preventive vaccine. More certain is the link between obesity and cancer. No prizes for guessing the best preventive strategy there.

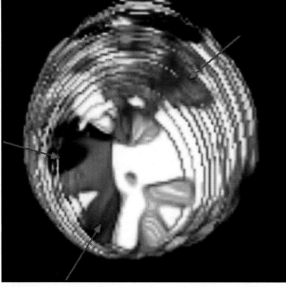

CTLM takes a series of images and reconstructs them in 3D to clearly show the shape and extent of breast cysts.

## Diagnostic advance
# Shining light on breast cancer

For many women the word 'mammogram' has negative associations, carrying with it images of radiation and painful breast compression. Now, US radiologist Dr. Eric Milne is pioneering a new breast diagnostic test called CT laser mammography (CTLM) that involves neither.

Dr Milne is professor emeritus of radiology at the University of California-Irvine, and chief radiologist at Florida-based Imaging Diagnostic Systems, the company that invented CTLM. Not only is this test more comfortable for women, it could also radically reduce the number of invasive biopsies performed to check suspicious tissue, which in many cases turn out to be benign. And it could be used to check the breasts of younger women whose dense breast tissue prevents mammograms from detecting lumps.

In one preliminary study, 120 women underwent both conventional mammography and CTLM. Had radiologists relied on just the CTLM scans, says Dr Milne, the number of biopsies ultimately performed would have plummeted from 80 to 40.

Typically, about 80 per cent of the lumps detected by mammograms turn out to be negative, resulting in unnecessary stressful and painful procedures for thousands of women, he says. Dr Milne presented his results at the European Congress of Radiology in Vienna in March 2003.

**How it works** Instead of standing while her breast is compressed between two X-ray plates, a woman lies on a table on her stomach with her breast placed through a hole. 'It looks perfectly comfortable and nothing touches the breast at all,' says Dr Milne. Instead of the X-rays that are used in conventional mammography, CTLM uses a laser beam not much bigger than a pencil to peer through the tissue.

The test relies on the theory that in order to grow and spread, malignant tumours require a blood supply. They therefore send out signals that spur the growth of new blood vessels, which are often visible long before the tumour is large enough to be seen. Haemoglobin in the blood absorbs the CTLM laser light more than surrounding tissue, making blood vessels emerge as bright, white images so that any new growth is obvious.

The laser circles the breast, then drops down slightly and makes another circle, collecting a series of images in 'slices', or tomograms, from the chest wall to the nipple. Those images are reconstructed

**RESEARCH ROUND-UP**

## Improving on the radiologist's eye

Computer-assisted diagnosis (CAD) is used in hospitals to help remove some of the human error and guesswork involved in reading mammography X-rays. A physicist at the Moffitt Cancer Center at the University of South Florida, Tampa hopes to achieve even greater accuracy with a software program that, in clinical studies on 350 women, pinpointed tumours with 100 per cent accuracy and determined which were malignant with 80 per cent accuracy. At present, human evaluation of mammograms cannot detect which suspicious areas, or calcifications, are actually cancerous and only 20 per cent turn out to be positive in resulting biopsies.

'If we can bring it down from 100 women having a biopsy to 50 having a biopsy, that's a big improvement already,' says Maria Kallergi Ph.D., associate professor and director of the imaging science research department at Moffitt. The software program, called computer-aided diagnosis for breast calcifications, examines calcium deposits and, using an algorithm that includes information on the patient's medical and family history, determines whether the deposits are likely to be benign or suspicious.

One day soon, getting screened for breast cancer could be a much more comfortable procedure – no more painful compression or X-rays.

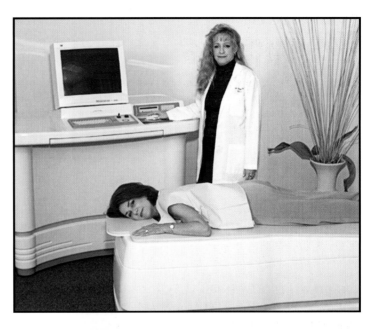

into a green-and-white, 3D computer image that a radiologist can immediately read. The entire scanning process takes about 15 minutes.

The image the scan produces is so clear, claims Dr Milne, that radiologists can tell whether a lesion is a harmless cyst or a tumour – something that's very difficult with mammograms. They're also cheaper than MRI scans, which also provide very clear, detailed pictures. In fact, Dr Milne claims CTLM may even cost less than a typical mammogram.

**Availability** In February 2003, trial results were submitted to the US Food and Drug Administration (FDA) for approval in a bid to market the device in the United States as an adjunct to mammography. The FDA was expected to rule on the application in late 2003. Investigative studies on the CTLM system are currently being carried out in three hospitals in Europe – in Vienna and Berlin. European CE Marking has already been granted, so it should become available in Europe soon.

Professor Stephen Duffy, from Cancer Research UK, believes the technique may prove useful for double-checking mammograms: 'Something non-invasive that was able to be done at the same time as a mammogram, and therefore reduce the numbers of women called back for further invasive checks, would be welcome.' However, he stresses the need for further research to prove its reliability.

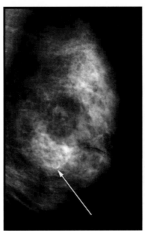
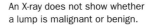

An X-ray does not show whether a lump is malignant or benign.

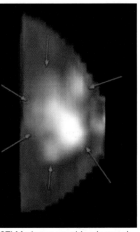

CTLM shows new blood vessel growth, which indicates cancer.

RESEARCH ROUND-UP

## Dense breasts likely a genetic trait

About 40 per cent of women have very dense breasts – defined as breasts with significant amounts of connective tissue and blood vessels – that make it almost impossible for doctors to locate potential cancers with mammography. Researchers also know that the risk of breast cancer in these women is 1.8 to 6 times higher than in women without dense breasts.

A study published in a September 2002 issue of the *New England Journal of Medicine* finds that having dense breasts is probably genetic. Australian and Canadian researchers evaluated 962 pairs of twins and found that identical twins, who share exactly the same genes, had similar breast densities, while fraternal twins, who share half their genes, had similar breast densities about half the time.

The next step will be for researchers to locate the specific gene or genes responsible, which could help to identify those women who have a high risk of developing breast cancer and potentially point the way to new treatments.

Key discovery

# Hormones to blame for obesity link to breast cancer

Researchers have known for years that overweight women have a higher risk of breast cancer but they were unsure of the reason for this link. A recent study has revealed that a form of the sex hormone oestrogen may be responsible.

The study, published in an August 2003 issue of the *Journal of the National Cancer Institute*, looked at eight separate investigations around the world comparing body mass index (BMI) and sex hormone levels in almost 3,000 women. Scientists discovered that obese patients had an 18 per cent higher risk of developing breast cancer than those with a healthy weight. They also found that as weight increased so too did oestrogen levels, in particular a type of oestrogen called oestradiol. Dr Tim Key of Oxford University's Cancer Research UK Epidemiology Unit, who led the research, said: 'We know that hormonal factors are central to the development of breast cancer. This study helps us to better understand the role obesity and certain hormones play in the mechanism that increases risk of the disease.'

Meanwhile, separate research led by University of Minnesota researcher Margot P. Cleary Ph.D. points to another possible culprit for the link between breast cancer and obesity: leptin, the so-called obesity hormone. Researchers discovered several years ago that as body weight increased, so did levels of leptin, which is secreted by fat cells. Researchers had identified leptin receptors – 'docking ports' for the hormone – on some cancer cells and found that adding leptin to these cells caused a significant increase in growth.

**How it works** Dr Cleary and her team, working together with researchers at the Mayo Clinic, tested the effects of leptin on breast cancer cells in the laboratory. In the presence of leptin, the number of cancerous cells rose by 150 per cent, compared to 50 per cent without leptin. The researchers

## RESEARCH ROUND-UP

### Fat consumption linked to leptin levels

More body fat means higher levels of leptin – the so-called obesity hormone, recently linked to an increased risk of breast cancer. But according to a small study at the University of Texas M.D. Anderson Cancer Center in Houston, women who switch to a low-fat, high-fibre diet can lower their leptin levels regardless of their weight. Measuring blood leptin levels could provide an additional marker for measuring breast cancer risk, along with body fat composition, oestrogen levels, and factors such as family history, number of pregnancies, and the age at which menstruation starts.

also identified leptin receptors on the breast cancer cells. Researchers found further evidence when they bred several groups of mice, some of which were genetically programmed to develop breast cancer but were deficient in leptin. The mice that should have developed breast cancer did not. The study results were published in a November 2002 issue of the *Journal of the National Cancer Institute*.

Both studies reaffirm the importance of maintaining a healthy weight in order to minimise breast cancer risk. In fact, the findings have served as an incentive for Dr Cleary, who has lost a few pounds herself.

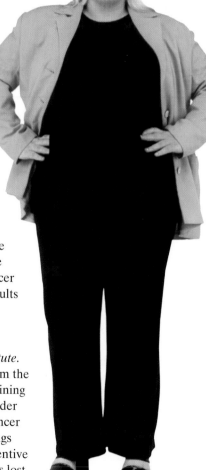

Key discovery

# Common virus the colon cancer culprit?

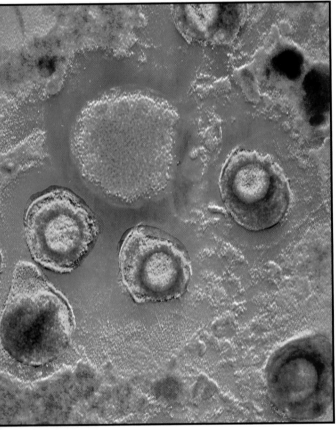

Many people are infected with the human cytomegalovirus, one of the herpes viruses, without knowing it. Scientists believe that the virus may increase the risk of colon cancer.

Colon cancer is the third most common cancer in men in the UK and the second most common in women, with over 35,000 new cases each year. Risk factors include a family history of colon cancer, the presence of polyps in the bowel, recurring chronic inflammatory infections, inherited gene mutations and, possibly, a diet that is high in fat and low in fibre. And, to add to the list, a US neurosurgeon has recently discovered that a common herpes virus may be linked to colon cancer. This finding could pave the way for new treatments or even a vaccine.

Dr Charles S. Cobbs, associate professor in the departments of surgery and cell biology at the University of Alabama at Birmingham Medical Center, was researching the role of chronic inflammation in brain cancer. The more he studied the topic, however, the more convinced he became that a persistent virus must be contributing to brain cancer. Dr Cobbs discovered that, indeed, there was; it was the human cytomegalovirus (CMV). Although this common virus rarely causes problems in healthy adults, it can lead to birth defects and severe infections in people with weak immune systems. The virus had been strongly linked to malignant glioma, the most prevalent and malignant type of brain tumour, and Dr Cobbs soon realized that it may also be linked to colon cancer.

**How it works** It turns out that CMV is ideal for causing cancer, says Dr Cobbs. Once it infects you, it never goes away, lying dormant until something – such as stress or reduced immunity – reactivates it. It also causes DNA mutations (a key step in turning a normal cell into a rapidly dividing cancer cell) and enables cells to move around (critical to cancer cells, which metastasize, or spread). Most importantly, once CMV infects a cell, it produces a protein-based 'invisibility cloak' to keep that cell hidden from immune system cells that could destroy it.

During his research, Dr Cobbs dug up journal articles from the 1970s hinting at the possibility of a link between CMV and colon cancer. To explore the theory further, he obtained specimens of colorectal polyps (precancerous cells), colorectal tumour cells, and normal cells from 28 people with the disease and tested them for CMV. He found two specific CMV proteins in about 80 per cent of the polyps and about 85 per cent of the cancer samples. The results of that study were published in a November 2002 issue of *The Lancet*.

The theory is that the virus may infect cells that already have a slight DNA injury. This turns what may have been a slow-growing mutation into a fast-growing cancer. 'If we show that's the case, then it would raise a lot of questions,' Dr Cobbs says. For instance, should people with a high risk of colon cancer be treated with existing drugs that block CMV infection? Or should a vaccine be developed to prevent CMV infection, much like the vaccine currently being developed to prevent infection with human papillomavirus, which causes cervical cancer? Those are all questions, notes Dr Cobbs, that future research will help to answer.

Progress in prevention

# Cancer benefits for miracle drug aspirin

The humble painkiller aspirin has been getting quite the wonder drug reputation lately. Research has found that it helps prevent not only heart attacks, strokes and possibly Alzheimer's disease, but lung, prostate, and colon cancer as well. And that's not all. Now it appears the bitter white tablets may have some effect against breast and ovarian cancer as well as other cancers.

**Breast cancer** A study that followed 27,616 women over six years found that those who took aspirin six or more times a week cut their relative risk of breast cancer by nearly a third. The results were published in the journal *Cancer Epidemiology Biomarkers and Prevention* in December 2002.

**Ovarian cancer** Another study, published in the October 2002 issue of *Obstetrics and Gynecology,* found that regular doses of aspirin prevented the growth of ovarian tumour cells – at least in the laboratory – by as much as 68 per cent. And when combined with a drug that blocks the action of certain proteins that encourage cancer cell growth, it decreased ovarian cancer cell growth by 84 per cent. Of course, test tube studies don't show what would happen in real women with cancer. Scientists stress that much more study is needed before anyone could point to aspirin as part of ovarian cancer treatment.

**Cancers of the throat and mouth** Scientists in Italy have discovered that taking aspirin for five years or more cuts the risk of developing cancers of the mouth, throat and oesophagus by two-thirds. Researchers from the Institute of Pharmacological Research in Milan analysed data from three separate studies involving 965 cancer patients and 1,779 people who were in hospital for other reasons, noting details about their smoking and drinking habits, diet and how often they took doses of aspirin. The research was published in the *British Journal of Cancer* in March 2003.

Dr Richard Sullivan, Head of Clinical Programmes for Cancer Research UK, says: 'Aspirin has to count as one of the greatest finds in the history of drug

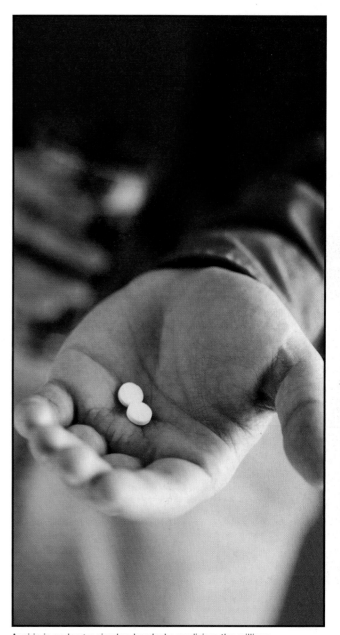

Aspirin is no longer simply a headache medicine: the millions of people who now take the medication to help stave off a heart attack or stroke may be doing themselves an extra favour by lowering their risk of certain cancers.

discovery. What began life as a simple painkiller now seems to have a wide range of beneficial effects for our health, and this new study adds to the evidence of a significant protective effect against cancer.'

However, he also cautions that much more research is needed into the effectiveness of the drug and the potential side effects of long-term use before people can start taking aspirin on a daily basis.

## Key discovery
# A cancer danger in your food?

Believe it or not, how you eat your bread may have an effect on your risk of cancer. Scientists have known for some time that a white, odourless substance called acrylamide causes cancer, at least in mice. The substance is used to make polyacrylamide, a chemical found in everything from cosmetics to plastics. It's also used in sewage and waste treatment and to purify drinking water.

In 2002, Swedish researchers made a disturbing discovery: even people who had no known acrylamide exposure showed signs of the substance in their blood. After further investigation, the researchers concluded that the source of the toxin was food.

**Suspect foods** It seems that acrylamide is formed as a result of the chemical changes that occur when foods are baked, fried or roasted (but not boiled). Many foods with the greatest amounts of acrylamide are also those that are the worst for you, such as French fries and crisps. These findings were reinforced by a separate investigation carried out by the UK Food Standards Agency (FSA) in May 2002 on a range of products, including chipped and fried supermarket potatoes, crisps, crispbreads, and several brands of cereal.

**No final answers yet** Not everyone agrees that acrylamide in food is a cancer threat. A study published in the *British Journal of Cancer* in January 2003 revealed that acrylamide in the diet might not be a cancer risk after all. Researchers from the Harvard School of Public Health in Boston and the Karolinska Institute in Stockholm, Sweden, evaluated the diets of 987 cancer patients and 538 healthy people but found no association between eating foods high in acrylamide (primarily crispbreads and fried potatoes) and increased risk of bladder, bowel, or kidney cancer. Another study published in July 2003 found similar results for additional cancers (oral, pharyngeal, oesophageal, laryngeal, breast, and ovarian).

These findings were greeted with interest, although many experts remain cautious about jumping to conclusions. Dr Lorelei Mucci, who led the research, admitted that acrylamide levels in certain foods are still not known and very high levels could contribute to cancer risk. Sir Paul Nurse, chief executive of Cancer Research UK, said: 'We know that acrylamide can be carcinogenic to animals, but this study suggests that either levels in food are too low to affect cancer risk, or that the body is able to deactivate the chemical in some way.' However, he urged that more research is needed to investigate the link between cancer and acrylamide.

The FSA stress that there's no cause for concern. They do not recommend that consumers stop eating any of these foods or change their cooking methods, but advise that, as part of a balanced diet, people should limit the amount of fried and fatty foods they eat.

Baked, fried, and toasted foods are often high in acrylamide, a known carcinogen.

# Debating the safety of our food

The acrylamide question is far from settled. On one side of the issue are consumer activists concerned that our food supply poses a serious cancer threat. On the other side are researchers who are finding little risk when they compare the amount of acrylamide some populations consume with their overall cancer risk.

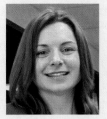

## SAFE

*Lorelei Mucci Ph.D. is a researcher at the Harvard School of Public Health. She is lead author of the study published in January 2003 that found no link between acrylamide in food and an increased risk of bladder, large bowel, and kidney cancer in humans.*

**Q** It seems that your study disputes what the animal studies found. How is that possible?

**A** Animal studies are based on amounts (of the toxin) several hundredfold higher than what humans are exposed to. Also, the way animals are exposed is different. Animals are injected with the chemical or they inhale it, as opposed to consuming it in their food supply. It's a little tricky to extrapolate those very high dosages to what we're seeing consumed through the diet of the average person.

**Q** So are you saying that acrylamide is not dangerous in the food supply?

**A** A lot of additional research needs to be done to confirm our findings, but it seems that we can tone down some of the high levels of concern that were raised. It is probably not responsible for the thousands of cancer cases that people said it was.

**Q** Are you still conducting research on this issue?

**A** Yes. We are correlating data examining the use of coffee and examining the risk to additional cancer sites [other parts of the body where the cancers are found].

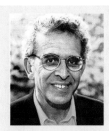

## UNSAFE

*Michael F. Jacobson Ph.D. is executive director of the nutrition advocacy organization Center for Science in the Public Interest, which is based in Washington, D.C. in the USA.*

**Q** The Harvard and Italian studies found no cancer risk from acrylamide. Does this make it a non-issue?

**A** The study provides no reassurance whatsoever that acrylamide is safe for humans. The researchers considered three cancers – bladder, colon, and kidney – but those are not the ones that acrylamide causes in animals. Moreover, the researchers' estimates of acrylamide exposure are flawed because they were based on a limited number of foods. We get acrylamide from a wide range of foods, and someone who eats a lot of fried potatoes may eat less bread, which is also a source of acrylamide. You have to look at things a lot more closely. Also, acrylamide *doesn't* cause that many cancers (fewer than 1 per cent). To detect something in an epidemiological study (like the Harvard and Italian studies), you need a blockbuster carcinogen like tobacco.

**Q** So how great a threat is acrylamide?

**A** The risk is significant, but it's not like smoking cigarettes or eating hot dogs or some of the other foods that have been linked with cancer. I've been looking at different ways to estimate risk, and the number varies between about 1,000 cancers per year and 25,000 per year. So it's not an enormous risk, and it's hard to expect that people are going to avoid French fries because of it.

**Q** So what should consumers do?

**A** Our general advice has been to eat less of the least nutritious, most contaminated foods, things like French fries, potato chips [crisps], corn chips, and coffee. Other foods, like Cheerios or bread, that have some acrylamide, I wouldn't say to cut out, because they have other nutritional benefits. The ultimate answer will be for scientists to figure out how to prevent or minimize its formation.

## Key discovery
# To cut your risk of cancer, shed a few pounds

The list of health problems linked with being overweight is getting longer: heart disease, high blood pressure, diabetes, insulin resistance, arthritis, depression. Now we can add cancer to that list, based on the findings of a seminal study of more than 900,000 American adults. The results, published in an April 2003 issue of the *New England Journal of Medicine,* can be summed up in one sentence: the more you weigh, the more likely you are to die from cancer – *any* cancer.

**How they did it** Researchers from the American Cancer Society used data from the Cancer Prevention Study II, which has tracked more than a million people since 1982. The study looked at factors such as the subjects' health and various lifestyle and physical characteristics, including weight. They also took into account other factors related to cancer, such as smoking, alcohol intake, and diet as well as race, educational status, and physical activity. They used the body mass index (BMI), which considers weight and height, to evaluate weight status. A BMI between 18.5 and 24.9 is considered normal, while one between 25.0 and 29.9 is overweight, and 30.0 or more is obese.

**What they found** Men with a BMI over 40 were 52 per cent more likely to die from cancer, while women whose BMI was more than 40 were 62 per cent more likely to die from the disease. Overall, the authors estimated, as many as 14 per cent of all cancer deaths in men

over 50 and 20 per cent in women over 50 are attributable to being overweight. Researchers believe an explanation for the link between obesity and cancer may lie in hormonal changes that result from being overweight, along with some mechanical changes that occur. For example, heavy people are more susceptible to acid reflux, or heartburn, which is a risk factor for oesophageal cancer.

The findings reinforce a study carried out by the International Agency for Research on Cancer (IARC) in France in 2002. Researchers estimated that 40 per cent of womb-lining cancers, 25 per cent of kidney cancers and 10 per cent of breast and colon cancers could be avoided if people kept their weight down. Obesity is particularly dangerous in postmenopausal women where it can increase the risk of breast cancer by as much as 40 per cent. The team calculated that obesity is responsible for 35,000 new cases of cancer each year in Europe.

The results of these studies have caused a stir in the UK, where obesity rates have risen sharply in the past decade due to poor diet and sedentary lifestyle. About 50 per cent of men and 35 per cent of all women in the UK are overweight and an estimated one in five people is obese. Experts are calling for a concerted effort to tackle obesity by governments, the media, schools and employers. Cancer Research UK recommend that people eat a healthy, balanced diet and take regular exercise to reduce their risk of developing cancer.

### As waistlines grow, so does cancer risk

The table shows by what percentage your risk for various cancers increases if you are overweight. A body mass index (BMI) of 18.5 to 24.9 is considered normal. A BMI between 25.0 and 29.9 indicates overweight and 30.0 or more is obese.

| CANCER | BODY MASS INDEX | | | | | |
| --- | --- | --- | --- | --- | --- | --- |
| | 25.0–29.9 | | 30.0–34.9 | | 35.0–39.9 | |
| | Men (%) | Women (%) | Men (%) | Women (%) | Men (%) | Women (%) |
| Colorectal cancer | 20 | 10 | 47 | 33 | 84 | 36 |
| Liver cancer | 13 | — | 90 | 40 | 352 | 68 |
| Pancreatic cancer | — | 11 | — | 28 | — | 41 |
| Prostate cancer | 0.8 | — | 20 | — | 34 | — |
| Kidney cancer | 18 | 33 | 36 | 66 | 70 | 70 |
| Breast cancer | — | 34 | — | 63 | — | 70 |
| Non-Hodgkins' lymphoma | 0.8 | 22 | 56 | 20 | 49 | 95 |

*Source:* New England Journal of Medicine

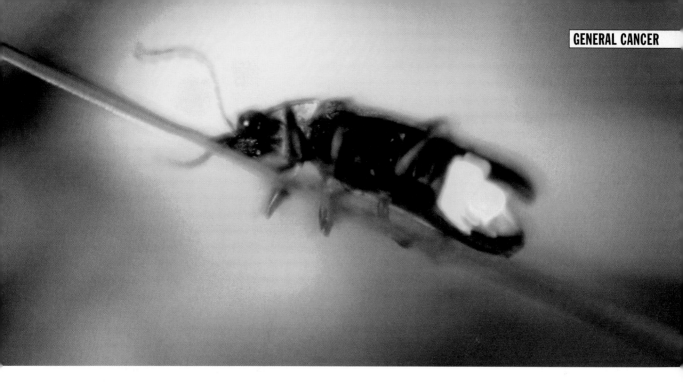

## High-tech help
# Fireflies' glow lights the way in cancer treatment

The chemical that helps fireflies glow may have a role to play in cancer treatment. The goal of most cancer treatments today is to kill cancer cells or, more accurately, to make the cells commit suicide. However, it's nearly impossible to know if such treatments work until weeks or months after they're used. Researchers from the University of Michigan Health System may now have found a way around that problem with the help of the gene responsible for a firefly's glow.

The researchers inserted the gene into mice with cancer, but first they manipulated the gene so that it was turned 'off' until cancer cells began to die. The cancer cells' death turned the glow gene 'on', causing the mice to emit faint traces of firefly light. Once perfected, the technique could be used to determine if cancer treatments are working days or weeks after they're administered, rather than months. The researchers' work was published in the December 2002 issue of the journal *Proceedings of the National Academy of Science*.

In Britain, researchers at University College London are using the firefly light gene to actually kill cancer cells. They first inserted the gene into cancer cells to make them glow. Then they added a photosensitizing agent to the cells which, when exposed to firefly light, destroys the cells. The technique is similar to an existing treatment called photodynamic therapy (PDT), in which cancer cells are injected with a photosensitizing chemical and blasted with laser light.

One problem with PDT is that the light source can pass through only a very thin layer of cells, so it's been used primarily to treat tumours just below the skin or on the outer parts of organs. With the firefly gene, the light source is implanted directly into the tumour cell, so even tumours deep within the body can be targeted.

**The cancer cells' death turned the glow gene 'on', causing the mice to emit faint traces of firefly light.**

More research is needed, but scientists hope that treatments based on the firefly gene may one day be used on patients. Researchers at the University of California at Los Angeles have already shown that this gene may be delivered to prostate cancer cells.

**147**

# Lethal anthrax toxin – the new cancer hero

The same deadly toxin that terrified the world in the autumn of 2001 may one day turn out to be an effective cancer treatment. Researchers at the US National Institutes of Health (NIH) found in tests on hundreds of mice that a genetically modified version of the anthrax toxin dramatically reduced, and even eliminated, certain cancers, without harming the mice. The study results were published in the January 2003 issue of *Proceedings of the National Academy of Sciences*.

**How it works** For decades, researchers have been investigating the use of biological poisons, including diphtheria toxin and ricin (a poisonous protein in the castor bean) for cancer treatment. It's not as crazy as it sounds. After all, what are chemotherapy drugs if not poisons? The idea to try anthrax came from a chance conversation between NIH scientists Stephen Leppla Ph.D. and Thomas Bugge Ph.D. Dr Bugge was telling Dr Leppla about his work with plasminogen activator systems, which are enzymes found only on cancer cells. Because of this, these enzymes make good targets for drugs and other cancer treatments. The two men wondered if plasminogen activators could somehow be used in conjunction with anthrax, which Dr Leppla had been studying for years.

Their brainwave was inspired by the way the anthrax toxin works. In order for it to do its damage, it has to hook up with an enzyme called furin, found on the surface of nearly all cells. Without this enzyme, anthrax is basically harmless. Pairing it with furin, though, is the equivalent of pulling the pin in a hand grenade.

So what would happen if the anthrax toxin were modified to hook up only with a plasminogen enzyme? To find out, the two scientists 'rewrote' a sequence of amino acids in one anthrax protein. The new sequence amounted to a change in instruction for the protein, telling it to combine only with a plasminogen activator called urokinase, which is produced in high levels by tumour cells.

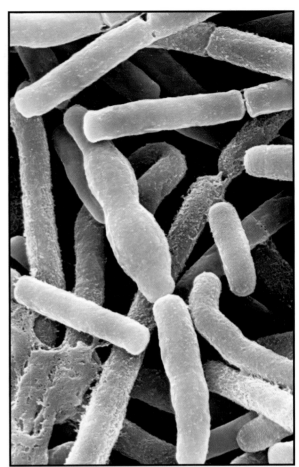

Anthrax killed five people when it was sent through the post in the United States. Now the deadly toxin is being unleashed on cancer.

The results were tremendous. In trials in mice, a single injection of the modified anthrax toxin shrank lung tumours by about 65 per cent and reduced soft-tissue tumours such as melanoma and fibrosarcoma, two forms of skin cancer, by about 92 per cent. The tumours shrank even more after two treatments. It had no effect on normal cells, however.

**Availability** The Danish biotechnology company OncoTac has licensed the technology, which may move into human clinical trials in 2004. Dr Elaine Vickers, of Cancer Research UK, found the results interesting but says there is need for more research: 'Molecules that are over-produced by cancer cells are very interesting as targets for developing new cancer treatments, hopefully with fewer of the side effects associated with more conventional therapies. However, it is essential that the molecule targeted by the treatment is exclusively overproduced by cancer cells to avoid damage to healthy tissue.'

Surgical solution
# First, remove the liver...

A team of Italian surgeons and researchers has given new meaning to the term 'out-of-body experience'. In one of the most unusual cancer treatments ever, they removed a patient's liver, transported it to a nuclear reactor and blasted it with radiation. Then they returned it to the operating room and reimplanted it in the 48-year-old patient. Doctors performed the 21-hour operation in December 2001 and the man was still cancer-free at his quarterly check-up in April 2003. 'The result is beyond our hope,' says physicist Tazio Pinelli Ph.D. of the National Institute of Nuclear Physics in Italy.

The patient's 14 tumours had not responded to chemotherapy and the cancer was so pervasive that conventional radiation would have destroyed the liver entirely. So Dr Pinelli and his team decided to try a procedure they'd been working on for more than 13 years, called boron neutron capture therapy, or BNCT. It's been tried in brain cancer patients but has had poor results.

**How it works** The organ – in this case, the liver – is infused with boron, an element that has both metallic and non-metallic properties. Cancer cells, which grow faster than normal cells, take up more boron atoms. When the neutron beam, or radiation, is turned on, the beam splits the boron atoms into destructive high-energy particles, which then kill the cancer cells. It would be difficult to provide this level of radiation while the organ is in the body because healthy tissue would be damaged.

The patient's liver was placed in a Teflon bag for its trip to the reactor. Meanwhile, the patient was kept alive on an artificial liver, just as he would have been during a traditional liver transplant. The liver was out of the patient's body for about two hours.

**Availability** Dr Pinelli and his team are preparing to conduct more surgery of this type in 2004. They hope that it may be used to treat cancers in other organs that can be transplanted, such as the lungs or pancreas. Nigel Hughes, chief executive of the British Liver Trust, hailed the results saying: 'The likelihood is that a patient with 14 liver tumours would not ordinarily last a year, so if this technique can extend life expectancy and improve quality of life, that is tremendous.' But doctors stress that the treatment is still in its infancy and, even if it proved effective, is likely to be used only in the most serious cases.

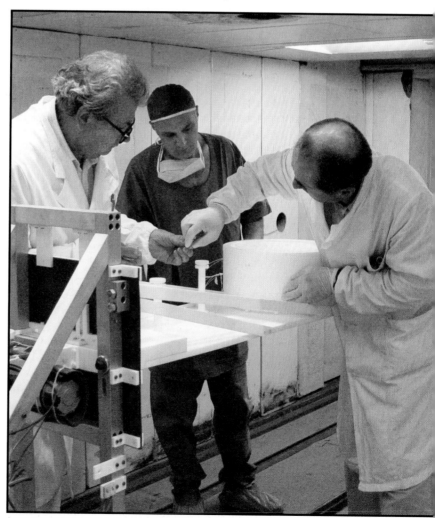

A cancerous liver has been removed and placed in a cylindrical Teflon bag, above. Soon the organ will be irradiated and returned to the patient.

## Drug development
# New target for old breast cancer drug

Seattle lawyer Randolph Urmston had never smoked and had no family history of lung cancer. So when he was diagnosed with the disease in 1997, it was an immense shock. Standard chemotherapy and radiation treatment did little to stem its progression. Then his doctor started him on the chemotherapy drug docetaxel (Taxotere), used to treat breast cancer. After four months of drug treatment, along with additional radiation therapy, the cancer disappeared. And it has stayed gone, a miracle that Urmston, now 58, attributes in part to the docetaxel.

Docetaxel has been used in the UK since 2001 to treat advanced non-small cell lung cancer (NSCLC), the most common form of the cancer, in patients who have failed to respond to other forms of chemotherapy. Now recent research in the USA has reinforced its effectiveness as a lung cancer treatment and it was approved by the US Food and Drug Administration (FDA) in December 2002

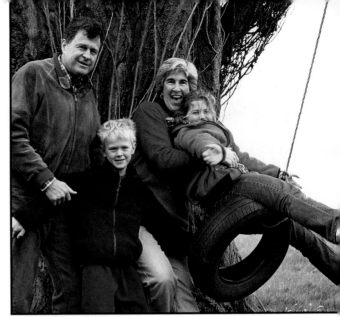

Seattle lawyer, Randolph Urmston, once again enjoying life with his family, knows that he was very lucky to survive his lung cancer.

for use in the primary treatment of the cancer (in combination with the chemotherapy drug cisplatin).

**How it works** Docetaxel prevents cancer cells from dividing by 'freezing' the cell's internal skeleton, which is made up of structures called microtubules. These microtubules assemble and disassemble as the cell divides. The drug encourages their assembly but blocks their disassembly, thereby preventing cancer cells from dividing.

The FDA based its approval on a clinical trial of 1,218 patients that compared the effect of docetaxel plus cisplatin or docetaxel plus carboplatin (another chemotherapy drug) to the standard chemotherapy combination of vinorelbine plus cisplatin. Patients in the docetaxel/cisplatin group had a median survival time of 10.9 months against 10.0 months for patients treated with the vinorelbine regimen. Overall, 31.6 per cent of the patients responded to docetaxel plus cisplatin, compared with 24.4 per cent of those treated with vinorelbine plus cisplatin. Although the improvements are small, in the case of lung cancer they can make all the difference. The disease is the most common cancer in the UK, killing nearly 35,000 people each year. Only five per cent of those diagnosed with the cancer survive beyond five years.

This is not the only time that an existing drug has been found to have new cancer-fighting properties. Recent research has revealed that the morning sickness drug thalidomide, which was banned in the 1960s because it was found to cause birth defects, may help to fight small cell lung cancer. A clinical trial funded by Cancer Research UK, currently in its third stage, has so far produced encouraging results.

RESEARCH ROUND-UP

### A natural cancer treatment

You won't find it on the shelf of your local garden centre but the natural plant extract called deguelin, used as an insecticide in Africa and South America, appears to prevent the growth of precancerous and cancerous lung cells without harming normal cells. The new findings, published in the February 2003 issue of the US *Journal of the National Cancer Institute*, suggest a possible nontoxic treatment for lung cancer.

The compound belongs to the same family as other health-enhancing plant compounds called flavonoids, found in tea, coffee and red wine. It appears to work by affecting a molecule called Akt, which is responsible for the survival of tumour cells. By blocking the cells' ability to send out survival signals, the compound causes them to commit suicide.

High-tech help

# Erasing the immune system and replacing it – to combat deadly cancer

Groundbreaking new research has come up with a new way to help patients with the deadliest form of skin cancer, melanoma. Replacing a patient's entire immune system with specially developed cells that attack the cancer has been shown to stop the cancer cells from growing or even destroy them altogether.

**How it works** Researchers from the National Cancer Institute, led by Dr Steven A. Rosenberg Ph.D., took immune system cells called T cells that were already attacking patients' tumours and grew massive numbers of them in the laboratory. While the cells were growing, the researchers used chemotherapy to destroy the patients' existing immune systems to make room for the new immune cells. Then, in the space of about 20 minutes, they infused more than 70 billion of these new tumour-attacking cells into the patients. (The new cells also defend the body against viruses and bacteria.) Researchers also gave the patients high doses of a protein called interleukin-2 (IL-2), which stimulates T cell growth.

Dr Rosenberg performed the procedure on 13 patients with metastatic melanoma, some of whom had only months to live despite previous highly aggressive treatment. The results, published in the online version of the US journal *Science* in September 2002, were astounding.

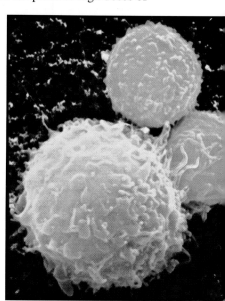

A cancer cell (pink) is attacked by two T cells (orange). Doctors have tried replacing cancer patients' entire immune systems with T cells.

One 16-year-old boy, who'd been given just two months to live, was still free of disease two years after the procedure. Overall, the treatment shrank the tumours by half in six of the patients, with no growth or appearance of new tumours, while four patients saw some of their tumours disappear entirely. Three of the original patients have since died, however. Side effects included relatively mild autoimmune disorders, with some patients developing white patches on their skin where the T cells destroyed the pigmentation, and one patient experiencing an inflammation of the iris.

**Availability** The T-cell therapy is still highly experimental, says Dr Rosenberg, and at least two years away from widespread use in cancer patients. Meanwhile, he and his team are testing it against breast, prostate and ovarian cancers. It may also eventually be used to treat some infectious diseases, such as AIDS.

## ALSO in the NEWS

### Relief from bone cancer pain

Once cancer gets into the bone, it results in excruciating pain that strong narcotics often can't help. Now, bone cancer patients may have another option for pain relief: radiofrequency ablation, which uses intense heat transmitted through the tip of a needle to kill nerve endings and much of the cancer tissue in the bone, alleviating pain. A clinical study of 43 patients conducted at nine medical centres in the United States and Europe found that 95 per cent of the patients treated with the procedure experienced significant pain reduction. Before the treatment, patients' pain averaged 7.5 on a scale of 1 to 10, with 10 being unbearable pain. Following the procedure, pain scores dropped by half, and after eight weeks the average score was 1.

In October 2002, the technology was approved in the USA for treating bone cancer patients. At present, it is only used in the UK for treating secondary lung cancer.

High-tech help

# Conquering pancreatic cancer with a Trojan horse

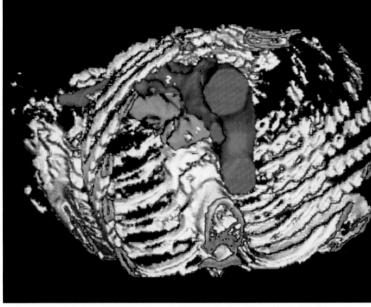

Pancreatic cancer (green) is notoriously difficult to treat. A new type of gene therapy makes the tumours more susceptible to cancer drugs.

Pancreatic cancer is one of the most difficult cancers to treat. The disease, which affects nearly 7,000 people in the UK each year, is almost always fatal because it is often found so late and because it is very resistant to traditional chemotherapy and radiation. So researchers are looking for new ways to destroy these cancers. Results from the first phase of a gene therapy trial suggest they may have found one.

While most gene therapy trials in cancer have focused on the use of genetically modified vaccines to bolster the immune system, this method, developed by Dr Ralph Weichselbaum and his research team at the University of Chicago, is designed to make the tumour cells more susceptible to chemotherapy and radiation.

**How it works** Certain white blood cells secrete a protein called tumour necrosis factor (TNF), which binds to areas on cancer cells aptly described as 'death receptors', spurring those cells to commit suicide. These proteins also make tumour cells more receptive to chemotherapy and radiation. More recent research suggests that TNF also blocks the blood supply to tumours.

In the gene therapy process, a genetically engineered virus containing the TNF gene (called TNFerade) is injected into the tumour once a week for five weeks. The virus is designed to have an 'on-off' switch, and it remains turned off until it receives a signal from a dose of radiation, delivered four hours after each injection. Once that signal is given, the virus spreads out into the tumour cells and infects them, dropping off its 'package' – the TNF gene – like a biological Trojan horse.

Results from a pilot study of 24 late-stage cancer patients (4 of whom had pancreatic cancer) were presented at the November 2002 meeting of the American Society of Clinical Oncology. Of the patients with pancreatic cancer, three had significant improvements in their tumours and were still alive and doing well a year or more after treatment. The fourth died before completing the treatment.

In spring 2003, another study involved 22 patients from eight centres. Five were being treated at Virginia Commonwealth University's Massey Cancer Center in Richmond by radiation oncologist Dr Theodore Chung. All were in the final stages of pancreatic cancer, with little or no hope of recovery. Four months after treatment the results were dramatic says Dr Chung. One patient was 'doing marvellously'. A second, whose tumour was too large to be removed surgically before the treatment, had it removed three months after the gene therapy. And an autopsy on the one patient who died showed that nearly all of the tumour had been destroyed. The patient was simply too sick to survive even after the treatment.

'Objectively, we cannot make any claims about how much better, if any, this treatment is compared with standard treatment until more studies are completed,' says Dr Chung. But hopes are high.

**Availability** From autumn 2003, TNFerade has been undergoing Phase II clinical trials in the US. In the UK, a similar study is being carried out on a gene therapy drug to treat breast cancer. Developed by Oxford Biomedica, the genetically modified drug, called Metxia, helps chemotherapy to work more effectively by targeting the tumour directly. Trials of a low dose of the therapy on four patients have shown it to be effective. The study is still at an early stage, but it is hoped that the therapy will eventually tackle other cancers, including pancreatic cancer.

## Surgical solution
# Microsurgery technique can preserve male fertility

When bicyclist Lance Armstrong learned he had testicular cancer in 1996, he banked his sperm before having one of his testicles removed and later was able to father three healthy children. But thousands of other men with testicular cancer aren't as lucky.

Generally, the testes are removed along with the tumour even before it's confirmed that the tumour is cancerous. In many such cases, the tumour isn't malignant, but the man's fertility is already compromised by the surgery. Now, a New York reproductive specialist has pioneered a new microsurgery technique that allows the removal of tumours while preserving the testes in some men.

**How it works** With the advent of high-resolution scrotal ultrasound, testicular tumours can be identified even before they're felt, notes Dr Marc Goldstein, professor of reproductive medicine and urology at Weill Medical College of Cornell University in New York City. Because the incidence of these tumours is 38 times higher in infertile men than in men without fertility problems, Dr Goldstein began doing ultrasounds on every infertile man he saw. 'I was picking up small tumours, but I didn't want to remove the testicles before I was sure they were cancerous,' he says.

To find out if the tumours were cancerous, he borrowed a technique from breast cancer surgeons, who use an ultrasound-guided needle to perform a biopsy on suspicious breast lumps. He combined the needle with the operating microscope and microsurgical tools that he uses for reversing vasectomies and discovered that using the three together enabled him to find and remove the tiny tumours – some as tiny as a grain of rice – without removing the testes.

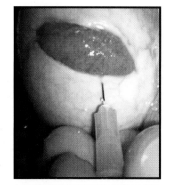

A new microsurgery technique lets doctors biopsy suspicious lumps – and even remove tumors – without removing the testicle.

Of the 65 men who underwent fertility evaluation in his study, 5 per cent had testicular tumours, half of which were benign. The study was published in the US *Journal of Urology* in September 2002.

These results reinforce similar work carried out by Italian researchers from 1988 to 1994 on men with tumours in the epididymus – the coiled tube leading from the testis. They used microsurgical techniques and also magnifying optical instruments to remove these tumours to avoid affecting the patient's fertility.

**Availability** Dr Goldstein is now teaching the technique to other surgeons. Once more doctors learn how to do the surgery, he says: 'It will change the way we approach testicular tumours.' He compares it to the situation with breast lumps: formerly, women who had lumps were automatically given mastectomies, but today, biopsies and lumpectomies are considered the norm.

# DIGESTION AND METABOLISM

## THERE'S VITAL NEWS FROM THE EXPERTS FOR PEOPLE WITH TYPE 2 DIABETES

People with Type 2 diabetes can reduce their risk of diabetes-related problems such as heart disease and eye, kidney and nerve damage by up to 50 per cent, according to a Danish study. The strategy includes exercising assiduously, eating properly and aggressive treatment of health threats such as high cholesterol with medication. British researchers warn that, if your spouse has developed diabetes, you should be extra careful of your own health, as you are twice as likely to develop it, too.

In other news, more people suffer from coeliac disease than previously thought. If you have abdominal pain and the symptoms worsen when you eat wheat products, you may be one of them. Also, a new type of drug to counteract Crohn's disease is in the final stage of testing, and a vaccine that targets the bacteria that

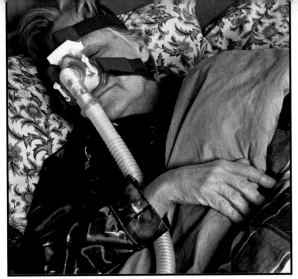

It's not pretty but it works: wearing a sleep mask like this one in bed can alleviate both sleep apnoea and nocturnal indigestion.

## High-tech help
# Breathing mask banishes two thieves of sleep

Barking dogs, car alarms and telephone callers with the wrong number may top your list of the most aggravating sleep disturbances, but they are mere nuisances compared with sleep apnoea and night-time indigestion. Either condition can make you toss and turn at night, leaving you groggy during the day – but when they strike together, they can make a good night's sleep doubly difficult to achieve.

Results of a recent study showed that one remedy – a treatment called nasal continuous positive airway pressure (NCPAP) – can reduce the symptoms of both conditions. The therapy involves a device that pumps air through a face mask that is strapped over a person's nose at night. The pump device is the most common treatment for obstructive sleep apnoea, in which sagging flesh in the throat disrupts normal breathing during sleep and causes people who have it to waken repeatedly with a gasp. An estimated 80,000 people in the UK suffer from obstructive sleep apnoea.

In the study, researchers asked 181 people to use NCPAP masks. All of them had both apnoea and nocturnal gastro-oesophageal reflux – night-time indigestion – in which stomach acid flows back into the oesophagus, the tube that leads from the mouth to the stomach. The 165 people who continued to use the pumps during the study had a 48 per cent improvement in their reflux symptoms, according to John O'Connor, assistant professor of medicine at Duke University Medical Center in Durham, North Carolina, and one of the authors of the study. The higher the amount of air pressure the machine exerted, the more the symptoms subsided. The 16 people who stopped using the devices had no reflux improvement.

The results were published in January 2003 in the US journal *Archives of Internal Medicine*.

**How it works** The NCPAP device treats apnoea by increasing air pressure in the throat, keeping tissues pressed back out of the airway and allowing easier breathing. It also increases pressure in the oesophagus, Dr O'Connor says. This keeps acid in the stomach where it belongs, or pushes it back if some slips through the valve that separates the oesophagus from the stomach.

A common factor in many people with the two conditions is obesity. 'Almost all patients with sleep apnoea are overweight and so are a significant proportion of those with reflux,' says Dr O'Connor. Being overweight sets the stage for floppier tissues in the throat and increases pressure in the abdomen, compressing the stomach and pushing acid upwards into the oesophagus.

If you have acid reflux but not apnoea, NCPAP treatment is probably not the best choice for you. Several medications are available that effectively treat reflux more conveniently than wearing a face mask at night. However, if you have apnoea as well as night-time indigestion, ask your doctor to refer you to a sleep clinic for assessment.

**Availability** The treatment is available in the UK at sleep clinics. If your symptoms are assessed and judged to be disabling, and the diagnosis is confirmed by a sleep study, you are likely to be offered the therapy to aid sleep.

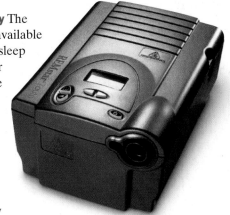

The mask is connected to a machine that provides pressure to keep airways open and the 'door' to the stomach closed.

Key discovery
# New study reveals more cases of coeliac disease

The bread aisle at the supermarket may harbour a more serious hazard than previously suspected. According to the findings of a large study into the prevalence of coeliac disease – a condition made worse by eating particular grains – the disease strikes one in every 133 Americans. This makes it about 100 times more common than previously thought, says Alessio Fasano, co-director of the Center for Celiac Research at the University of Maryland, who took a leading role in the study.

In the UK, coeliac disease was until recently thought to be rare, but more and more doctors are now starting to recognize the condition in their patients. The average incidence in the UK is estimated to be one in 1,000 people. The condition is also known to run in families.

Coeliac disease is an autoimmune disorder – a condition in which the immune system attacks the body, in this case destroying the fingerlike projections in the small intestine known as villi. But it is unique in being the only autoimmune disease that has an identified environmental trigger. That trigger is gluten, a protein that is found in wheat, barley, rye and possibly oats – though most otherwise fit and healthy adults with the condition seem to be able to tolerate a small quantity of oats in their diet.

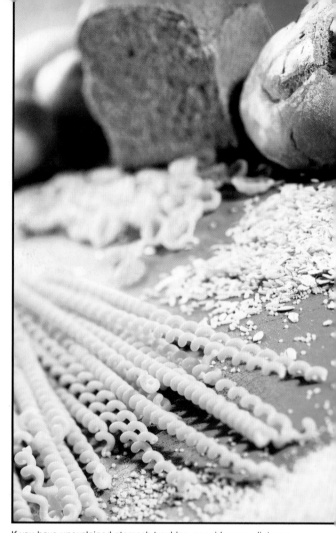

If you have unexplained stomach troubles, consider your diet as a possible cause. More people than previously thought are sensitive to gluten, a protein found in many grains, including wheat.

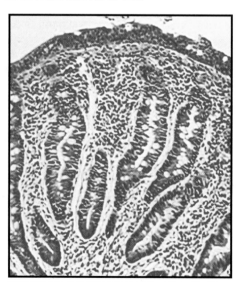

Nutrients are absorbed into the blood through villi, finger-like projections in the small intestine.

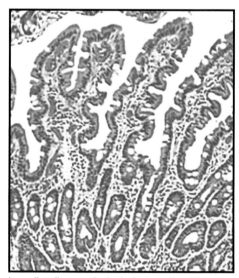

In coeliac disease, the body destroys the villi, leading to poor absorption of nutrients.

When someone with coeliac disease consumes gluten, the immune system turns against the small intestine. The consequent damage can interfere with the absorption of nutrients from food, resulting in malnutrition. Symptoms may include diarrhoea, constipation and abdominal pain – but the condition is just as likely to be free of symptoms.

The new study, whose results were published in the February 2003 issue of *Archives of Internal Medicine*, involved more than 13,000 children and adults from across America. Some of the subjects were known to be at risk of coeliac disease: either they had symptoms, or they had a relative with the disease, or they had a condition associated with coeliac disease, such as short stature, arthritis, osteoporosis or infertility.

According to the findings, 0.75 per cent of people – or 1 in every 133 people without the specified risk factors – have coeliac disease. That percentage rises to 4.5 among people who have a close relative such as a parent or sibling with the disease. It is also higher for people with osteoporosis – about 2.5 per cent. And it is even higher (4 per cent) for people who are short in stature and those with unexplained infertility (6 per cent). Malnutrition caused by the disease can lead to any of these conditions.

In the 1950s, coeliac disease was considered to be almost exclusively a childhood condition, but many more adults than children are now being diagnosed. Coeliac symptoms can manifest themselves at any age, and statistics demonstrate that most coeliacs are diagnosed when they are between the ages of 30 and 45.

**Testing for coeliac disease** Since coeliac disease often causes no symptoms and can be hard to diagnose, people with a family history of the disease or another condition associated with it are advised by Dr Fasano to ask their doctors for a test. The disease can be diagnosed by a blood test, though a positive test requires a tissue sample from the small intestine to confirm the diagnosis. The treatment is straightforward: avoid gluten.

If unusually short children are diagnosed with coeliac disease before puberty, they can make up their lost height once they adopt a gluten-free diet. A woman who is infertile may be able to get pregnant once the disease is corrected. And, if people with coeliac disease change to the correct diet before early adulthood, Dr Fasano says, they have a good chance of reversing the osteoporosis that the disease causes.

# ALSO in the NEWS

## 'Good' bacteria in the gut are linked to a natural antibiotic

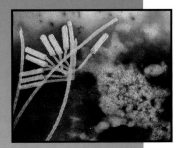

It is well known that 'good' bacteria in the digestive tract help to fight off 'bad' bacteria such as listeria, which are associated with food poisoning. But good bacteria offer other benefits to health, according to a new laboratory study. It seems that, in mice, the good bacteria stimulate cells in the intestine to make a protein that acts as a natural antibiotic. Humans do not produce the protein, called angiogenin-4, but we do make a number of other 'protein antibiotics' that may be regulated by friendly bacteria, says researcher Lora Hooper, of Washington University in St Louis, Missouri. 'I'm sure this is just the beginning of the story,' she adds. The findings were reported in the online version of *Nature Immunology* in January 2003.

## Milk linked to Crohn's disease

Milk may be wreaking havoc in your intestines, according to UK research published in the *Journal of Clinical Microbiology* in July 2003. The study found that Crohn's disease – an inflammatory bowel condition causing diarrhoea, weight loss and tiredness – may be linked to a bacterium in cow's milk called *Mycobacterium avium paratuberculosis* (MAP). The bacterium was detected in 92 per cent of Crohn's patients compared with only 26 per cent of people in a control group. 'The rate of detection of MAP in individuals with Crohn's disease is highly significant and implicates this pathogen in disease causation,' wrote the study's authors. Earlier tests revealed that MAP can survive current pasteurization procedures.

The medical charity Action Research, which backed the study, has called for more stringent pasteurization to kill the MAP bug, as well as tests for MAP in dairy herds and improved hygiene on farms. One of the study authors noted that MAP may also contribute to irritable bowel syndrome.

Drug development

# Movement of harmful cells blocked by Crohn's drug

By 2005, people with Crohn's disease may be able to gain the upper hand over their condition with a new type of drug that blocks the movement of harmful cells in the intestine before they can do their work.

Crohn's is a type of bowel disease that typically strikes young people, causing inflammation and damage throughout the digestive tract. Although experts remain uncertain about what triggers the inflammation, it is the source of serious symptoms – including bleeding, diarrhoea and pain – and may require surgery.

The new drug, natalizumab, acts like a guided missile, targeting specific immune cells implicated in the disease. Drugs currently used to treat Crohn's, including steroids, affect the entire immune system.

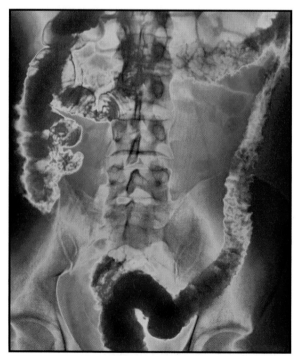

Crohn's disease often strikes the small intestine or the colon. It can affect different parts of the digestive tract at the same time.

Natalizumab showed promise in the results of a study published in the *New England Journal of Medicine* in January 2003. In the study, 248 people with Crohn's were divided into four groups and given either two doses of placebo (dummy pills), one dose of natalizumab and one dose of placebo, or two doses of natalizumab, either at a lower or higher dosage. Those who had two doses of natalizumab saw a decrease in symptoms more often than those who received placebos. And all the groups that received the drug scored better on an index that measured the severity of their disease.

In the same issue of the journal, another study reported success in treating multiple sclerosis (MS) with natalizumab. In MS, the protective myelin sheath on nerves is destroyed or damaged, forming lesions (sclerosis) in the brain. The resulting disruption of nerve function can cause blindness, difficulty of movement and other symptoms, according to where the lesions occur.

In the MS study, 213 patients had either a placebo or one of two different dosages of natalizumab, all given monthly for six months. Those who received the medication developed only about one-tenth as many new lesions as those who received the placebo. The groups treated with natalizumab also had about half the number of relapses as the placebo group and they reported greater well-being.

**How it works** In people with Crohn's disease, immune cells called lymphocytes trigger and prolong inflammation after they enter the gastrointestinal tract from the bloodstream. On the surface of the cells are molecules that help the lymphocytes find their way to the area and stay there, says Subrata Ghosh, a professor at London's Imperial College and leading author of the study. Natalizumab blocks the molecules, preventing migration of the cells to the inflamed intestine and giving the area a chance to heal.

Natalizumab will probably be used for patients who have severe problems with Crohn's and have failed to respond to conventional medications, Dr Ghosh says.

In MS, the drug works by blocking the same type of molecules on the surface of immune system cells, and thereby prevents the cells from entering the brain from the bloodstream.

**Availability** If tests go well, natalizumab is expected to be available in Britain as a Crohn's treatment in 2005. Availability as an MS treatment will take longer.

## Progress in prevention
# A healthier and longer life for people with diabetes

New evidence has emerged that adopting a healthier lifestyle can prolong the life of people with Type 2 diabetes.

An eight-year study in Denmark looked at 160 people with Type 2 diabetes, the most common form of the disease. The patients also had early signs of kidney disease and were at increased risk of developing cardiovascular disease, as most people with diabetes are. In fact, some 80 per cent of people with diabetes are ultimately killed by a heart attack.

Half of the participants in the Danish study were given conventional treatments such as insulin to control high blood sugar and blood-pressure-lowering drugs such as ACE inhibitors. The goal was to get the patients' readings within the limits recommended by

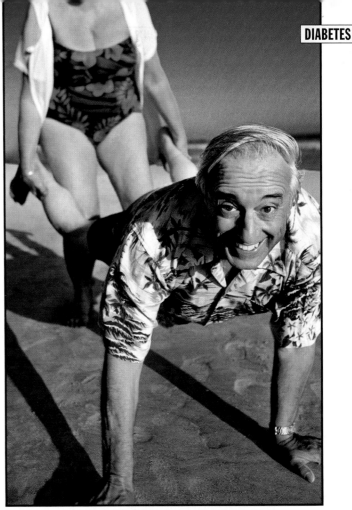

Regular exercise is one of the things that can help to keep the complications of diabetes at bay. And who says it can't be fun?

**RESEARCH ROUND-UP**

## Obesity may be to blame in Type 1 diabetes increase

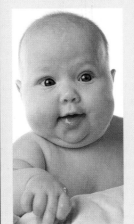

Type 2 diabetes, typically associated with being overweight, is becoming increasingly common in children in both the UK and the USA. And there has also been a rise in the incidence of Type 1 diabetes, which is caused by the destruction of insulin-producing beta cells in the pancreas. In the USA, the incidence of Type 1 diabetes per 1,000 children has doubled or even trebled since 1960.

A study published in October 2002 in the journal *Diabetes Care* suggests that the obesity epidemic linked to Type 2 diabetes may also be responsible for

the increase in Type 1. European researchers studied data on 499 children diagnosed with Type 1 diabetes before they reached the age of 15 and compared it with data on 1,337 healthy children in the same population. They found that children with diabetes were significantly taller and heavier from the time they were about one month old until the age of six than those without the disease. They also found that breastfeeding the children for any length of time cut the risk of diabetes by one-quarter, duplicating findings from other studies.

Although the researchers cannot explain the link between weight and Type 1 diabetes, an analysis in *Child Health Monitor* suggests it may be related to how much children are fed in their early years and to the fact that increased weight may put more strain on insulin-producing beta cells.

# ALSO in the NEWS

## When fructose is not so sweet

If you are bothered by unexplained rumblings and pain in your stomach, the culprit could be the fruit juice in your refrigerator. Fruit juice is high in fructose, a sugar that is not digested as well as other sugars, says Peter Beyer, associate professor in dietetics and nutrition at the University of Kansas Medical Center.

Beyer and his fellow researchers gave 15 healthy adults 25g of fructose on one day and 50g on another. (A 1 litre of juice can contain about 55g.) At least half the people tested suffered gas, bloating and a gurgling stomach after the 25g dose, he says, and even more had those problems – plus mild diarrhoea – after the larger dose. The researchers presented their findings at a meeting of the *American College of Gastroenterology* in October 2002.

If you have this sort of problem regularly, try drinking only small amounts of juice at a time, and drink juice only with meals to help your body absorb the fructose better, Beyer suggests.

If you suspect that you have a fructose intolerance, ask your doctor about having a hydrogen breath test. This simple test is designed to find out whether fructose is being properly digested by your small intestine or whether it is travelling undigested to your colon. When the bacteria that naturally reside in the colon eat the fructose, they produce hydrogen gas, which can then be measured in your breath.

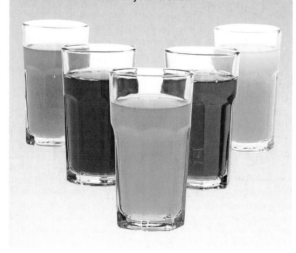

the Danish Medical Association – for example, total cholesterol below 4.94mmol/l (190mg/dl) and blood pressure less than 135/85mm/Hg. In Britain the acceptable upper limit for total cholesterol is slightly higher at 5.2mmol/l (200mg/dl).

The other 80 people who took part in the study pursued goals that were 'much more ambitious', according to Oluf Pedersen, chief physician at the Steno Diabetes Centre in Copenhagen and senior author of the study.

The 'ambitious 80' study subjects ate large quantities of fish and vegetables and less saturated fat. They exercised regularly. The smokers among them attended classes to help them give up smoking. They received regular education and counselling from a doctor, a nurse and a dietitian. They took more frequent and higher doses of medication such as statin drugs to lower cholesterol and ACE inhibitors to lower blood pressure. In addition, they took vitamin and mineral supplements and low-dose aspirin for heart health.

At the end of the study, the participants who had followed the intensive therapy were more than 50 per cent less likely to have cardiovascular disease than the people in the other group. Also, their risks of eye, kidney and nerve damage from diabetes had fallen by more than 50 per cent.

### Keep in regular touch with your doctor

To achieve the same sort of improvements in your blood sugar and cholesterol levels and blood pressure, you need continued support, education and motivation from your doctor, Dr Pedersen explains. You should visit your GP every few months for a check-up, which could include a physical examination and blood tests. Discuss which risk factors need most serious attention.

As well as taking regular medication to keep their risk factors under control, 'Type 2 diabetic patients should take their disease as a challenge and do their very best to change their lifestyle,' recommends Dr Pedersen.

Among diabetics who are obese, a vital factor in prolonging life is loss of weight. According to Diabetes UK: 'For every kilogram of weight loss after a Type 2 diagnosis, there is a 3-4 month increase in life expectancy.'

To support obese patients who are trying to lose weight, a Lifestyle Change Programme was launched by the National Health Service in northwest England in 2002. Its approach accords with the findings of the Danish study.

Key discovery
# Having a partner who is diabetic is a risk factor

Vowing to have and to hold your spouse 'in sickness and in health' takes on new meaning for couples when one of the pair has Type 2 diabetes. According to a British study of nearly 500 people, those married to someone with Type 2 diabetes are more than twice as likely to develop the disease as people whose spouses don't have it.

The spouses who took part in the study also showed an increased risk of the abnormal blood sugar levels that lead to diabetes, and they had higher levels of triglycerides, a type of blood fat known to raise the risk of heart disease. The study was conducted at London's Royal Marsden Hospital and its findings were published in the March 2003 issue of the journal *Diabetes Care*.

Diabetes is not unique in this respect. Research published in 2002 in the *British Medical Journal* showed that partners of people with asthma, depression or peptic ulcers had a 70 per cent increased risk of developing the condition themselves.

**Birds of a feather?** One reason for the finding is that people tend to choose partners who are similar to them in body type and ethnicity, says Tahseen Chowdhury of the Royal London Hospital, a co-author of the study. Being overweight increases the chances of developing the disease, as does being a member of certain ethnic groups.

A more important explanation, however, is that spouses have a tendency to share similar diet and exercise patterns. Eating healthy foods and taking plenty of exercise are critical for avoiding and treating Type 2 diabetes. If one spouse has bad habits, the other is likely to have them, too. Dr Chowdhury suggests that, when either spouse has diabetes, treating it should be a family affair. 'Spouses of patients with diabetes should be very vigilant with their own health,' he says, advising regular medical check-ups. Children of parents with diabetes are also at higher risk and need to adopt healthy lifestyle habits to avoid developing the disease.

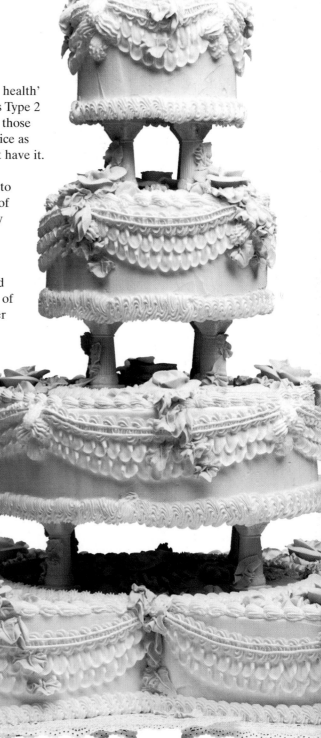

## High-tech help
# Virtual stomach offers hope of better pills

When you swallow an extended-release or timed-release tablet, it vanishes into your stomach, where it eventually breaks down and releases its contents. A new computer simulation offers insights into exactly what happens to that pill during its fantastic unseen voyage.

A team of researchers led by James Brasseur, professor of mechanical engineering at Pennsylvania State University in the USA have created a 'virtual stomach', which may some day help drug companies to make their extended-release tablets more effective or reveal which drugs should be taken with which kinds of meals.

**How they did it** The virtual stomach, which is operated by a huge cluster of computers, produces animated, two-dimensional outlines of a stomach on a computer screen. A small coloured pill can be electronically 'dropped' into the stomach, where it drifts about, slowly leaking a cloud of medication as it dissolves.

To program the computer model, Anupam Pal, the Pennsylvania State post-doctoral student who developed the simulation, fed the computer with information that had been taken from magnetic resonance imaging (MRI) scans of the human stomach. He also used films of dog and cat stomachs made with X-ray machines, as well as measurements of pressure in human stomachs. AstraZeneca, a pharmaceutical company, is supporting the development of the computer model.

**What it shows** The simulation has led to interesting discoveries about delayed-release medications and about how the stomach works, Dr Brasseur says. For instance, the vigorous muscle motions that mix the contents occur only in the bottom one-third of the stomach. The upper part acts mainly as a holding chamber, although it squeezes material down towards the bottom. Think of a fruit smoothie in a liquidizer: at the top, the slush is relatively calm; the real churning happens at the bottom, where the blades are whirling. Researchers were also surprised by the extent to which a tablet's density influences how it moves in the stomach. When the pill is in the calmer, upper part of the stomach, it does not break down quickly. But when a denser – and therefore less buoyant – tablet falls into the more active, lower portion, the stomach fluids shifting back and forth rub away at the tablet and can quickly wear down its surface, says Dr Pal.

When the researchers simulated a stomach filled with a smooth, soft food such as mashed potato and dropped in a virtual tablet that was only slightly denser than the stomach contents, the tablet quickly fell to the bottom section, where it was more rapidly broken down. In the future, drug manufacturers may be able use this information to control the absorption of drugs by adjusting the density of pills and recommending that they be taken with particular kinds of foods.

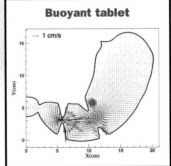

**Buoyant tablet**

A diagram of the stomach with a tablet that floats. Pills that float rather than sinking take longer to break down. Food affects how fast a tablet sinks.

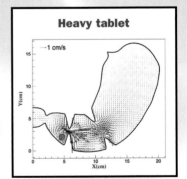

**Heavy tablet**

A diagram of the stomach with a tablet that sinks. Denser tablets fall to the bottom of the stomach more quickly and are therefore broken down faster.

## Drug development
# A new vaccine to ward off peptic ulcers

In the early 1980s, a couple of Australian physicians discovered that spiral-shaped bacteria named *Helicobacter pylori* were the real culprits behind most peptic ulcers – not stress or diet, as doctors and the public alike had previously thought. (Peptic ulcers are sores in the lining of the stomach or the beginning of the small intestine.) Antibiotics that destroy *H. pylori* have become a standard treatment for ulcers. Even better would be a vaccine that could eliminate the bug in people who have it and prevent infection in people who don't – especially since strains of the bacteria are emerging that are resistant to many common antibiotics.

Just such a vaccine is undergoing trials in the USA. In 2003, Antex Biologics, a Maryland-based biopharmaceutical firm since taken over by Bioport, announced two clinical studies designed to evaluate the effectiveness and safety of its vaccine, called Helivax.

Although most people who harbour *H. pylori* show no symptoms, in some people it causes ulcers. In fact, about 80 to 90 per cent of peptic ulcers are caused by *H. pylori*.

The bacteria weaken the mucous coating that protects the stomach lining, allowing acid to damage it. Infection by the bacteria also puts individuals at a two to six times higher risk of stomach cancer – whether or not they develop an ulcer – and it may also play a role in inflammatory bowel disease, says Vic Esposito, a spokesman for Antex.

**How it works** Previous attempts to develop an *H. pylori* vaccine have been hampered by the fact that the bacteria are hard to grow in the laboratory. Researchers have typically focused on cloning specific proteins from *H. pylori* and using them to teach the body's immune system to recognize and fight the bacteria. But Antex has found a way to mass-produce the bacteria in 400-litre tanks. They are grown to a certain point, then killed, and the whole cells are used in the vaccine. This is similar to the approach used in vaccines against polio, hepatitis and flu viruses.

**The ulcer vaccine would be similar to the vaccines used to protect people against hepatitis, polio and influenza.**

Tissue samples taken from participants in earlier studies showed that the vaccine causes the immune system to produce antibodies in the stomach and small intestine to work against the bacteria.

**Availability** The present trials are scheduled to be completed by mid-2004. If all goes well, the vaccine could be available in the USA in 2007.

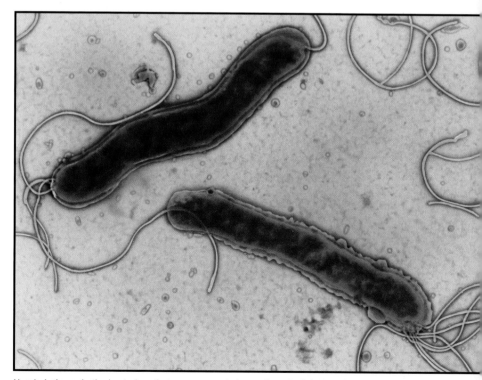

*H. pylori*, above, is the bacterium that causes most ulcers. About half the people in the world are infected with it. While most people exhibit no symptoms, in particular individuals the bacterium triggers ulcers. A new vaccine could eliminate *H. pylori* for good.

# EYES AND EARS

## GLASSES AND TRADITIONAL CONTACT LENSES MAY ONE DAY BECOME OBSOLETE

Thanks to new technology in laser eye surgery, night vision problems that can plague people undergoing LASIK can be avoided. If you're not interested in LASIK, you may wish to consider having permanent contact lenses implanted instead: for many people, these are a safer, more effective alternative to laser surgery.

Older adults who need cataract surgery – which can leave people with vision bad enough to require glasses – could get perfect sight with a new kind of lens that can be adjusted after it's surgically implanted. And the world's first artificial cornea brings new hope for those who've lost vision due to corneal blindness, and mean no more waiting for a donor cornea.

Doctors are also making progress in treating some hitherto intractable hearing problems.

High-tech help

# New lens set to clarify fuzzy night vision

If you can't see where a carpet ends, you may trip. And you'll have trouble driving at night if you can't make out where one object ends and another begins. This aspect of vision is known as contrast sensitivity. Cataract surgery cannot correct it effectively, but a new artificial lens may hold a solution by providing the equivalent of 'high-definition TV' clarity.

The TECNIS Z9000 lens uses so-called wavefront technology to correct tiny aberrations in the spherical shape of the eye. A German study of 37 patients who had the TECNIS lens in one eye and another lens in the other found the TECNIS lens significantly improved contrast sensitivity, according to Professor Ulrich Mester from the Universität des Saarlandes in Sulzbach, Germany.

A US study carried out in 2002 at the Oregon Eye Institute in Portland found the TECNIS lens improved vision during night-time driving as well as reducing glare from headlights. 'The amazing result was that the people who were looking through this modified lens could see as well with glare as those with the standard lens could see without the glare,' said Dr Mark Packer, clinical assistant professor at the Institute. The new lens should be available in Europe in 2004.

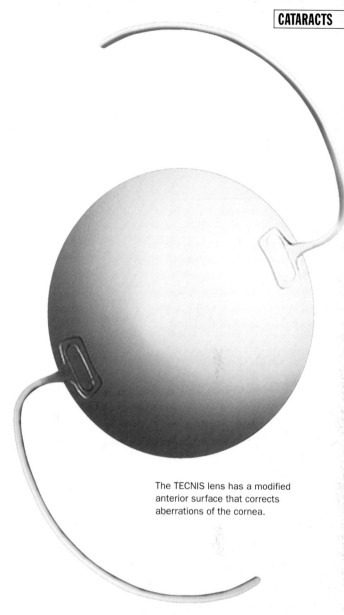

The TECNIS lens has a modified anterior surface that corrects aberrations of the cornea.

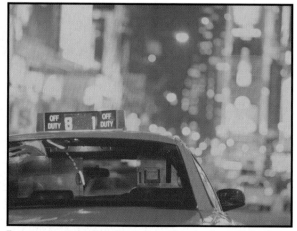

To someone who suffers from a loss of contrast sensitivity, the taxi pictured here would appear grey and hazy.

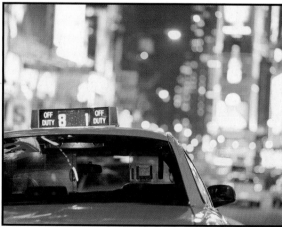

To anyone who has been fitted with the implantable TECNIS lens, the same cab would appear to be sharper and more distinct.

High-tech help

# Sharpening vision with a shape-shifting lens

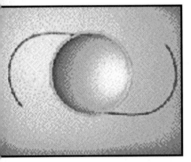

The Light Adjustable Lens can be adjusted using lasers *after* it's been implanted in the eye.

There's a little secret most people don't know about cataract surgery, one of the most common surgical procedures in the UK. Although the surgery is extremely successful at restoring normal vision, about half of the people who have it still need to wear glasses afterwards. But a new lens under investigation may change that.

During cataract surgery, doctors remove the cloudy lens, usually leaving intact the membrane, or capsule, that encloses the lens. They then insert an artificial lens into the empty capsule through the same tiny slit they used to remove the contents. This gets rid of the cataract and also helps to correct vision because a lens of the appropriate optical 'power' is used. However, as the eye heals, it may

change shape slightly, which will cause the artificial lens to be either too powerful or not powerful enough. A new type of lens, called the Light Adjustable Lens (LAL), solves this problem as it can be adjusted *after* it has been implanted.

**How it works** The LAL is made of silicone embedded with light-sensitive molecules called macromers. After the lens is implanted and the eye heals, the strength of the lens can be adjusted by shining a beam of ultra-violet light into the centre or the edges of the lens. The light reacts with the macromers to change the lens' shape according to where the light is aimed and on the intensity and duration of the light delivered. The LAL can be adjusted several times as needed. Once perfect vision is achieved, the prescription is 'locked in' by blasting the entire surface of the lens with light.

'I think it's the breakthrough of the decade in my field,' says Dr Robert K. Maloney, a Los Angeles-based ophthalmologist and spokesperson for the American Academy of Ophthalmology.

Dr Maloney sees additional applications for the lens, such as providing 'super vision' – even better than 20/20. 'You would literally have vision like an eagle,' he says. It could also be used to eliminate the need for reading glasses, often required as people move into middle age and develop presbyopia (difficulty focusing on nearby objects), because it could be adjusted to provide a kind of bifocal effect.

**Availability** Human clinical trials on the LAL began in early 2003 in Mexico. The first lens was implanted in a blind person to test its safety, and the second lens was given to a patient who was undergoing cataract surgery. After surgery, that patient was tested and found to be still slightly nearsighted; however, the lens was successfully adjusted afterwards to rectify this.

During the first phase of testing, the LAL is scheduled to be implanted in about 25 eyes. It is hoped that the lens will soon be available in Europe. In the USA, it is awaiting approval by the Food and Drug Administration (FDA). When that is granted, it is likely to become available there by 2006.

## How the lens works

During cataract surgery, doctors remove the eye's lens and replace it with a new one. But since the eye changes shape as it heals, the 'power' of the lens may need adjusting.

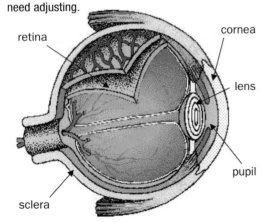

retina

cornea

lens

pupil

sclera

High-tech help

# First artificial cornea approved

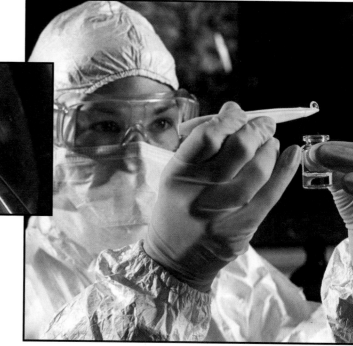

An estimated 10 million people throughout the world suffer from corneal blindness, yet only 100,000 corneal transplants are performed each year because of the difficulty in obtaining corneas. Soon, that may no longer be an issue. The International Lions Eye Institute in Perth, Australia – the leading eye institute in the Southern Hemisphere – have developed the world's first soft artificial cornea called AlphaCor.

**How it works** The artificial cornea is a curved, flexible plastic disc. The central part is transparent, just like a lens, while the rim is soft like a sponge, which enables the patient's own eye tissue to grow onto it and hold the lens in place. Recipients of transplanted donor corneas often need to take strong drugs to suppress their immune system so it doesn't reject the new lens as foreign tissue. However, these drugs aren't necessary when the artificial cornea is implanted.

Developed in Australia, the AlphaCor can reverse corneal blindness with no need for a donated cornea.

The implantation procedure is similar to that for a donor cornea. Part of the existing cornea is removed and the AlphaCor is inserted through a tiny slit at the top of the eye, which is stitched closed after the operation. Then a flap of tissue taken from the conjunctiva (the outer layer of the white of the eye) is used to cover the surface of the front of the eye to make a kind of natural bandage. After three months, the flap of tissue and a thin layer of cornea are removed, exposing the AlphaCor and allowing light to enter the eye. Most patients have some, if not all, of their sight restored.

In clinical trials conducted in Australia and Asia, the artificial cornea worked better than a human corneal graft for some high-risk patients and caused fewer clinical complications. In one trial, in which AlphaCor was implanted in 41 patients, more than 80 per cent had some vision restored within a year after the surgery.

**Availability** The Lions Eye Institute hopes to expand its clinical testing programme into Europe, America and Asia. AlphaCor has been approved for use in Europe but it will be available only from surgeons accredited through the ArgusConnect programme. To locate one of these doctors, see the company's web site at www.argusbiomedical.com.

---

**RESEARCH ROUND-UP**

## Putting your eye where your mouth is (or vice versa)

A team of Japanese doctors from the Kyoto Prefectural University of Medicine successfully restored the sight of several patients by growing an artificial cornea from membranes taken from the patients' mouths. It took three weeks to turn a 2mm square of membrane into a cornea, growing it on a bed of tissue obtained from a placenta. The surgery was successful in eight patients but failed in a ninth because of the effects of another illness. A major benefit is that the patient does not require drugs to prevent rejection of the graft. The results were presented at the Japanese Society for Regenerative Medicine meeting in March 2003.

High-tech help
# Sign language glove offers a helping hand

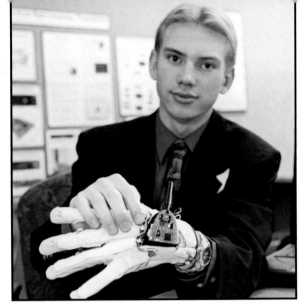

Ryan Patterson displays his award-winning invention, which he hopes will offer more independence to deaf people.

Secondary school student Ryan Patterson was sitting in a Burger King restaurant in Colorado when he observed a deaf teenager trying to order. The teenager communicated the order by sign language to an interpreter, who relayed it verbally to the clerk. 'That would be a bummer – to be unable to go out on your own and order food,' Patterson thought. Soon afterwards, he read about a deaf student who attended school with a translator accompanying her everywhere she went. This gave Patterson a brainwave.

Using little more than a leather golf glove, a circuit board, a laptop computer, and some basic electronic parts (costing under £150), Patterson designed a sign language translator for his school's science fair. The device translates finger-spelling sign language into words on a computer screen.

**How it works** Ten sensors placed along the fingers of the glove send data to a microprocessor, which transmits the information wirelessly to a small portable receiver. The screen – about the size of those on mobile phones – displays the words. The invention won Patterson the grand slam of science competitions, including the Siemens Westinghouse Science and Technology Competition and the Intel International Science and Engineering Fair. In late 2002, *Time* magazine named his glove one of the top inventions of the year, and in April 2003, *Teen People* listed him as one of 20 'teens to watch'.

'It's really cool to be honoured like that,' says Patterson, a blond young man who looks as if he'd be more comfortable on the ski slopes than in a laboratory.

After completing his first year at the University of Colorado-Boulder in the spring of 2003 (where he's studying electrical and computer engineering), he planned to spend the summer refining and improving his invention.

**Availability** Although Patterson has patented his invention (just beating a similar patent from Japanese electronics giant Hitachi), manufacturers have yet to approach him, and the glove exists only as a prototype. One reason is the cost: producing it would be very expensive as it is now designed, he says. By the time he has finished with it, though, that should just be one more problem resolved.

# ALSO in the NEWS

## The earlier the better for cochlear implants

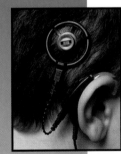

Cochlear implants – small electronic devices surgically implanted deep in the inner ear (accompanied by a transmitter, as shown on the right) – can provide a sense of sound, although not actual hearing, to someone who is profoundly deaf. They have long been controversial when used in children, with some people in the deaf community concerned that their use would harm the deaf culture and many insisting that implants should not be considered until children turn 18 and can make their own decisions. But research from the University of Texas in Dallas suggests there may not be time to wait. The study, which examined the brain activity of children with normal hearing and deaf children who received cochlear implants at varying ages, found that deaf children should receive the implants by the age of 3½. If they receive them any later, the researchers found, the neurological pathway for hearing doesn't fully develop.

## High-tech help

# With special contact lenses, more drug meets the eye

If you've ever tried to put drops in your eyes, you know how frustrating the process can be. Half of the medicine goes sliding down your nose, while the other half might, if you're lucky, make it into your eye for a minute before being washed away via your tear ducts into your nose and from there into your bloodstream, where it can sometimes cause serious side effects. For instance, timolol (Timoptol), used to treat glaucoma, can cause heart problems. Overall, only about 5 per cent of eye medications go where they need to go.

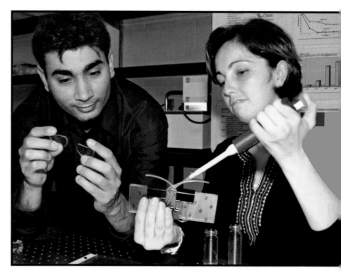

Derya Gulsen (right) injects a specially designed glass mould with a solution containing drug-loaded nanoparticles to create the prototype lenses held by Dr Anuj Chauhan (left).

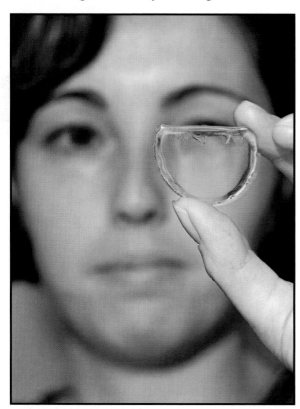

The prototype of a drug-laden lens (obviously larger than a real lens would be). The disposable contact lenses would be a new and improved way to deliver drugs to the eyes.

Now, researchers at the University of Florida think they may have found a way to slowly release drugs into the eye using specially designed contact lenses. Although the idea of delivering drugs in this way is not new, previous attempts failed because they involved soaking the lenses in the drug solution and then inserting them into the eye. This method resulted in many of the same problems as with eyedrops, says Anuj Chauhan Ph.D., who is developing the drug-containing lenses.

**How it works** Dr Chauhan's approach encapsulates tiny amounts of the drug within nanoparticles, or oil-based particles, within the plastic of the contact lens. Because the particles are so tiny, they do not interfere with vision, and because the drug is encapsulated, it seeps out over time, providing a steady dose of medicine. The idea is that the lenses – which could also be used to improve vision – would be disposable after being worn for up to two weeks at a time. Dr Chauhan presented his research at the American Chemical Society's national meeting in March 2003. A spokesman for the Royal National Institute for the Blind (RNIB) said: 'The RNIB welcomes all scientific advances that lead to improvements in the treatment of eye conditions, but we do stress that this research is currently at a very early stage.'

**Availability** So far, Dr Chauhan has demonstrated that it is possible to produce a drug-containing lens, but it will be at least 10 years before a commercial product is available, he predicts.

Surgical solutions
# New laser treatment for glaucoma

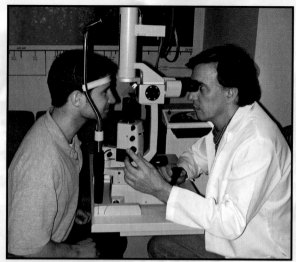

A patient undergoes the new laser treatment for glaucoma.

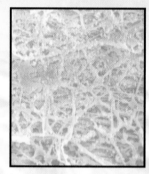

Clogs in the eye's meshwork cause fluid back-ups. Pulses of light shake the meshwork, dislodging stuck particles.

About a quarter of a million British people have the insidious eye disease glaucoma, the leading cause of blindness in the UK. The most common form, called primary open-angle glaucoma (POAG), affects one in 200 of the population aged over 40 and comes on silently, with no swelling or pain – just a slow buildup of pressure and the equally slow destruction of the optic nerve. Treatments typically involve daily medications, most of which have significant side effects, or surgery, which is often effective for only a short time and usually can't be repeated when the pressure builds again. But now a new laser treatment may provide another option.

Glaucoma results from a buildup of fluid in the eye. Normally, fluid travels through various parts of the eye and drains through a spongy meshwork, called the trabecular meshwork, where the cornea and iris meet. If the fluid passes through this drain too slowly, pressure builds and can eventually cause damage to the optic nerve that can lead to blindness.

The most common laser surgical procedure, argon laser trabeculoplasty (ALT), releases the pressure by making small burns in the mesh, causing the drain holes to stretch. But it's effective in only about 60 per cent of patients, and for half of them, the effects wear off within a few years. Because the lasers emit such powerful beams, they can burn the eye tissue and leave permanent scars, so patients can undergo the procedure only once or twice.

**How it works** The new procedure, developed by a small company called SOLX who are based at the Photonics Center at Boston University, relies on a different kind of laser, called a titanium sapphire laser. Instead of stretching the meshwork, the laser emits quick pulses of energy to shake it, rather like shaking out a blanket after a day at the beach. The motion dislodges any particles that may be blocking the flow of fluid and normalizes pressure without damaging the eye.

'If you produce minimal change in the eye, you have the possibility of retreatment,' says Dr Francisco Fantes, professor of ophthalmology at Miami University's Bascomb Palmer Eye Institute.

One study of 100 patients conducted by researchers in Madrid, Spain, found that the SOLX procedure, called gonioscopic laser trabecular ablation (GLTA), reduced pressure in the eye more than ALT did. Another study of patients who had already had ALT produced similar results. Those who had GLTA were able to cut the amount of medication they required by 72 per cent. If they were taking only one drug before the surgery, they didn't need it afterwards.

Another new laser procedure approved by the US Food and Drug Administration in October 2002 is selective laser trabeculoplasty (SLT). Like the GLTA laser, it uses a low-intensity laser and can be repeated several times. But the GLTA laser can penetrate deeper into the eye, says Dr Fantes, making it more effective. Studies have found that GLTA penetrates almost 90 per cent of the trabecular meshwork, compared to about 15 per cent for SLT, making it better able to clear out any 'clogs'. Additionally, GLTA patients required significantly fewer medications after surgery than SLT patients.

**Availability** SOLX was approved for use in Europe in August 2003. Dr Fantes hopes that soon GLTA will be considered a first-stage treatment for POAG instead of drugs.

# ALSO in the NEWS

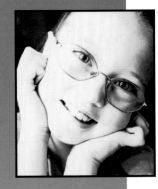

## Acne drug shows promise for eye disease

Researchers suspect that the acne drug isotretinoin (Accutane) may be able to prevent not just pimples but also a certain type of blindness. Researchers at the University of California, Los Angeles, injected the drug into mice bred to have the same genetic defect that causes Stargardt's macular degeneration, an inherited form of blindness that usually begins in late childhood. It occurs when pigment builds up on the eye.

For some reason, Stargardt's mice raised without light don't go blind, so researchers decided to try Accutane because of one of its side effects: it prevents the eyes from getting enough light. Two months after the treatments began, the pigment had stopped accumulating in the mice's eyes, with no negative effects on their daytime vision. The findings were published in an April 2003 issue of the *Proceedings of the National Academy of Sciences.*

Researchers warn, however, that people with Stargardt's should not start asking their doctors to put them on Accutane. Without human studies to determine effective dosages, taking the drug could not only be worthless when it comes to eyesight but could even be harmful. Stay tuned for more research.

## Expert study suggests fewer hours of patch-wearing for children with squints

Many children with squints suffer from an eye condition called amblyopia – more commonly known as a 'lazy eye'. The usual treatment is for the child to wear a patch over the good eye forcing the other one to work properly. But children are often reluctant to wear the patch for the recommended six hours a day because this often leads to teasing at school. However, a new US study has found that wearing a patch for two hours a day is just as good as six hours in treating a lazy eye, so children don't need to wear the patch to school. The study, sponsored by the US National Eye Institute, tested 189 children with moderate amblyopia. Half wore patches for two hours a day and the others for six hours. After four months, more than 75 per cent of children in both groups had improved vision. Ann McIntyre, principal orthoptist at Moorfields Eye Hospital, agrees with the findings but says it is important to monitor treatment.

## Kids who wear glasses really are smarter

A study has revealed that the amount of reading and studying that children do may have an effect on their eyesight. Research that was published in *Investigative Ophthalmology & Visual Science* in December 2002 found that nearsighted (myopic) children spend an average of two hours more a week studying and reading for pleasure but they spend less time playing sports than non-myopic children. Not surprisingly, nearsighted children also scored higher on a test of basic reading and language skills than children with normal vision. And the difference is not related to more electronic game playing and television watching either. Both sets of children spent the same amount of time playing video games and watching TV. However, before you blame that book and snatch it from your child's hands, you should check your own eyesight. The researchers found that by far the largest risk factor for myopia in children was myopia in one or both parents.

## Questioning yearly eye examinations for people suffering from diabetes

People with diabetes are susceptible to diabetic retinopathy, in which blood vessels in the retina are damaged. It is the leading cause of blindness in adults up to age 74, but if it is caught early, vision loss can be prevented or delayed. That's why people with diabetes are advised to have vision screenings at least once a year, although there's never been any research confirming that annual visits are really worthwhile.

Now, a study published in a January 2003 issue of *The Lancet* suggests that people with diabetes who have no signs of retinopathy in one examination, have had diabetes for less than 20 years and are not taking insulin could go up to three years before having another screening. Researchers evaluated 7,500 patients with Type 2 diabetes in Liverpool. People who have had the disease for more than 20 years and those who use insulin are more likely to develop retinopathy and so should be screened at least once a year, the researchers reported.

Alternative answers

# Good vibes are sweet music to Ménière's patients

Imagine knowing that at any time, you could lose your hearing and become so dizzy you collapse on the floor, vomiting. Driving and even walking would be risky, since the spells come without warning.

That prospect is reality for people who suffer from Ménière's disease, an abnormality of the inner ear that causes severe dizziness, a roaring sound in the ears, fluctuating hearing loss, and the sensation of pressure or pain in the affected ear. An estimated one in 1,000 people in the UK are affected by this disease. Now, a physician at the University of Rochester in New York has discovered that using a simple £30 vibrating apparatus can be more effective than surgery for treating the condition.

**How it works** Ménière's disease results from a buildup of fluid in the inner ear, but no one really knows what causes the build-up. The disease is difficult to treat. About 20 to 30 per cent of patients fail to respond to conventional medical treatment (mainly, drugs to reduce fluid volume) and require ear surgery. Even with surgery, 20 to 40 per cent of patients don't improve.

Dr Paul Dutcher, associate professor in the division of otolaryngology at the university, wondered why two forms of surgery for the condition – one that removes a middle ear bone and another that involves drilling through the bone and opening up a fluid-containing sac in the inner ear – produced similar results. He realized that the only common factor was drilling the bone. The drilling causes the skull to vibrate and those vibrations may knock loose tiny particles that wind up in the inner ear, clogging the system and resulting in fluid accumulation. 'It's basic plumbing,' he says.

To test his theory, Dr Dutcher got patients to lie in the same position as they would for surgery, then used an oscillator (an instrument that creates vibrations) over the middle ear bone of the affected ear. He used the device on patients for 30 minutes once a week for four weeks, with the result that 70 to 80 per cent of the patients improved. He presented the results of a small pilot study on 29 patients in September 2002 at the annual meeting of the American Academy of Otolaryngology-Head and Neck Surgery Foundation.

**Availability** Since his presentation, Dr Dutcher has heard from several other US physicians who are trying his technique. He cautions that it will be another five years or so before enough data is collected to prove that it definitely works. However, several of his patients who had the procedure are still doing well two years after the treatment, and even those who experienced relapses responded to another course of treatment. Dr Jim Cook, ENT consultant neurotologist at the Leicester Royal Infirmary, says the procedure sounds promising as it involves minimal intervention but more research is required before it will become available in the UK.

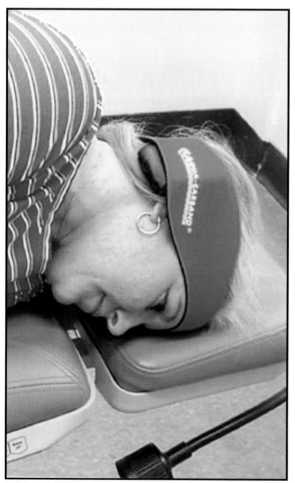

In this novel Ménière's treatment, an oscillator (the black device under the headband) seems to knock loose particles in the ear.

High-tech help

# Jamming the signal to switch off tinnitus

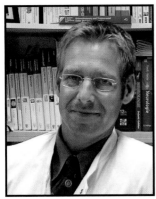

Dr Christian Gerloff invented a possible new tinnitus treatment.

If you have ever been to a loud rock concert, you may have experienced an annoying ringing in your ears afterwards. But people with a condition called tinnitus live with constant or intermittent phantom sounds – from ringing and buzzing to whirring or roaring – all the time. It often occurs for no apparent reason, although previous exposure to loud noise increases the risk.

Traditionally, tinnitus is treated with psychological training procedures (also referred to as retraining), in which patients are taught to cope with the noise so they can continue to live normally. Although most patients report some improvement after retraining, says tinnitus expert Dr Christian Gerloff, of the University of Tübingen in Germany, the noise rarely disappears completely.

A preliminary study conducted by Dr Gerloff and his colleagues has now found that rather than being imaginary, in most cases, tinnitus emanates from abnormal activity in a part of the brain. 'It means that, in some patients, tinnitus can be something like an acoustic phantom perception,' he says. This is similar to phantom pain experienced by amputees. 'In other words, the noise is not generated in the ear but directly inside the brain, like an illusion.'

To turn off that signal, Dr Gerloff and his team conducted a small pilot study in 14 patients with intractable, chronic tinnitus. They used a procedure called transcranial magnetic stimulation to stimulate regions of the brain involved in processing auditory input in order to interfere with the electrical activity in those portions of the brain. By doing so, they were able to temporarily 'jam' the signal causing the noise, disrupting the tinnitus for several seconds in most of the patients.

Results of the study were published in the *Annals of Neurology* in February 2003. The finding could lead to new treatments for the condition, says Dr Gerloff. But first, he says: 'Controlled clinical trials are necessary to evaluate whether this method can permanently reduce and thus cure tinnitus.'

## Magnet therapy

By using a magnet to stimulate a region of the brain called the left temporoparietal cortex, doctors were able to temporarily reduce tinnitus symptoms. There was no reduction when other areas of the brain were stimulated.

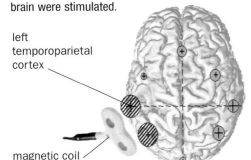

left temporoparietal cortex

magnetic coil

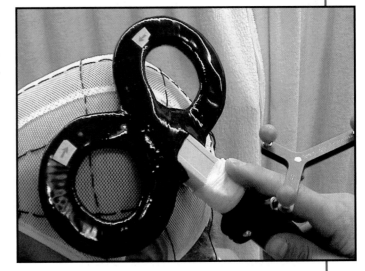

Surgical solution

# Implantable lenses – they're getting better and better

Each year around 100,000 people in the UK undergo laser eye surgery to correct their vision. But many others don't qualify – often because they're too nearsighted or their eyes have some factor that makes them poor candidates for the surgery. Recent US research has found that permanent implantable contact lenses (ICLs) not only provide a solution for such cases but may actually be a safer and more effective alternative to LASIK surgery for those who suffer moderate to severe myopia (shortsightedness). Known as phakic intraocular lens implantation, the procedure has been available in the UK for a few years although it is pending approval in the United States.

**How it works** The lens is slipped into the eye over the existing lens through a tiny slit that closes on its own once the implant is inserted. Although

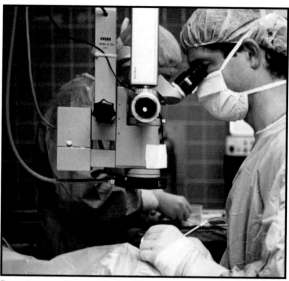

Recent research suggests the ICL may be more effective than laser surgery and could one day make LASIK a thing of the past.

procedure involves a small incision, it leaves the cornea intact, thus avoiding some of the side effects, such as a corneal haze, of LASIK surgery. The lens can also be removed at any time, if necessary. A study by Dr John Vukich, surgical director at the Davis Duehr Dean Medical Center in Madison, Wisconsin, and published in *Cornea: The Journal of Cornea and External Disease* in May 2003, compared the results of LASIK surgery with ICLs made by US company STAAR Surgical. It found that over 50 per cent of ICL patients with moderate to severe myopia achieved 20/20 vision or better as compared to only 35 per cent of LASIK patients. The ICLs also had fewer adverse effects.

One drawback is that the ICL cannot offer perfect vision for those with significant astigmatism – a defect in the shape of the cornea. However, a new specialist implantable lens could solve this problem. The Toric Implantable Contact Lens (TICL), also produced by STAAR Surgical, appears to reduce astigmatism and correct myopia and hyperopia (farsightedness) in one procedure. A US clinical trial carried out in 2002 on a patient with significant astigmatism who was barely able to see his fingers, found that 24 hours after having a STAAR TICL implanted, his vision improved significantly, to the extent that he could drive a car without glasses.

**Availability** ICL surgery costs about £1,000 per eye and is available at private eye clinics. The STAAR TICL has received European approval and should be available soon.

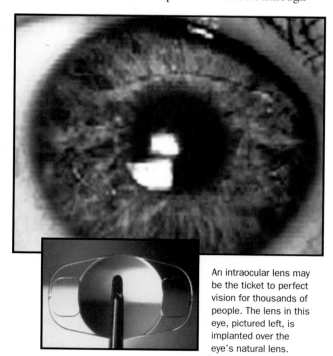

An intraocular lens may be the ticket to perfect vision for thousands of people. The lens in this eye, pictured left, is implanted over the eye's natural lens.

High-tech help
# The next wave in LASIK surgery

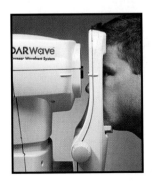

Some people choose not to undergo LASIK surgery for fear of night glare, a common side effect. But a new technology could provide a solution. At the European Society of Cataract and Refractive Surgeons conference held in February 2002, a number of presentations focused on a medical device that is used in a procedure called wavefront-driven customized ablation. In US clinical trials, nearly 80 per cent of people who underwent the new laser surgery had better vision than that achieved with LASIK.

**How it works** The device, called LADARWave, uses special technology to measure and adjust tiny defects in the shape of the cornea, called higher-order aberrations. Experts believe that these aberrations contribute to common night vision problems, including glare and halos around lights such as headlights.

The LADARWave transmits a ray of light into the eye that reflects off the back of the retina, out through the pupil and into the device, where the light is captured and arranged into a unique map of a person's corneal aberrations. This map is used to guide the laser during the surgery, ensuring more precise reshaping of the cornea – and better eyesight. The new surgery can be used to correct the vision of people who

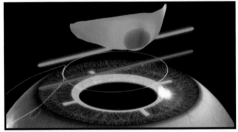

Prior to surgery, the LADARWave makes a detailed three-dimensional map of the cornea.

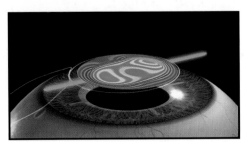

The map makes it possible to correct tiny flaws in the shape of the cornea to provide better vision.

have already had LASIK and it can even be performed on some people who would not generally qualify for LASIK.

**Availability** Approved in October 2002 by the US Food and Drug Administration, this new technology is just beginning to become mainstream in Europe. It is already available at some private clinics in the UK, but whilst many are excited by its potential, some European surgeons say more research is needed.

RESEARCH ROUND-UP

## Throw away those reading glasses

An estimated 23 million people in the UK require reading glasses as they become increasingly longsighted with age. Ageing causes eyes to lose flexibility, as the lenses become harder and less elastic, while the muscles surrounding them grow stiff. This condition, called presbyopia, makes it more difficult to focus on close tasks, such as reading, sewing, or computer work. But a new form of surgery could change this.

Called conductive keratoplasty (CK), the painless procedure uses a needle-like probe to deliver radiofrequency energy to the cornea. The non-dominant eye (everyone has one eye that's stronger

than the other) is overcorrected, making it slightly nearsighted. It's like creating bifocals from your eyes: one eye to see far, the other to see near.

In a US study of 70 people, 70 per cent had perfect eyesight after the surgery and it improved the vision in almost 90 per cent. The three-minute procedure became available in the UK in early 2003 and costs between £1,000 and £1,500. Dr David Allamby from the Horizon Eye Laser Centre in Manchester expects it to become more popular than laser correction. 'It's like winding the clock back five or 10 years. The only thing is, in a few years' time, patients may have to wind it back again.'

# HEART & CIRCULATORY SYSTEM

## THE WORLD'S DEADLIEST AND COSTLIEST CONDITION IS HEART DISEASE

The challenges of treating and preventing it have spurred scientists to make amazing life-saving advances. Heart repair without opening the chest? Doctors can now use robots to operate through pencil-size holes. A pacemaker without the pacemaker? Researchers are recruiting heart cells to do the job themselves. Early detection of heart disease with a simple blood test? It's a reality.

Prevention, still the best cure, means among other things keeping your cholesterol under control. A drug called Ezetrol not only provides a new mechanism for lowering cholesterol, it can also be combined with existing drugs to really bring those readings down.

There are new breakthroughs for the rest of your circulatory system too. People who have sickle cell disease may soon be able to prevent painful episodes by inhaling nitric oxide gas. And there's a new and painless way of

## Key discovery
# Sea worm may provide blood substitute

If you're ever unlucky enough to need a blood transfusion in an emergency medical situation, you may not be thrilled to hear a doctor say: 'Give this patient a unit of sea worm blood.' But it is certainly better than hearing: 'We're out of blood.'

HIV/AIDS, Mad Cow Disease, and a host of other health threats have cut the world's blood supply to uncomfortably low levels. The situation has sent scientists scrambling to come up with a safe substitute. In June 2003 French researchers unveiled a most intriguing candidate: the common lugworm, a sand-burrowing sea creature often used for bait. It turns out that its blood is strikingly similar to human blood. In laboratory tests with mice, infused sea worm blood did what a blood substitute is supposed to do – that is, deliver oxygen to organs – without triggering any immune system reactions. The results were encouraging enough to merit more study, including tests on humans.

Medical experts worldwide consider it a matter of when, not if, artificial blood will replace the real thing in emergency rooms and accident scenes and even during non-emergency surgery. Various blood substitutes, some of them derived from cow's blood, are currently being researched all over the world. One of them, HemoPure, is already in use in South Africa and has been approved for use in dogs in the UK.

Consider the advantages of blood substitutes: unlike donated human blood, they require no refrigeration, have a shelf life of two years or more, carry no risk of viral disease and can be available in unlimited quantities. There's also no chance of mixing up blood types: artificial blood is one-type-fits-all.

**A longstanding quest** A person who has lost blood has an urgent need: to keep oxygen moving from the lungs through the vessels to the organs. The blood component charged with this task is the protein haemoglobin, which is why most potential blood substitutes focus on getting haemoglobin into the bloodstream. One reason the now 50-year-old quest for artificial blood has been so frustrating is that haemoglobin is unstable when freed from its usual confines inside blood cells. It tends to fall apart, so it can't carry any oxygen, and its fragmented remains can poison the kidneys. Also, free (that is, non-cell-bound) haemoglobin will bind with nitric oxide in blood vessel walls, preventing that gas from keeping the vessels relaxed. That raises blood pressure to dangerous levels.

With the cow-based blood substitutes, modern biotechnology has solved those problems by modifying the cows' haemoglobin molecules so that they hold together in the bloodstream for at least 24 hours – long enough to get a patient through an emergency. (Any blood substitute is a temporary solution; eventually everyone needs real human blood.) The modified haemoglobin molecules are also bigger, so they can't enter blood vessel walls and react with the nitric oxide there.

**The lugworm advantage** Lugworm haemoglobin is already 50 times larger than human haemoglobin. That fact makes the French investigators hopeful for a medical miracle – a haemoglobin source that doesn't need to be modified but just collected, purified and used. If the idea proves viable after more advanced testing, it is envisaged that sea worm 'farms' could eventually be created in coastal areas to harvest enough of the little sea worms to create a life-saving substitute blood supply.

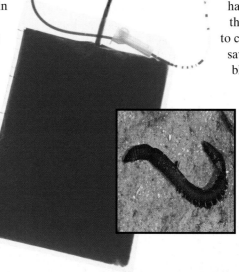

The common lugworm, or sea worm, could prove a source of the blood substitute scientists have long sought.

Diagnostic advance
# Diagnosing heart disease from a drop of blood

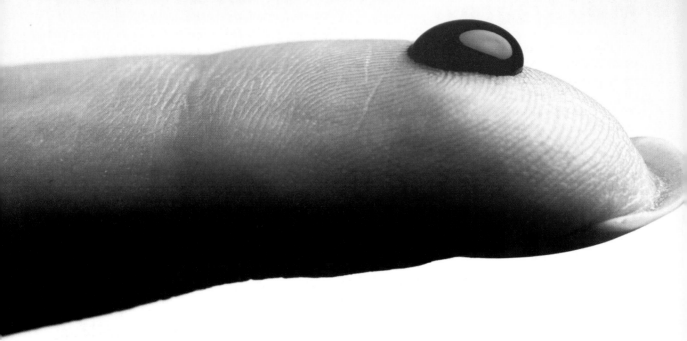

You have probably been told plenty about what puts you at risk for heart disease: smoking, obesity, high blood pressure, elevated cholesterol levels and more. But how do you know for sure if you actually *have* heart disease?

So far, the most useful diagnostic tool has been angiography, which involves injecting dye into the coronary arteries through a long, narrow tube inserted up through the groin so that X-rays can reveal any blockages. But this procedure is invasive, not to mention expensive. Wouldn't it be infinitely better if you could be tested for heart disease simply by giving a blood sample?

UK researchers from Imperial College, London and the University of Cambridge think so, and they revealed just such a diagnostic test in November 2002. The test is so quick, cheap and dependable that its inventors envision a day in the near future when entire populations can be routinely screened for heart disease. By providing early warning of heart attacks in the making, the test could save thousands of lives a year in the UK alone, the researchers estimate.

The new test is referred to by the unwieldy name of proton nuclear magnetic resonance-based metabonomics. From the patient's point of view, it's very simple – giving a bit of blood and waiting for the results. But what's done with the blood sample in the laboratory is more complex. Modern imaging equipment (nuclear magnetic resonance, or NMR) is used to analyse the sample at the molecular level. In study results published in November 2002 in the journal *Nature Medicine,* the technique had a 92 per cent success rate at spotting which samples came from people with heart disease and which didn't.

**How it works** The key to finding heart disease in a drop of blood lies in a new method of analysis that the researchers call metabonomics. It focuses on molecules called metabolites (glucose and cholesterol are well-known examples). Researchers use high-frequency radiowaves to measure the magnetic properties of these molecules in the blood sample. Then they feed the data into a computer program that turns the information into a pattern, or 'fingerprint'. Heart disease can be seen as a recognizable metabonomic pattern.

**Availability** Larger and more rigorous studies must be completed before metabonomic tests have any chance of replacing angiography. Researchers began work on these at Papworth Hospital, a cardiology centre near Cambridge, in 2003.

If the test passes muster, it could be ready for widespread use on patients as early as 2005. And that may be just the beginning. In theory, any kind of disease that yields a metabonomic fingerprint could be diagnosed with the new technique. Researchers are already looking into the feasibility of using metabonomics to diagnose diabetes, osteoporosis, arthritis and Alzheimer's disease.

## FingerPrint technology

FingerPrint technology provides a cheap, rapid, noninvasive alternative to angiography for the diagnosis of heart disease.

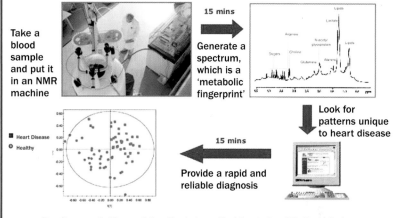

Take a blood sample and put it in an NMR machine

15 mins

Generate a spectrum, which is a 'metabolic fingerprint'

Look for patterns unique to heart disease

15 mins

Provide a rapid and reliable diagnosis

■ Heart Disease
○ Healthy

*Results generated by a collaboration between the laboratories of Dr. David Grainger (Cambridge University), Professor Jeremy Nicholson (Imperial College, London), and Dr. Peter Schofield (Papworth Hospital NHS Trust), supported by TCP Innovations Limited, Metabometrix Limited, and FingerPrint Diagnostics Limited*

# ALSO in the NEWS

## A life-saving device for the home?

In addition to the latest digital camera or stock-quoting cell phone, Americans now have another electronic gadget to add to their homes, although this one has a more serious purpose. Automatic external defibrillators (AEDs) – the hand-held machines that shock stopped hearts back into action – won US government approval for home use in November 2002. By June 2003, the manufacturer was announcing Father's Day specials that knocked 15 per cent off the list price of the already popular machines. Approval came after similar devices had become standard issue for airports, sports venues, and other public places where fast action can revive victims whose hearts unexpectedly stop beating. Since most cardiac arrests happen in the home, it was a logical step to approve the equipment for home use. But it may be some time before the British can add AEDs to their mod cons. The British Heart Foundation (BHF) said it would need to review all the data before suggesting that people should have defibrillators in their homes and it will be studying the outcome of the US initiative. The UK charity does support the placement of defibrillators in the community where they are manned by community responders who have been trained to use them. Perhaps, in time, the UK will follow America's lead. For now, the BHF recommends that people learn how to perform emergency life support, including mouth-to-mouth resuscitation and chest compressions. As a victim's chances of survival shrink by 20 per cent with each passing minute, your skills could mean the difference between life and death.

Key discovery

# Heart cells learn to keep the beat

The 600,000 heart patients worldwide who are fitted with pacemakers each year are probably grateful that a machine can keep their hearts beating when their bodies can't. But if there were a way to avoid implanting an electronic device in their chests, they'd probably choose it without hesitation. Now a team of researchers has successfully tested a new technique that reprograms certain heart cells to take over pacemaking chores, and it's just a matter of time before such an alternative is available.

Dubbed the biopacemaker when laboratory success (in guinea pigs) was announced in late 2002, the technique would also provide more versatile pacemaking that could adjust to changes in physical exertion levels in a way that pacemaker implants can't. Such a biopacemaker is also a potentially important option for patients who are at too great a risk of infection from conventional pacemakers.

**How it works** When the human heart is working properly, two types of cardiac cells supervise the heartbeat by emitting electrical impulses to trigger contractions in all the other heart cells. When these 'pacing' cells are diseased, damaged or otherwise incapacitated, the heartbeat falters and fatal circulatory collapse looms. Traditional mechanical

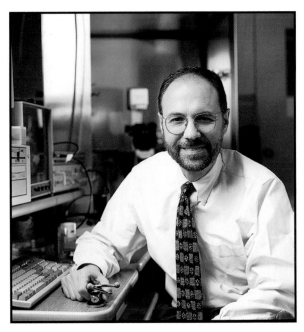

Dr Eduardo Marban and colleagues at Johns Hopkins University Hospital pioneered the work on the so-called biopacemaker.

pacemakers have saved the day by emitting the carefully calibrated electrical impulses that create a heartbeat. But the biopacemaker researchers, from Johns Hopkins University Hospital in Baltimore, solved the problem in an entirely different way: they used gene therapy to stimulate other, healthy heart cells to help to 'conduct' the rhythm section.

The researchers speculated (correctly, as it turned out) that all adult heart cells have the capacity to perform pacing duties. So why don't they? Because a steady supply of potassium to the heart suppresses the innate pacing function in all but the designated

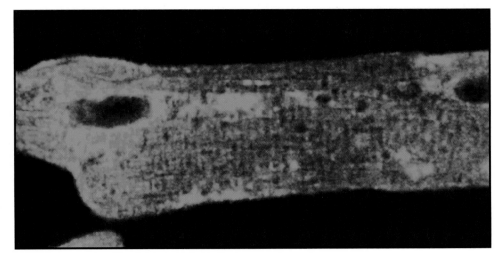

This guinea pig heart cell is producing green fluorescence protein (GFP), a sign that it has taken up the instructions to become a pacemaking cell. The virus that delivered the instructions also delivered the GFP instructions.

pacer cells. This is a good thing in healthy hearts, since too many 'conductors' increase the chances of mistakes by the 'orchestra'. When the pacing cells stop working, however, substitutes are needed. Regular heart cells can be prompted into performing back-up pacing duty by altering their potassium levels. That's where gene therapy comes into play.

The researchers injected each guinea pig's heart with a virus that served as a vehicle to carry a specially encoded gene into the protein segments of the DNA responsible for pumping potassium into heart cells. The gene reduced the potassium levels in the cells and, sure enough, that freed them up to fire off the electrical jolts that qualified them as bona fide acting pacemaker cells.

**Availability** It's a long road from manipulating guinea pig cells to coming up with a viable bio-pacemaker that will work safely in humans. The most optimistic guess is that it will be four years before a human treatment is ready.

**RESEARCH ROUND-UP**

## Is test a better way to discount false heart attack fears?

You feel pressure in your chest and you're sweating and feeling panicky. You're sure you're having a heart attack – but are you really? Almost four out of five people rushed to emergency rooms with heart attack symptoms are not actually having heart attacks. Now there is a new blood test which can be used to help them to rule out false alarms. The test is known as albumin cobalt binding (ACB) and is marketed by Ischemia Technologies Inc.

When heart tissue is starved of oxygen, as it is during a heart attack, a blood protein called albumin changes properties, binding less easily to cobalt, a metallic element. For the ACB test, emergency room personnel simply add a bit of cobalt to the patient's blood sample. The chemical reaction that takes place provides a good indication of whether a heart attack has taken place.

ACB can be used only negatively – that is, to rule out heart attacks rather than to confirm that one has occurred. Also, it isn't foolproof, which is one reason it has been approved for use only in conjunction with two existing tests – an electrocardiogram, which measures the heart's electrical activity and a test for toponin, another blood protein.

The three tests appear to make a good team. One US study showed that when the ACB test was added to the other two, doctors were able to rule out heart attacks 70 per cent of the time, up from 50 per cent. The more efficient diagnosis means that precious emergency room resources can be better directed to where they're needed most.

The ACB test, approved in the USA in February 2003, was presented at the British Society of Cardiology meeting last April.

## Exercising harder – not longer – helps the heart

As experts debated whether to recommend a half-hour or a full hour of daily exercise, new research showed that it may not matter. When it comes to staving off heart disease, a five-year study of 9,758 men aged 50 to 59 revealed that what counts most is not how long you exercise, but how hard.

The participants in the study, published in *Circulation* in May 2002, were from Northern Ireland and France. When their leisure-time physical activities were measured it was found that the greater the intensity of exercise, the lower the chances of a coronary event. Those who merely walked or cycled to work reaped no benefit.

The British Heart Foundation recommends that for optimum heart health you should aim to build up to and then maintain a constant level of fitness. Exercise should be taken for 30 minutes at least five days a week. The exercise should be enough to raise the pulse and pro-duce mild breath-lessness. Aerobic exercise such as *brisk* walking and swimming are useful as well as tennis, rowing or bad-minton. Press-ups, squash and weight-lifting are not recom-mended as they put too much strain on the heart. Always warm-up before you exercise.

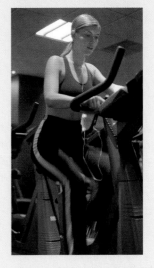

Surgical solution

# A da Vinci masterpiece – robotic heart surgery

As life-saving as a heart operation can be, the prospect of having your chest cracked open so that surgeons can get in there and go to work is daunting, to say the least. But the day is coming soon when heart surgery will routinely be a closed-chest procedure, with a few tiny holes substituting for a football-size chest excavation site, while precision-guided computerized robotic arms are used instead of human hands.

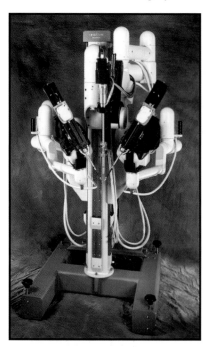

A robot's arms, with instruments attached, perform heart surgery as a doctor controls them.

That day got much closer in November 2002, when the first research results based on actually performing the robotic procedure were announced. The verdict: all 15 'open-heart, closed-chest' operations performed at Columbia-Presbyterian Medical Center in New York City were carried out without major complications. Just one required follow-up surgery five days later.

The advantages of robotic heart surgery go beyond easing the dread factor. According to the study, the closed-chest patients were out of the hospital two to four days earlier than what's typical for conventional open-heart surgery patients, and they were strong enough to return to work 50 per cent sooner. There's less pain during recovery and less scarring as a lifelong souvenir of the surgery. The procedure itself did take a bit longer but that's expected to change as surgeons become more familiar with the technique.

**How it works** Robotic heart surgery is the latest application of the da Vinci Surgical System, an extraordinarily high-tech piece of medical equipment. It allows the surgical team to insert a camera through a pencil-size chest incision and two remote-controlled robotic arms through two other equally small holes. Surgical materials are inserted as needed through a fourth hole. The instrument-wielding robotic arms perform the actual operation, controlled with joysticks by a surgeon as he views the image at a nearby console. So, yes, mere mortals are still in charge but the da Vinci system allows a degree of precision and steadiness unmatched by human hands.

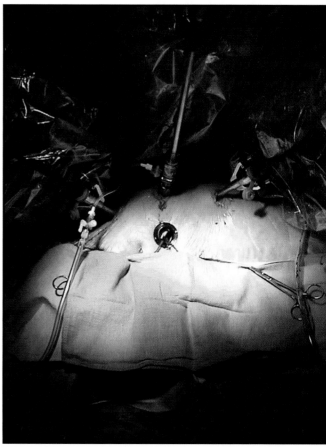

Robotic assisted cardiac surgery significantly reduces the trauma – and the recovery time – for the patient.

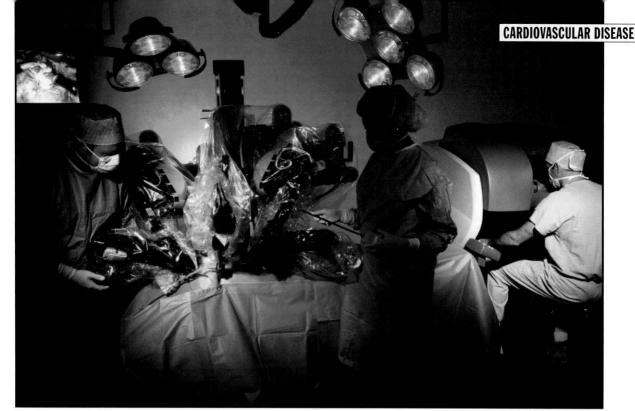

The doctor seated at the control console is performing surgery on a patient lying about 8ft away. His hand and wrist movements are translated precisely by instruments – held by tiny mechanical wrists – inside the patient.

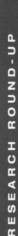

**Availability** The Columbia-Presbyterian study was a major step towards making robotics the norm for heart surgery. The procedure performed in this case was the closure of an unwanted opening between the heart's two upper chambers, a congenital condition called atrial septal defect. The innovative technique has been adapted for bypass surgery and has already been used successfully in Britain.

In May 2003 a patient at St Mary's Hospital, London, became one of the first to undergo a totally endoscopic robotic coronary artery bypass. This life-saving procedure reroutes blood flow around clogged arteries near the heart, bypassing any dangerous blockages.

The technique has only so far been used on patients requiring a single vessel bypass, but surgeons hope that in the future it could be used to perform double and triple bypasses. As the technology improves and surgeons build up experience of the technique it will probably have many other medical applications.

Formal evaluations (clinical trials) of robotic bypass surgery in terms of effectiveness and safety were nearing completion in 2003.

RESEARCH ROUND-UP

### Green isn't your cup of tea? Try black

Green tea has gained a lot of attention lately for its heart benefits, but a new study of tea drinkers brings good news for those who prefer the darker version of the world's most popular beverage. After examining the health records and sipping habits of more than 3,000 men and women in Saudi Arabia, researchers found there was a clear correlation between black tea consumption and a lower risk of heart disease.

In the study, published in the January 2003 issue of the journal *Preventive Medicine,* people who drank at least six cups of black tea a day reaped the most heart-health benefits. Six daily cuppas may be a tall order even in a tea-loving country such as Britain. Still, the study authors point out that even lesser amounts will deliver some flavonoids, the plant chemicals believed to be responsible for tea's beneficial effect. Flavonoids, abundant in both black and green tea, help to protect the cardiovascular system by acting as antioxidants, which neutralize cell-damaging molecules called free radicals.

Belinda Linden, from the British Heart Foundation, points out that a healthier lifestyle is the key to avoiding heart disease. 'Including flavonoids in your diet is just one step in the right direction,' she says.

Surgical solution

# Drug-coated stent popularity balloons

A new way to unclog blocked coronary arteries took a giant step closer to becoming common practice in April 2002, with the eagerly awaited approval of a drug-coated stent, known as the Cypher stent. Cardiologists began using words such as 'remarkable' and 'revolutionary' to describe the stents – tiny wire mesh tubes that prop open coronary arteries and also emit a drug that helps to prevent the stent itself from becoming clogged.

There is good reason for the enthusiastic adjectives. The go-ahead for the new stents means that a much higher percentage of people with serious heart disease will be able to avoid open-heart surgery as well as heart attacks.

**Bypassing bypass surgery** In the past, if arteries near your heart were blocked or narrowed, making you a prime candidate for a heart attack, your only choice was to undergo bypass surgery, in which doctors remove a blood vessel from else-where in the body and use it to reroute blood flow around the blockage. A more recent and far less invasive option is balloon angioplasty. Instead of opening up the chest, doctors guide a narrow balloon-tipped tube up from the groin and into the blocked artery, then inflate the balloon to expand the artery so blood can flow freely.

Angioplasty works as well as bypass surgery but only temporarily, as the arteries soon collapse or narrow again. To avoid that problem, doctors began leaving behind a tiny, cylindrical, hollow tube

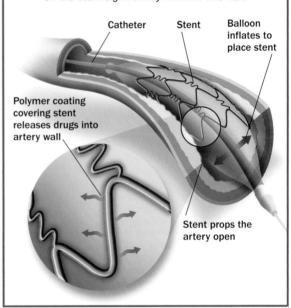

## Angioplasty advances

Stents, the tiny mesh-like tubes placed in arteries to keep them open after angioplasty, become blocked again in 20 to 30 per cent of patients. A drug coating on the stent significantly reduces this risk.

Catheter    Stent    Balloon inflates to place stent

Polymer coating covering stent releases drugs into artery wall

Stent props the artery open

called a stent to prop the artery open, much like scaffolding in a mine tunnel. That helped, but not enough, as the stents themselves tended to become blocked with scar tissue, a process called restenosis.

Because restenosis often makes repeat procedures necessary, less invasive angioplasty remained a distant second to very invasive bypass surgery as the treatment of choice for coronary artery disease. The drug-coated stents are expected to change that.

The Cypher stent is treated with a drug called sirolimus (also called rapamycin), which inhibits the proliferation of cells that create the scarring. A 2002 study published in the *New England Journal of*

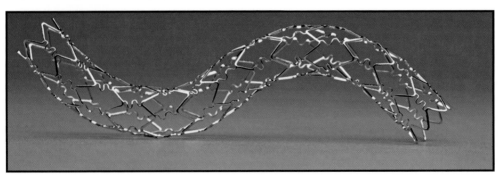

The Cypher stent is coated with a drug to prevent the stent from becoming clogged inside the artery.

*Medicine* credits the drug coating with drastically reducing restenosis in heart patients with stents. More importantly, among the study subjects, the rate of 'major cardiac events' (such as heart attacks) after receiving a stent dropped from 28.8 per cent to just 5.8 per cent if the stent was drug coated.

**More angioplasties on the way** Not all drug-coated stents are approved for use in the UK, and research is being undertaken to test other types and determine their efficacy. Cardiologists predict that because of the reduced restenosis rate with drug-coated stents, physicians will be more likely to recommend angioplasty rather than bypass surgery to heart patients with serious coronary artery blockage.

Cost seemed to be a drawback for a while, since drug-coated stents are more expensive than the uncoated ones. But evidence published in the *American Heart Journal* in March 2003, then updated at a meeting of the American College of Cardiology, showed that the newer stents are more economical in the long run than regular stents and that angioplasty with any kind of stent is more cost-effective than bypass surgery.

## RESEARCH ROUND-UP

### A slice of rye for your health

Fibre is a famous ally of older adults, but now we know which fibre source is the seniors' best friend. The winner is whole grain cereal fibre, especially in the form of dark bread. University of Washington researchers, in a study published in an April 2003 issue of the *Journal of the American Medical Association,* found that eating two slices of fibre-rich, whole-grain bread a day, such as wheat, rye or pumpernickel, reduces the risk of heart disease.

An Australian paper, published in the *European Journal of Nutrition* in January 2002, found that five large cohort studies, carried out between 1996 and 2001, agreed with this finding. The researchers concluded that the more whole grains you eat, the more your risk of coronary heart disease is reduced.

The finding is an eye-opener for two reasons. For one thing, it shows that fibre from grains is better for the heart than fruit or vegetable fibre. The other reason is that whole grain cereal fibre benefits your heart even if don't start eating it until late in life.

Progress in prevention

# Low doses of blood thinner ward off killer clots

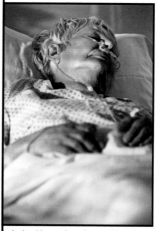

In bed-bound patients, blood clots in the legs pose a threat.

Along with hospital-acquired infections, medical errors and bad food, there's another danger you need to consider when you or a loved one is hospitalized: deep vein thrombosis (DVT), blood clots that form in the leg after a long period of inactivity. DVT becomes particularly dangerous when a blood clot breaks loose, travels through the bloodstream to the heart, and finally lodges in the lung, causing an often fatal condition called pulmonary embolism.

DVT affects one in 5,000 of the UK general population per year. But this increases to one in 2,000 for those who have been recently hospitalized.

Now, a major study published in an April 2003 issue of the *New England Journal of Medicine* has found that a long-term, low-dose course of the blood thinner warfarin can help prevent recurrence of these blood clots without negative side effects.

Currently, people who have had a blood clot or embolism are treated for six months with higher doses of warfarin. The drug is then stopped because of fear of bleeding complications, which is most likely why those people have a 6 to 9 per cent risk of experiencing another blood clot within the following year.

The participants in the study received warfarin for up to four years, with no negative results and a 64 per cent reduction in DVT compared with those who didn't receive the drug. The news was deemed so important that not only did the journal release the results on its web site several weeks prior to publication, but experts who gathered to discuss the prevention and treatment of DVT in March greeted the announcement with applause.

The value of the treatment was so obvious that the study's sponsor, the National Institutes of Health (NIH), stopped the study early so that all participants could benefit from it.

**The ABCs of DVT** Deep vein thrombosis made headlines several years ago with reports of 'economy class syndrome' – blood clots in the leg suffered by people crammed into cramped airline seats during long flights. More recently, in April 2003, NBC news reporter David Bloom, 39, died of a pulmonary embolism while covering the war in Iraq. Experts speculate that a clot may have formed because of the cramped travelling conditions Bloom suffered, coupled with dehydration.

Other risk factors for DVT include orthopaedic surgery, cancer, chronic heart or respiratory failure, varicose veins, smoking, and use of birth control pills and hormone replacement therapy. But the risk is higher for people in hospitals and nursing homes, says Dr Samuel Z. Goldhaber, who directs the Venous Thromboembolism Research Group at Brigham and Women's Hospital in Boston, which conducted the NIH study. 'The rate increases with age and with additional medical illness,' he says. It also rises with obesity and, unfortunately, the number of obese people in the UK, as in other Western countries, is steadily increasing.

Despite these facts, studies find that doctors often don't take the necessary precautions to prevent such dangerous clots from forming, says Dr. Goldhaber, including treating patients with blood thinners *before* they develop clots, asking them to wear special compression stockings to increase blood flow in the legs and also making sure that they move regularly.

You can't blame just the doctors, though. 'Not only the doctors but also the patients and their families have some responsibility,' Dr Goldhaber says.

So, if you feel a cramp in your leg that gets worse and doesn't go away, or you have any unexplained shortness of breath or chest pain – common symptoms of DVT – tell your doctor about it. And if you have a relative who's confined to bed, ask the health care provider: 'What are you doing to prevent DVT in my loved one?', suggests Dr Goldhaber.

Also, take matters into your own hands on long car or plane trips, doctors advise. Get out of that cramped seat occasionally and walk around. On long-haul flights it is also a good idea to stay off the alcohol and make sure you drink plenty of water.

## Key discovery
# Say 'nuts' to high blood pressure

Here's the kind of health news everybody likes to hear: tasty, dry-roasted soy nuts can reduce your blood pressure and therefore lower your risk of heart disease. These snacks really can make a substantial difference. According to research presented to the American Heart Association in November 2002, eating a sizeable portion each day can reduce your blood pressure readings as much as some prescription blood pressure medications.

Soy nuts aren't nuts, of course. They're simply roasted soybeans that taste and crunch like nuts. Plenty of research over the years has solidified soy's reputation as a heart-healthy food. Recently, the attention turned from soy's cholesterol-lowering benefits to its effect on blood pressure. In the second half of 2002, a Spanish study found that substituting soy milk for cow's milk significantly lowered blood pressure. Canadian research found evidence that eating soy in any form – milk, beans, tofu – helps reduce blood pressure, at least in men.

**What the study shows** The soy nut study focused on women – specifically postmenopausal women, who are at much higher risk of heart disease than younger women. The researchers, from Boston's Beth Israel Deaconess Medical Center, put 60 such women on the same diet for eight weeks, except that half the women ate 58g of roasted soy nuts each day instead of the equivalent amount of protein (about 25mg) from other sources. Then the soy eaters switched with the non-soy eaters, and they all followed the diets for another eight weeks.

The results of the research seem to support the effectiveness of soy: while in the soy nut group, women experienced a much more significant drop in blood pressure on average than those who were not eating soy. Those whose blood pressure was too high at the start of the study lowered it by 10 per cent while eating soy nuts daily. Those with normal blood pressure readings at the start of the study saw a 5 per cent drop.

No one is certain why soy helps to lower blood pressure. It's rich in plant chemicals known as isoflavones and much research has attributed soy's heart-saving benefits to these chemicals. But the Canadian study found that soy products that are low in isoflavones (such as soy-based hot dogs and ice cream) also seemed to lower blood pressure in men, indicating that other beneficial mechanisms may be at work. The Spanish researchers point out that soy milk is rich in the amino acid arginine, which converts in the body to nitric oxide, a chemical that relaxes blood vessels.

**How to enjoy soy nuts** Soy nuts were launched in UK health food shops by Harvey Mercer in 2002 and should soon be available from supermarkets as well. You can eat them straight out of the bag, use them as croutons on salads or put them into soups or casseroles.

RESEARCH ROUND-UP

## Want high blood pressure? Then hurry up!

Are you the type who sounds your horn at red lights so they'll change faster? If so, you'd better check your blood pressure. After following more than 3,000 men and women for 15 years, researchers found that impatient people are two to three times more likely than their more laid-back counterparts to develop high blood pressure, a risk factor for heart disease. This is the first time impatience has been linked to high blood pressure independently of other characteristics of the 'Type A' personality, such as agressiveness and competitiveness. Also noteworthy was the relatively young age (18 to 30) of the volunteers when the study began in 1985, meaning that a hurry-up attitude in your youth could lead to high blood pressure before middle age.

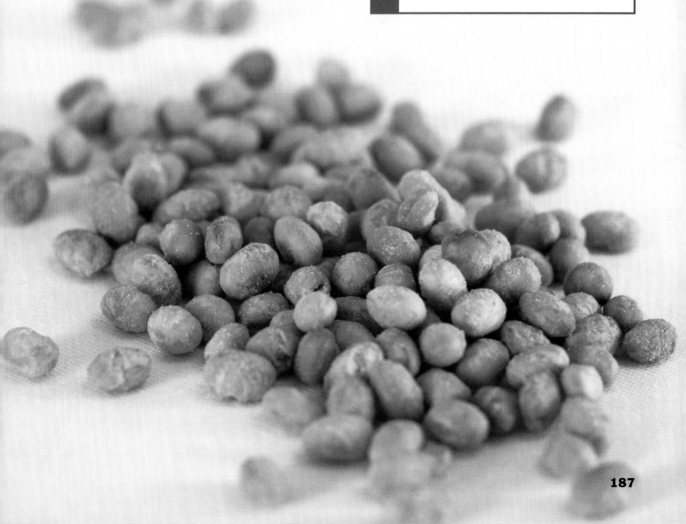

# Blood pressure – do diuretics work best?

A huge North American study that spanned eight years and looked at more than 33,000 hypertension patients in 623 medical centres in the United States, Canada and the Caribbean made a finding that has upset some specialists. The oldest, simplest and cheapest blood pressure-lowering drugs turned out to be the best choice more often than newer drugs. The study authors recommended that the older drugs, called diuretics, be considered first for treating high blood pressure.

The study (known by its acronym, ALLHAT) drew immediate fire from cardiologists and hypertension specialists who objected to the idea of any blood pressure drug being singled out as a first choice. Many also doubted that ALLHAT had made a good case for diuretics' superiority. The ALLHAT team held firm and the diuretics-first advice was included in the US 2003 guidelines for treating high blood pressure. The British Hypertension Society agrees: its guidelines state that a low dose thiazid diuretic should be the first port of call in uncomplicated cases of hypertension.

Right: one of the study's authors and a prominent critic of its conclusions explain their sides of this medical controversy.

The drug types compared in the **ALLHAT** study are **diuretics,** which ease the pressure on blood vessel walls by drawing water from the bloodstream; **calcium channel blockers,** which expand arteries to ease blood flow; and **ACE inhibitors,** which loosen artery walls by blocking a chemical that would otherwise stiffen them.

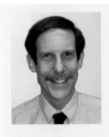

## FOR

*Dr Barry Davis Ph.D. was an ALLHAT study author who had full responsibility for the integrity of the data and the accuracy of the data analyses in the published version. He is a physician/statistician at the School of Public Health of the University of Texas Health Science Center at Houston.*

**Q** Why should diuretics be the first choice for controlling hypertension?
**A** In our study, diuretics were shown to be superior to calcium channel blockers and ACE inhibitors in preventing one or more forms of cardiovascular disease. Also, JNC-VII, the new guidelines for controlling high blood pressure, have recommended diuretics as a first choice after considering the totality of all the evidence from ALLHAT and other studies.

**Q** What does such a recommendation accomplish that's better than leaving doctors to use their best judgment based on the individual patient?

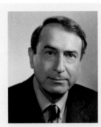

## AGAINST

*Dr Michael A. Weber is past president of the American Society of Hypertension. Professor of medicine and associate dean for research at the College of Medicine of the State University of New York Downstate Medical Center in Brooklyn, Dr Weber has published much commentary critical of the ALLHAT study.*

**Q** Why shouldn't diuretics be the first choice to treat high blood pressure, as ALLHAT concluded?
**A** With many patients, diuretics may not be the best option. We can't over-generalize from ALLHAT. The average age of the subjects was close to 70, and there were a large number of African-American patients, for whom diuretics work well. But there's good evidence, that for white people under the age of 65, diuretics do not have a meaningful blood pressure-lowering effect. So I know that if I have a white patient who is not elderly, diuretics aren't going to get the blood pressure down. Also, people with diabetes and those who have heart or kidney conditions do better with drugs like ACE inhibitors or angiotensin-receptor blockers.

**Q** Didn't the study show that people on diuretics fared better against heart disease in the long run?
**A** In the two most important areas – fatal or non-fatal heart attacks and death – there was absolutely no

**A** JNC-VII looked at the totality of the evidence. For mostly every patient (except those who cannot tolerate a diuretic), the evidence is fairly compelling that diuretics are better. Many guidelines for treatment are based on looking at all the available evidence, which individual doctors can't always do.

**Q** Didn't all the blood pressure drugs tested turn out to be equally effective at preventing heart disease in general?
**A** The drugs tested in ALLHAT were equivalent in preventing coronary heart disease and total mortality. But diuretics were

better at preventing heart failure and other forms of cardiovascular disease. Heart failure is a very serious condition in terms of mortality and cost.

**Q** Don't most people with hypertension need more than one drug anyway?
**A** Yes, so diuretics should be part of the regimen.

**Q** How could professionals disagree so vehemently over this issue?
**A** There is not much disagreement among most professionals. The inclusion of the ALLHAT findings

in the JNC-VII guidelines is a good indication of ALLHAT's broad acceptance. The problem is that those who question ALLHAT's results are very vocal. Their reasoning is not clear. The evidence from the largest hypertension trial ever conducted speaks for itself.

**Q** What are people who are concerned about blood pressure supposed to make of all this?
**A** If they are not on a diuretic, they should ask their doctors why they aren't. The cheapest antihypertensive drugs are the best.

difference between the ACE inhibitor and the diuretic, despite the fact that the study didn't use the ACE inhibitor in an optimal way.

**Q** But then the tie was broken, so to speak, by the diuretics' performance in preventing heart failure.
**A** That's passionately disputed by experts in the field. Making a diagnosis of heart failure is difficult, and even more so in this study, because a diuretic can hide the symptoms of heart failure. So we don't really know what the true incidence of heart failure was. Heart failure is serious. People tend to die from it very soon. So if there was really a dramatic decrease in heart failure rates for those on the diuretic, it should have been reflected in the death rate. It wasn't.

**Q** Does it matter that diuretics are less expensive?
**A** It's doubtful whether diuretics are in fact cheaper. Unlike the other blood pressure drugs, diuretics have metabolic effects. For example, they cause the body to lose potassium, and they can increase uric acid, which can lead to gout. And they increase blood sugar, which increases the likelihood of diabetes. To make sure everything is safe, we must do regular blood tests. If we find problems, they must be treated. So when you total it all up, we're not at all sure that diuretics are the cheaper treatment, even though they are less expensive to buy.

**Q** How could professionals differ so much on a topic like this?

**A** Actually, there are few instances where you have a unanimous point of view on how to treat a condition. The controversy in this case comes from the suggestion that there is one drug that will trump all. There's no such thing. Most people with hypertension will need a combination of drugs, so debates about which is the best single drug are inappropriate.

**Q** What are health consumers to make of all this?
**A** The most important thing is that we've made better progress in treating hypertension. We have a good selection of medicines that can control high blood pressure. Physicians often prefer newer drugs because they are effective and so well tolerated, but diuretics still have a role to play.

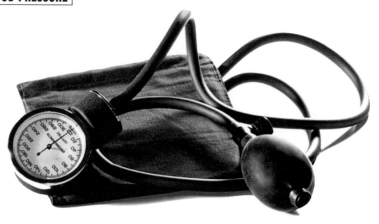

## Progress in prevention
# US panel sounds off on a 'silent killer'

It has been estimated that in the UK more than half of the 10 million people aged over 65 have high blood pressure. It has been called the 'silent killer' because it produces few symptoms and many people are unaware they have it. Yet high blood pressure is the number one risk factor for heart attack, stroke, heart failure and kidney damage. Regular monitoring is the key to identifying the condition in the early stages, which could literally save your life.

Standard practice has categorized anyone with a blood pressure of 140/90 or above (130/80 for diabetics) as having high blood pressure (hypertension) that requires intervention. In the USA, however, recent research has led doctors to devise a new category called 'pre-hypertension' for people whose blood pressure reading falls between 120/80 and 139/89, even if they don't have diabetes. The doctors reckon that people in this category are on their way to developing high blood pressure, and need to take preventive measures straight away. The US guidelines are part of a report issued in 2003 by a panel of experts (the Joint National Committee on the Prevention, Detection, Evaluation, and Treatment of High Blood Pressure) from more than three dozen health organizations.

Not all hypertension experts agree with the new category, arguing that it will cause unnecessary anxiety among people who are essentially healthy. UK blood pressure treatment guidelines do not recognize pre-hypertension and consider any reading between 130/85 and 139/89 to be 'high normal', which requires no action.

You should have your blood pressure measured regularly.

**Regular check-ups** Regardless of what they think of the 'pre-hypertension' category, all hypertension specialists would agree that regular monitoring is important. Ideally, adults should have their blood pressure measured routinely at least every five years until the age of 80 (when it should be measured annually). Anyone who has ever had a high-normal or high reading should also be monitored annually. People with diabetes are more at risk and need to be monitored more frequently.

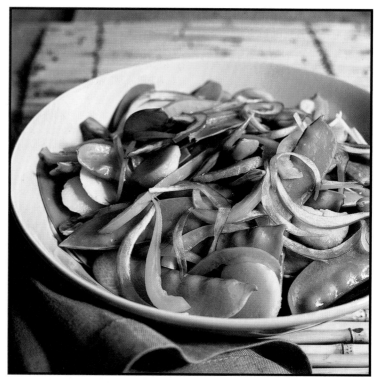

A diet rich in fruits and vegetables is one important part of a preventive approach as it has been proven to be effective at lowering high blood pressure.

## Getting blood pressure under control

People who have been diagnosed with hypertension should take the following into account when tackling the condition:

- **Diuretics are your first-choice drugs** This is discussed on page 188-9. But a number of special high-risk complications and other conditions call for the use of other blood pressure-lowering medications, such as alpha blockers, calcium channel blockers or ACE inhibitors.

- **Concentrate on the top number** If you are over 50, the top number in a typical blood pressure reading – for example, the 140 in a 140/90 reading – is a more important risk factor for heart disease than the bottom number. It's the measurement of systolic blood pressure, when the heart has contracted and sent a surge of blood into circulation. Get that number down, and the other number (your diastolic blood pressure) will follow.

- **You'll probably need at least two drugs** More is often better when it comes to blood pressure medication. People with hypertension will usually need at least two different drugs to get their blood pressure under control – that is, at least back down to less than 140/90. People who have high blood pressure as well as diabetes or chronic kidney disease need to get their blood pressure all the way down to 130/80.

**A preventive approach** There are plenty of non-pharmacological measures you can take to lower your blood pressure, or prevent it from becoming too high in the first place. The British Hypertensive Society recommends:

- losing excess weight
- taking regular dynamic physical exercise. (such as a brisk 20-minute walk each day);
- increasing your daily intake of fruit and vegetables (7 portions a day)
- consuming less salt (5g maximum per day)
- limiting your alcohol intake.

Although in most cases hypertension is symptomless, in severe cases it can cause headaches, shortness of breath, dizziness and visual disturbances. Anyone who experiences any of these symptoms should see their GP immediately.

## Drug development

# New cholesterol-lowering drug can boost the action of statins

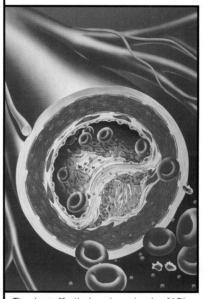

The drug effectively reduces levels of LDL cholesterol which causes arteries to narrow.

Statin drugs such as atorvastatin (Lipitor) or simvastatin (Zocor), have achieved near-wonder drug status because of their cholesterol-lowering prowess. In the UK, the number of statin prescriptions is increasing by 30 per cent each year. Even so, it is thought that as many as 60 per cent of people with statin prescriptions fail to reach their target cholesterol levels and thus remain at serious risk for heart disease and possibly a heart attack. However, a new hope has dawned with the recent approval of a drug called ezetimibe (Ezetrol).

Ezetimibe is not a statin substitute by any means. Rather, it belongs to an entirely new class of cholesterol-lowering drugs that not only reduce cholesterol on their own but also work in tandem with statins to get much better results than either drug could on its own. In studies, ezetimibe taken alone lowered 'bad' (low-density lipoprotein, or LDL) cholesterol by an average of 15 to 20 per cent.

Besides pushing down LDL levels, ezetimibe also lowers triglycerides (another dangerous blood fat) and raises levels of artery-cleansing HDL (high-density lipoprotein, the 'good' cholesterol). According to research released in 2003, the drug even appears to reduce counts of C-reactive protein, a marker for inflammation, which is now considered a significant risk factor for heart disease.

Again, all of these benefits are magnified when the drug is teamed with statins.

**How it works** The reason ezetimibe complements statins so well is that it attacks the problem from a different angle. Statins work in the liver, where they slow down the body's cholesterol-making factory by inhibiting an enzyme that stimulates cholesterol production. Ezetimibe, however, works in the intestines to prevent the absorption of cholesterol (without impairing the absorption of fat-soluble vitamins), so it's eliminated from the body before it can clog arteries.

**Availability** Ezetimibe is available on its own, and a combination tablet of ezetimibe with simvastatin is likely to be available in 2004. Talk to your doctor about it if your cholesterol levels are high even though you've been taking statin drugs.

### Game of ACAT and mouse points the way to unclogged arteries

A new discovery paves the way for a drug that could virtually eliminate atherosclerosis (hardening of the arteries). Studies in mice have pinpointed an enzyme responsible for converting the cholesterol made by the body into forms that circulate through the blood, including artery-clogging LDL (low-density lipoprotein). Mice genetically altered to lack the enzyme, called ACAT2, were found to be virtually free of athero-sclerosis. A drug that blocks ACAT2 could perhaps produce the same results in humans.

Pharmaceutical companies had already developed ACAT-inhibiting drugs but later research revealed that there are two forms of the enzyme. ACAT1 exists throughout the body, while ACAT2 is concentrated in the liver and small intestine – the areas where cholesterol is made and absorbed. That may explain why knocking out ACAT2 now seems a more promising choles-terol-lowering strategy than targeting both forms of the enzyme.

The authors of the study, who published their results in the *Proceedings of the National Academy of Sciences* in February 2003 , believe that a future drug which can target ACAT2 without disturbing ACAT1 will be a huge step forward in heart protection.

## Key discovery
# Sickle cell pain relief – only a breath away?

In the near future, children and other people with sickle cell disease may be able literally to breathe away its frequent pain attacks with an inhaler. New research carried out at Children's Hospital in Boston showed that inhaling nitric oxide, a chemical known to improve circulation, noticeably soothed youngsters' pain.

The findings point to an entirely new way to treat the devastating genetic blood disorder, as well as an alternative to morphine and other strong pain medications that are often needed. That would be a long overdue blessing for the 12,000 or more Britons, mostly of African descent, who inherit the genetic flaw that distorts red blood cells – the normally rounded cells that carry oxygen throughout the body

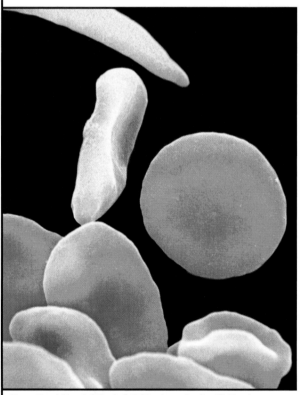

Normal red blood cells and sickle-shaped cells. Sickle shapes result from abnormal haemoglobin, the pigment in red blood cells.

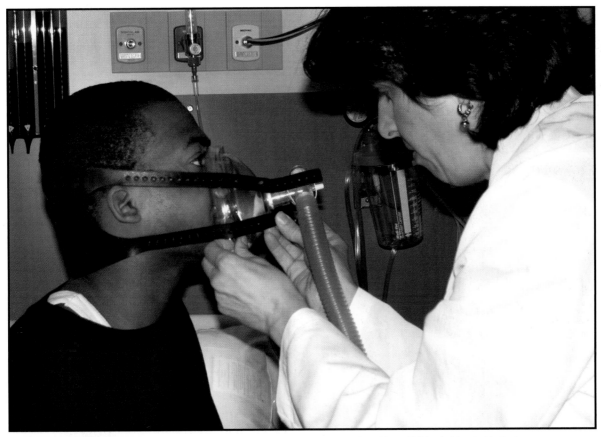

An 18-year-old patient suffering from sickle cell disease is treated with inhaled nitric oxide at Children's Hospital in Boston.

– into a sickle shape, like a quarter-moon. The jagged cells create traffic jams in the bloodstream, blocking small blood vessels, holding up oxygen delivery to tissues, and leading to organ damage over time. In the short run – as early as infancy – it can provoke 'crises', acute episodes of blood flow restriction that cause pain severe enough to send many to the hospital.

Nitric oxide promises to resolve or perhaps even prevent these crises by getting to the cause of the pain (poor blood flow) rather than merely treating the pain itself.

**How it works** Sickle cell patients are deficient in the very substance they need most: nitric oxide, a chemical that widens blood vessels and improves blood flow. That's because sickle cells are fragile and are often destroyed prematurely. When that happens, the oxygen-carrying haemoglobin proteins inside them are released to float free in the blood-stream, where they destroy any nitric oxide they encounter. Inhaling nitric oxide gas seems to raise blood levels of nitric oxide enough to widen blood vessels and clear the traffic jam. That certainly appeared to be the case at Children's Hospital, when 20 sickle cell patients aged 10 to 21 were given face masks to breathe through for four hours during a crisis episode. Half breathed nitric oxide and half breathed regular room air.

According to the results of the study, published in March 2003 in the *Journal of the American Medical Association,* those who inhaled nitric oxide reported a greater decrease in pain than the others, especially after the fourth hour of treatment.

**Availability** Although the results are encouraging, approval of nitric oxide as a treatment for sickle cell crises will require larger studies involving more patients. One such trial is being developed at King's College Hospital in London. 'But the treatment is currently expensive, costing about £500 a day', said senior lecturer Dr David Rees. Meanwhile, nitric oxide inhalation already has a positive track record. It's currently used to treat respiratory failure and pulmonary hypertension, a rare condition marked by narrowing of the blood vessels in the lungs.

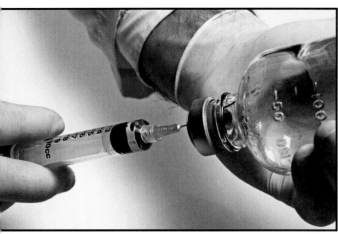
An injection of glycerine solution may be a safer, cheaper way to remove unsightly thread veins. It works by dehydrating cells.

## Key discovery
# Injections of glycerine – the solution to thread veins

Getting rid of unsightly leg veins with a simple injection has become safer, quicker and cheaper, thanks to a new glycerin solution that makes them disappear without a trace, often in just one session. Best of all, glycerine injections are relatively pain-free – unlike saline injections, which cause so much discomfort that they tend to discourage many people from seeking any treatment at all, .

The glycerine solution – essentially sugar water – has been used for many years in Europe in a formulation that incorporates chrome. But the use of glycerine on its own is more obscure. That could soon change. In June 2003, Dr Mitchel Goldman, a dermatologic surgeon from San Diego who pioneered the current formula, published results based on his own clinical experiences. After injecting

small varicose veins in one leg of each of 13 patients with glycerine and the other leg with STS (sodium tetradecyl sulfate, another superior alternative to saline), Dr Goldman found that glycerine cleared away veins more quickly and with less temporary bruising, swelling and discoloration.

**How it works** Any agent used in sclerotherapy (vein removal by injection) destroys the unwanted vein by killing the cells that form the vessel wall. It's that simple: no wall, no vein. Saline gets the job done by acting as a chemical irritant, which is one reason it's so painful ('barbaric' is the word Dr Goldman uses). STS is a detergent that works by stripping the cells of their proteins. Glycerine, on the other hand, dehydrates the cells to death. Since it's thicker than the other substances, glycerine is less likely to be drained away through the vessel and more likely to work slowly and effectively right where it's put.

According to Dr Goldman, glycerine works best for small varicose veins – thread veins – about the width of a pencil point. For problem veins up to the width of the pencil itself, STS is still the treatment of choice. By using the right agent for the right vein – and treating the entire vein 'complex' that's generating the unwanted surface veins – the job can be completed in one or two sessions instead of the multiple return visits traditionally required.

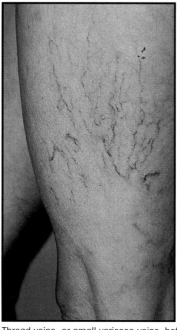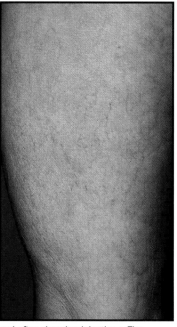
Thread veins, or small varicose veins, before and after glycerine injections. The treatment is beginning to be used in the USA and could become popular here.

**Availability** Glycerine is available to dermatologists and the treatment is beginning to gain popularity in the USA. In the UK, however, it is currently not widely available, although this could change as news of the procedure's success spreads. Thread vein treatment is considered cosmetic and is unlikely to be available on the NHS.

# ALSO in the NEWS

## Smokers' studies reveal new ways to treat early atherosclerosis

Research involving smokers, who are at increased risk for heart disease, has revealed three new ways to treat narrowing blood vessels before the problem can lead to something more serious. In two separate studies from Ireland and the USA, published in early 2003, a drug called allopurinol, a supplement called taurine and vitamin C were each shown to reverse an early stage of atherosclerosis, or hardening of the arteries. In this stage, called endothelial dysfunction, the artery walls lose so much flexibility that they can't expand to accommodate any increase in blood flow. The condition is common in – but not limited to – smokers.

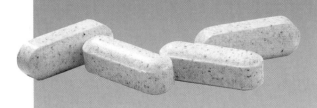

In the Irish study, smokers with this condition who were given 2g vitamin C or 1.5g taurine (an amino acid abundant in fish) for five days demonstrated measurable improvement in blood vessel function. In the US study, smokers were given one 600mg dose of allopurinol, a prescription drug that is commonly used to treat gout, then they were given a drug that stimulates artery expansion. The allopurinol clearly improved the arteries' ability to respond.

The fact that smokers were recruited as ideal models of endothelial dysfunction points to a fourth strategy for healthy arteries: don't smoke.

# Gene therapy could save patients' limbs

Early success with an experimental gene therapy may mean that people with severe circulatory problems in their legs will be able to avoid surgery – and possibly amputation – in the future.

Today, if you suffer from artery-blocking atherosclerosis in your lower body, you have much the same options as people with blocked coronary arteries: angioplasty (opening arteries by inflating tiny balloons inside them) or bypass surgery (rerouting blood around the blockage by grafting a blood vessel from elsewhere in the body). Unfortunately, not all people respond to treatment, and as many as 40 per cent of those with severely blocked vessels must eventually undergo amputation. In the future, however, some of those people may be able to keep their limbs intact, thanks to a groundbreaking new approach.

In early 2003, doctors from the Jobst Vascular Center in Toledo, Ohio, announced that they had treated atherosclerosis of the leg by stimulating the growth of new blood vessels with gene therapy. They did it by injecting 51 patients' muscles with a genetically engineered growth factor called non-viral fibroblast growth factor Type 1, or NV1FGF. The growth factor in turn instructs certain cells to create small new 'feeder' blood vessels that allow blood to flow around the blockage.

The treatment did not cause any serious side effects and patients showed signs of improvement. 'Many of the patients who were studied in the trial had ulcers on their feet that had been there for a long time,' says Dr Anthony Comerota, director of the Jobst Vascular Center. 'Many patients were in constant pain. After treatment with NV1FGF, their pain diminished, their ulcers healed, and the blood pressure in their ankles increased.' The next step: a larger, Phase II study that will compare the progress of gene therapy recipients with that of patients who get placebo (dummy) injections.

This very new and exciting field is also being researched in the UK.

# MUSCLES, BONES AND JOINTS

## MORE AND MORE ACTIVE ADULTS WITH TENDON PROBLEMS ARE SEEKING THEIR DOCTORS' HELP

Thanks to advances in the past year, orthopaedic surgeons now have three new minimally invasive ways to answer the call. One uses no more than an empty hypodermic needle to rid the tendon of pain-causing scar tissue. Another pulses low-energy shock waves through the skin to promote healing. And if surgery is required, it can now be done with gentle heat therapy through a tiny incision.

Pain is being tamed on other fronts as well. A drug called Humira eases arthritis symptoms in as little as a week. For people suffering from fibromyalgia, a compound called milnacipran has proven astonishingly effective in US studies and may be available in a few years' time. Another distressing condition, lupus, may succumb to a dramatic new treatment, which involves completely rebuilding the immune system after first destroying it down to the last cell. Drastic as it sounds, the treatment has already worked for several volunteers.

Last but not least, Forteo, the world's first bone-growing drug, promises to slash the risk of fractures for women with osteoporosis.

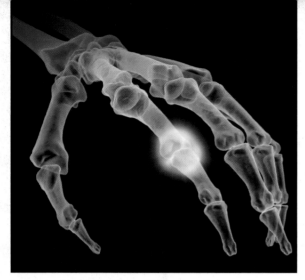

In rheumatoid arthritis, inflamed joints cause pain, swelling, and stiffness. If left untreated, severe joint damage may result.

## Drug development
# New rheumatoid arthritis drug will spare the immune system

A new rheumatoid arthritis drug that appears to be highly effective and eliminates the need to take immune-suppressing medicine with it (as happens with other similar drugs in this category) will soon be available in the UK. Adalimumab (brand name Humira) is already licensed in the United States and is likely to become available for use in the UK by early 2004.

The new drug is what is known as a 'monoclonal antibody'. Such drugs are laboratory-produced copies of antibodies. Others are already in use for rheumatoid arthritis, but because they're partially derived from mouse proteins, they are attacked by the human immune system, which means that patients who are prescribed them have to take immune-suppressing medication as well as the drugs.

With adalimumab, which is derived only from human proteins, that is not necessary. In no fewer than four major US studies, the drug worked wonders in alleviating rheumatoid arthritis symptoms and slowing the disease's progression. A significant number of patients reported pain relief after taking it for just a week.

## TOP TRENDS

### FOR AGEING BOOMERS, LIFE'S A SPRAIN

It is a laudable aim – to keep fit in middle age. But as men and women in their forties and fifties strive to stay forever young, they are often putting their bodies under enormous strain. Doctors' waiting rooms are filling up with the limping wounded, displaying joint, tendon and muscle woes emblematic of the first generation that has ever made a real effort to stay fit and active on an ageing frame.

Of all sports injuries, ankle sprain is the most common. It occurs at a rate of about one injury per 10,000 population every day. A person's chances of reinjuring a formerly sprained ligament soars each time they get out on the court or the running track – even if the original injury happened decades before.

Arthritis Research Campaign has advice for the middle-aged fitness fiends: make sure you warm up properly before taking exercise; build up slowly; and listen to your body – it's unreasonable to expect yourself to be able to do what you did when you were 20. A physiotherapist can give you strengthening exercises to do and there are various supports you can wear from elastic bandages to semi-rigid ankle supports.

### IF ONLY GIRLS WERE LIKE BOYS

Doctors have known for some time that women and girls are far more prone to a torn anterior cruciate ligament (ACL) – a serious knee injury – than men and boys are. Orthopaedic researchers are now convinced that typical 'female' movements during sports are responsible for the difference.

The main problem, they say, is that girls tend to jump in a more stiff-legged way than boys do. When they land, their knees absorb more of the shock. Girls also tend to do their cutting and shifting – the quick lateral moves which are common on the court or field – while standing more upright, which tends to put even more strain on their knees.

However, it appears that there is now a way to prevent such injuries and it involves retraining the body in the way that it reacts and moves. Recent Scandinavian research examined how introducing a neuromuscular training programme affected the incidence of ACL injuries in female team handball players over three seasons.

The women were given five, 15-minute training sessions involving balancing exercises that focused on neuromuscular control and on their planting and landing skills. The study found that the training was effective in preventing ACL injuries.

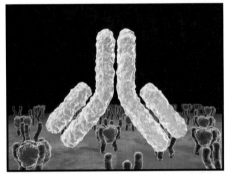

A build-up of TNF proteins (purple) in the joints causes painful swelling in rheumatoid arthritis.

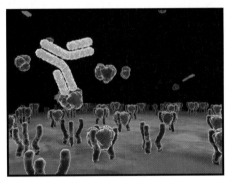

Adalimumab is a manmade antibody (yellow) that is almost identical to antibodies found in the body.

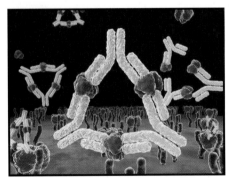

The antibody targets the troublesome proteins, blocking them by binding to them.

Because it is made only from human proteins, adalimumab doesn't provoke an immune response.

**How it works** Rheumatoid arthritis is treated differently from the more common osteoarthritis because its cause is completely different. The joint damage isn't the result of wear and tear (as with osteoarthritis) but of an immune system that runs amok, attacking the body's own tissues. Adalimumab blocks these misguided immune attacks by inhibiting a renegade protein called TNF – short for tumour necrosis factor. TNF is largely responsible for the inflammation that causes so much pain, swelling, stiffness, and even deformity in the joints of people with rheumatoid arthritis.

TNF inhibitors, including adalimumab and the older 'semi-human' monoclonal antibodies, are powerful drugs that not only reduce pain and inflammation but also slow and even halt structural damage to the joints. They are turning out to be star players among the cast of monoclonal antibodies and may some day in the future be used against other chronic inflammatory diseases.

They are also being studied as possible treatments for congestive heart failure, while adalimumab in particular is currently being evaluated as a possible treatment for juvenile rheumatoid arthritis, Crohn's disease and psoriasis.

**Availability** Adalimumab is likely to be available in the UK from early 2004. In the USA it's taken by self-administered injection every other week.

**RESEARCH ROUND-UP**

## Steroid shots safe for arthritic knees

Synthetic hormone-based drugs called steroids can provide months of pain relief when injected directly into arthritic knee joints. But even though steroids, such as prednisolone and hydrocortisone, have been in use for decades, there's always been a concern that repeated treatments could harm the joint and make the arthritis worse in the long run. Now, after conducting the first long-term study of the safety of steroid injections to relieve knee arthritis pain, Canadian researchers report that even repeated steroid injections don't appear to be harmful.

In a well-designed study of 68 women and men with severe osteoarthritis of the knee, researchers from the University of Montreal found that people injected every three months with 40mg of the steroid triamcinolone acetonide showed no more joint degradation after two years than those who received shots of salt water.

This evidence suggests that steroids may be safe in the long term for arthritis pain. The study, which was published in the February 2003 issue of *Arthritis & Rheumatism*, also confirmed that steroid shots reduce pain and stiffness and increase the range of movement of arthritic knees.

Key discovery

# Broken hips – prevention is proved better than cure

A 75-year-old woman loses her balance and falls, fracturing her hip. Her family sees to it that she gets good medical care, and after a hospital stay, she comes home. But she never regains her previous level of mobility, her health deteriorates and she dies some months later.

Sadly, this story is all too familiar – one in five people (mostly elderly) die within the first year after a hip fracture. With hip fractures accounting for 20 per cent (and rising) of all UK orthopaedic beds it is clear that a way of improving a patient's outcome needs to be found.

There has been considerable research into rehabilitation strategies including physiotherapy, quadriceps-strengthening exercises and neuromuscular stimulation and yet a Cochrane review in 2002 concluded that the available evidence is insufficient to show whether any of the techniques are actually any good.

Perhaps the answer is to avoid the hip fracture in the first place – prevention being better than a cure. In a study published in the *British Medical Journal* in January 2003, German researchers looked at the effect of encouraging residents of nursing homes to use hip protectors. They found that by using this simple measure the incidence of hip fractures was reduced by 40 per cent.

**How it works** A hip protector is a padded plastic shell worn over the hip – a bit like a shin pad. Hip protectors effectively prevent hip fractures but compliance is generally poor due to appearance and comfort. The German study focused on residents of nursing homes in Hamburg who had a high risk

of falling. The residents were divided into an intervention group (459) and a control group (483). Staff at the nursing homes were given a single session educating them in the use and benefits of hip shields and they then educated the residents.

Participants in the intervention group were each given three hip protectors. After 15 months, taking into account residents who had died or moved away, it was found that 4.6 per cent of the intervention group and 8.1 per cent of the control group had suffered hip fractures. The researchers concluded that the introduction of a structured education programme along with the provision of free hip protectors in nursing homes could increase the use of protectors and so reduce the number of hip fractures.

If more people could be persuaded to use hip protectors the benefits for an overburdened NHS are obvious – as well as for the older generation.

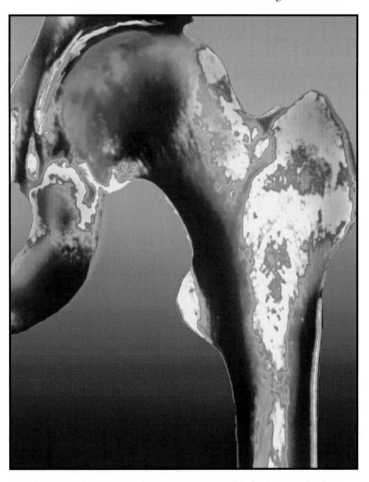

Of all fall-related fractures, hip fractures are responsible for the most deaths and significantly reduce the quality of life. To lower your risk, you can exercise to improve your balance and lower body strength, but if you are particularly vulnerable to falling, start wearing hip protectors.

Drug development

# Fibromyalgia drug shows promise

The long nightmare may be nearing an end for the million-plus Britons suffering from fibromyalgia. For years, they've endured the relentless pain, fatigue and mood-lowering effect of this chronic condition, with no approved medicines to help. As late as the 1990s, the syndrome was not even officially recognized. The pain relievers that were offered to control fibromyalgia symptoms had a distinct disadvantage: they didn't work.

Now, pharmaceutical researchers are convinced they have found a drug that does: milnacipran. According to study results announced in 2003 by American drug developer Cypress Bioscience, the drug is poised to give fibromyalgia patients back their lives. About half of 125 study participants were given milnacipran once or twice a day for 12 weeks. The others received a placebo (an ineffective substance used for comparison).

At the end of the study period, the patients were rated for their levels of pain, mood and fatigue. Those who received milnacipran showed a 'statistically significant' improvement over those given placebos. Seventy per cent reported an overall improvement in their symptoms, and 37 per cent reported that the intensity of their pain was cut at least in half. As a final survey question, all of the subjects were asked: 'How do you feel?' Seventy-five per cent of those on the drug said they felt much better than at the beginning of the study, while most of the placebo group felt the same or worse.

**How it works** Fibromyalgia pain isn't like most pain, and milnacipran doesn't work like most pain relievers. When you think of pain, you usually assume it's due

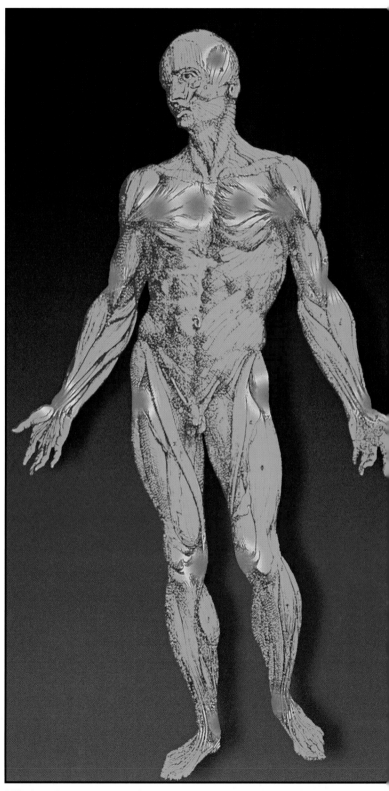

Difficult to diagnose and treat, fibromyalgia causes pain at 'tender points' in the body. A patient may be diagnosed with fibromyalgia if they have significant pain in at least 11 of 18 tender points when a doctor presses them lightly.

## Hard science took the 'mush' out of fibromyalgia

Daniel Clauw's research may lead to the first drug for fibromyalgia.

If Dr Daniel Clauw had listened to his colleagues early on in his career, he probably wouldn't now be doing cutting-edge research into fibromyalgia. He certainly would not have headed up the key study of the drug called milnacipran, which looks set to become the first ever fibromyalgia treatment available in the United States.

'As a young junior faculty member, I began to see fibromyalgia as a real problem that, like all real problems, could be understood by applying scientific principles,' says Dr Clauw, director of the University of Michigan's chronic pain and fatigue research group. 'People tried to dissuade me, though. They said it was a poor career choice – too unpredictable, too mushy.' It wasn't until just a few years ago that fibromyalgia was recognized as a disease. Previously, it was considered at best a collection of unrelated complaints and at worst a figment of overactive imaginations. Perceptions had to change before a drug could be found to treat the disease.

As Dr Clauw predicted, science itself started to turn things around. 'Research used techniques where you could see objective evidence of the pain that people were reporting,' he says. 'As these studies accumulated, there was more acceptance that there was a real problem.' Armed with a growing consensus that the disease was real, as well as evidence from Dr Clauw and others that the neurotransmitters noradrenaline and serotonin were a promising treatment focus, pharmaceutical companies such as Cypress Bioscience and Pfizer went in search of a treatment.

But they didn't look in the lab; they looked to Europe. 'Basically, they scoured the world for existing drugs that fitted the criteria they were looking for,' Dr Clauw says. 'We ended up testing milnacipran after Cypress licensed the compound from a company in France, where fibromyalgia isn't recognized as a disease. The French don't even have a word for it.'

Long-term fibromyalgia sufferers might feel a twinge of bitterness. While much of the medical community was pooh-poohing their condition, the drug that could help them was already approved and in use as an antidepressant in 20 countries. But any bitterness will surely turn to relief if milnacipran is approved in the USA in 2005 as predicted. And they'll also be grateful that Dr Clauw stuck to his guns and specialized in fibromyalgia research.

'I viewed it as an opportunity to accomplish something,' he says. 'And with milnacipran, that appears to be the case.'

to some kind of damage or inflammation in specific parts of the body. Fibromyalgia, however, is a malfunction in the way the entire nervous system processes pain. As one expert puts it: 'It's as if the volume control in the central nervous system is turned way up and stuck there.' Milnacipran adjusts the levels of key brain and nerve chemicals called neurotransmitters to turn the volume down.

Milnacipran belongs to a new class of drugs called selective serotonin and noradrenaline reuptake inhibitors, or SNRIs. If that sounds a lot like the well-known class of antidepressant drugs called SSRIs (selective serotonin reuptake inhibitors), it's no coincidence. Depression and fibromyalgia have a lot in common – their symptoms overlap, and they're both characterized by imbalances in brain chemicals. Essentially, scientists have adapted the antidepressant strategy of adjusting levels of the brain chemicals serotonin and noradrenaline. The result: a pain-relieving, mood-elevating, fatigue-fighting fibromyalgia drug.

**Availability** The drug milnacipran was discovered by French company Pierre Fabre Médicament and is currently marketed in Europe as an antidepressant. In the UK milnacipran is not licensed for any use. However, if the current American studies to confirm its effectiveness against fibromyalgia go well and the drug is shown to have acceptable levels of side effects, it could be approved for use in the US by mid-2005. Hopefully licensing of the drug in the UK will occur soon afterwards. A similar drug, pregabalin, being developed by Pfizer, has also shown good results and could be available in the USA at about the same time.

**Drug development**

# Attacking lupus by restarting the immune system

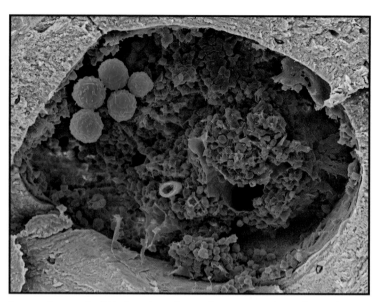

Because they survive high-dose chemotherapy, bone marrow stem cells may be the key to a new lupus treatment that involves wiping out the immune system.

The idea has to be intriguing for the one in 1,000 people in Britain who have lupus, the often painful, tissue-destroying disease that can seriously damage joints and key organs. Since lupus is an autoimmune disease, caused by a constantly malfunctioning immune system, why not simply wipe out the entire immune system and start a better one from scratch?

That seems outrageous? Maybe not. A team of researchers from Johns Hopkins Bayview Medical Center in Baltimore tried it on 14 lupus patients and reported that, nearly four years later, three of the patients had been essentially cured, two more were mostly symptom-free, and six others were controlling their disease much better than before.

> **For this study, one huge dose of the drug was used to obliterate the immune system – and hopefully the disease along with it.**

The chosen weapon of mass immune system destruction was cyclophosphamide (Cytoxan), a chemotherapy drug used to kill cancer cells. Cyclophosphamide is already used as a lupus treatment, but is administered in low doses (called 'pulses') over six months. For this study, however, one huge dose of the drug was used to obliterate the immune system – and hopefully the disease along with it.

**How it works** A person's immune system can recover from this drastic approach because stem cells, the multipurpose 'starter' cells found in bone marrow, are resistant to chemotherapy. After the chemical blast, these surviving cells immediately go to work to rebuild a new, disease-free immune system. In fact, a key feature of the study was the researchers' decision not to help the reconstruction process by removing bone marrow before the treatment and reintroducing it afterwards.

Other research using high-dose chemotherapy for lupus has used this method – removing stem cells before administering the immunosuppressant drug and then replacing them afterwards – and there is evidence to show that this method is successful.

However, some experts argue that there is a chance of reintroducing diseased cells together with the set-aside stem cells. The Johns Hopkins researchers, on the other hand, did not remove the stem cells and trusted in the cells' ability to survive on their own. It appears that their leap of faith has paid high dividends.

It's doubtful that most lupus patients will be willing to have their immune systems demolished – even temporarily – based on a study involving only 14 people. But the crash-and-reboot strategy holds out promise for a future lupus cure. It could also potentially help with other autoimmune diseases, such as rheumatoid arthritis.

**Availability** The next step will be a larger study comparing megadose chemotherapy with standard treatments in 100 lupus patients at medical centres in Philadelphia, Baltimore, and Madison, Wisconsin. The researchers began signing up volunteers in 2003 and expected to continue enrolment into 2004.

Drug development

# Bone-growing drug gets the green light

Osteoporosis, the progressive systemic skeletal disease characterized by low bone mass, results in over 200,000 fractures each year in the UK. There's no shortage of treatments for the bone-thinning condition but all of the current options are geared towards slowing bone loss rather than encouraging new bone growth. And that approach puts a limit on long-term benefits.

Things changed in November 2002, when a bone-growing drug called teriparatide (Forteo) became licensed for use in the USA. Forteo actually reverses the disease's damage by speeding up the formation of new bone tissue. One major drawback is that the drug is not available in pill form, only as an injection – a daily shot in the thigh or abdomen. Also, Forteo carries a warning from the US Food and Drug Administration (FDA) because it appeared to cause bone tumours in laboratory mice when they were given large doses of the drug over an extended period. No such problems emerged during the human trials, however. The benefits of Forteo are clear. Not only has it been shown to grow bone tissue and boost bone density better than other established drugs, it also has been shown to reduce fractures.

In 2001, a multinational study published in the *New England Journal of Medicine* showed that postmenopausal women with osteoporosis who were injected with 20mcg of Forteo a day for

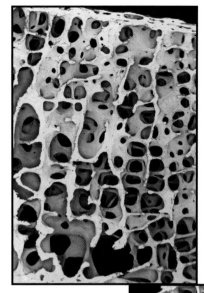

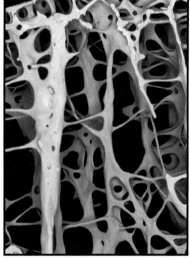

In osteoporosis, dense bone (left) becomes brittle and porous (below). It can lead to fractures, often of the hip, spine, or wrist. The new drug Forteo is the first to increase the rate of bone formation. Weight-bearing exercise (such as walking) is another way to boost bone density.

---

RESEARCH ROUND-UP

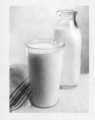

## Milk at 10, strong bones at 50

Kids who ignore the age-old parental command to 'drink your milk!' may live to regret it. New findings show that women over 50 who drank less than a glass of milk a day as girls have significantly lower bone density and twice the risk of fractures compared with those who drank a glass or more a day. It also appears there is no undoing past damage: in the study, the added risk existed no matter how much milk the women drank as adults or how much calcium they took.

Childhood and adolescence are key bone development stages that require sufficient calcium intake. Calcium supplements taken during those years help, but you have to keep taking them to sustain the benefits.

Milk, on the other hand, appears to impart bone-strengthening benefits that last well past menopause, even if you don't drink it as an adult. The study, published in the January 2003 issue of the *American Journal of Clinical Nutrition,* stops short of concluding that the more milk you drink in childhood, the more benefits you receive. But it clearly shows that drinking your milk while your bones are growing pays big dividends later – when you're trying to save them.

18 months reduced their risk of new vertebral fractures by 65 per cent. That was a much better performance than the 40 to 50 per cent (at best) reduced risk achieved with other drugs. Forteo also cut the risk of fractures elsewhere in the skeleton by more than 50 per cent.

**How it works** Your bone mass is ever changing, with bone cells constantly being destroyed and replaced. As long as the balance of old and new cells is maintained, bones remain dense and strong. With age, however, the breakdown process often outpaces new bone formation. That leads to weaker, 'airier' bones that can fracture easily. Indeed, the word *osteoporosis* means 'porous bone'.

> **Forteo stimulates bonegrowing cells known as osteoblasts.**

All osteoporosis treatments slow the pace of bone breakdown. That does improve bone density, because the new bone cells that are still being created naturally get a chance to catch up in their job of filling in the 'airy' parts. However, overall bone mass continues to shrink, which is why the strengthening effect of those drugs tends to plateau after a year or two.

Forteo works differently. It is a genetically engineered form of a human hormone called parathyroid. By mimicking the action of this hormone, the drug increases calcium levels in the blood while decreasing phosphorus levels. That combination stimulates bone-growing cells known as osteoblasts, giving people with osteoporosis a much-improved chance of avoiding fractures and posture problems.

**Availability** When Forteo was first licensed, it was approved primarily for post-menopausal women who had a high risk of fractures, but US doctors can prescribe it for anyone who has osteoporosis. The drug has already been licensed in Europe and its makers Eli Lilly hope that it will be licensed in the UK in 2004.

## The more you lift, the stronger your bones

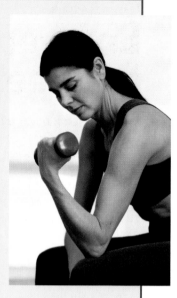

If you are a woman and have gone through the meno-pause and want to protect your bones from osteoporosis, you may have heard the advice from experts to undertake 'regular weight-bearing exercise'. Both the National Osteoporosis Society and Arthritis Research Campaign recommend it, but what sort of level of weight should you lift? Now, new US research shows that when it comes to lifting weights to fortify bones, more is definitely better.

In the study, published in the January 2003 issue of the journal *Medicine & Science in Sports & Exercise*, 140 women aged 44 to 66 performed eight different weight-training exercises three times a week. The researchers encouraged the women to use a weight load that was 70 to 80 per cent of their 'one-repetition maximum' – that is, the heaviest weight with which they could do an exercise once.

When a study subject's one-repetition maximum increased because she'd become stronger, the amount of weight she lifted for that exercise was increased accordingly. The women who made the most progress reaped the most bone-density benefits, especially in the hip area – the most troublesome fracture site for women with osteoporosis.

One note of caution: trying to find your one-repetition maximum on your own could lead to injury, fitness experts say, especially if you're an older person. Unless you're training with an expert, the surest way to make progress is to start with lighter weights and increase the weight to the point where you can just barely complete 12 repetitions.

## Key discovery
# Light up and feel the pain

Just when you thought there couldn't possibly be more harmful effects to attribute to tobacco, a team of British researchers has discovered a surprising one: smoking hurts. At least that's one interpretation of a new study led by Dr Palmer from Southampton General Hospital. The study revealed that smokers are at higher risk for muscle and joint pain than nonsmokers. Even ex-smokers among the study subjects complained more of pain than those who had never smoked, raising the possibility that there's something about tobacco smoke that causes long-term damage to muscle tissue or neurological responses.

The researchers uncovered the tobacco-pain link by surveying more than 12,900 Britons about their smoking habits as well as their experiences with lower-back, neck, arm and leg pain. After analysing the data, they found that both smokers and ex-smokers reported more overall pain than lifetime nonsmokers and were much more likely to have experienced episodes of pain severe enough to interfere with their normal activities. Most striking of all was that subjects who were still smoking were 50 per cent more likely to have experienced muscle or joint pain in the previous year than people who had never smoked. The study was published in the January 2003 issue of *Annals of Rheumatic Diseases*. Previous studies have also connected smoking to increased pain.

**How it works** The fact that there's an association of some kind between smoking and pain doesn't necessarily mean that smoking causes the pain. But there are at least two ways that it could, the researchers point out. The nicotine in tobacco could increase pain perception with its stimulant effect.

And smoking could actually damage musculo-skeletal tissue, possibly by reducing the blood supply to the tissue or interfering with the delivery of vital nutrients to muscles and joints.

The researchers went beyond previous studies on pain and tobacco by 'correcting' the data to allow for the fact that people in physically demanding blue-collar jobs are more likely to experience pain and to smoke. But it's also possible that the type of person who takes up smoking may be the same type of person who's prone to musculoskeletal pain, or that those who have more frequent pain may be more likely to take up smoking as a result. The researchers urged further study to find out if the link is coincidental. In the meantime, you have plenty of reasons not to light up.

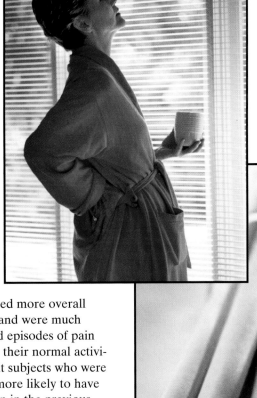

Earlier studies have shown that smokers have a much higher incidence of chronic low back pain. Now a large study indicates that smokers have more muscle and joint pain, and more pain overall.

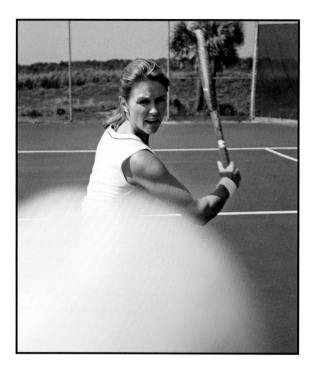

**Alternative answers**

# Serving up a new solution to tennis elbow

It happens to even the fittest of recreational sports buffs: one day they're blasting shots like Serena Williams at her best, and the next day they're watching from the sidelines because a minor tendon tear has put them in too much pain to play. If the joint injury is serious, they might consider orthopaedic surgery. But common cases of 'tennis elbow' and other tendon injuries are best taken care of by rest and patience. Patience can wear thin, though, especially if the pain refuses to go away. After several months or more of being sidelined, anyone with a chronic tendon problem is probably wishing for a treatment that's less drastic than surgery but more aggressive than doing nothing.

The answer has been found at the tip of a needle. Making use of recent advancements in ultrasound imaging, a new technique helps doctors solve tendon problems by aiming an empty hypodermic needle at them. Radiologist Dr Levon N. Nazarian and sports

medicine specialist Dr John McShane treated more than 300 people with 'ultrasound-guided needle therapy' – with good results. In January 2003, the doctors reported to the Radiological Society of North America's annual meeting in Chicago that pain was reduced and function restored in 65 per cent of those treated. What's more, because a needle probe is so much less invasive than surgery, recovery time was typically much shorter.

**How it works** Tendons attach muscle to bone. They're sinewy and elastic but prone to tears when overused or misused, especially if they belong to an older person. A typical tendon injury is tennis elbow (lateral epicondylitis), where the tendons of the elbow are inflamed. Unlike bone, injured tendons create scar tissue as they heal. That hard, dense tissue continues to cause pain as it's dragged across the bone when the muscle contracts.

Traditional treatment involves injecting a corticosteroid drug into the joint to reduce inflammation, but it's only a temporary solution. However, the new technique uses a needle point as a scraping tool to break up the scar tissue and clear the way for healthy new tendon tissue to form. That's essentially what's involved with arthroscopic surgery (which requires an incision), but in this case, it can be done with a mere needle puncture because ultrasound provides real-time imaging to help guide the doctor's needle directly to the scar tissue.

**Availability** Dr Nazarian recommends ultrasound-guided needle therapy for chronic tendon problems that don't warrant surgery but cause persistent pain. Currently, the procedure is being performed only at Thomas Jefferson University Hospital in Philadelphia, where the researchers developed it, and by a handful of doctors elsewhere who have learnt the technique. But Dr Nazarian anticipates more widespread availability as knowledge of the procedure spreads.

'It's not brain surgery,' he says. 'Any facility with somebody who knows how to handle an ultrasound machine and somebody competent to wield a needle inside a tendon can do it.'

Since the technique is based on already accepted practices – namely, ultrasound and the removal of scar issue – it needs no formal approval. But doctors usually don't rush to adopt a new procedure until it passes muster in a rigorously controlled clinical study. Dr Nazarian and Dr McShane have submitted an application for funding for just such a study, which could take place this year.

## High-tech help
# Gentler shock waves offer painless tendon treatment

For several years, professional athletes were flocking to Canada to take advantage of a nonsurgical therapy that uses low-energy shock waves to quickly heal tendon injuries. But now they can stay home and get the same results – and so can thousands of ordinary men and woman who are looking for a fast and painless way to end tendon problems such as tennis elbow, jumper's knee and chronic tendinitis.

Shock wave therapy, which has been used in Canada and Europe for years, is beginning to become more available in Britain. Its big advantage is that nothing pierces the skin – not a surgical tool, not a probe, not even a needle. Patients feel only a slight tapping sensation as shock waves are pulsed at the damaged area. With brand names, such as Sonocur, it is a much lower energy treatment than the older versions of shock wave therapy (originally used to break up kidney stones). That makes for a more patient-friendly treatment, usually consisting of three short sessions, with no need for the general anaesthesia that the painful high-energy treatment often required. The lower-energy shock waves also do a better job of healing tendons.

**How it works** Low-energy shock waves (actually high-pitched soundwaves) are directed at the damaged area at a rate of four blasts per second. 'The treatment works by the high pressure from the shock wave breaking down calcifications associated with chronic tendinitis,' says Carsten Uth, a physio-therapist working with the equipment at a clinic in Chelsea, London. 'This kick starts a healing process in the tissue and new blood vessels are created supplying the area and helping the body to heal itself. Pain caused by the injury or inflammation is also reduced (although researchers aren't sure how). As Mr Uth says, the treatment is not designed to relieve pain but to stimulate healing, which should leave healthy and strong tissue.

Mr Uth has used the equipment for about two years and finds the success rate is about 80 per cent. 'The patients I see are usually tennis players, golf players and runners. The condition often means they cannot do a sport they have been doing for years. Results are usually seen about six weeks after the last session and the majority of patients can take up their sport or other activity following the treatment.'

**Availability** The equipment is not yet widely used in physiotherapy clinics – possibly because of its expense. Shock wave therapy is available on the NHS for tendon and ligament injuries but only at a few hospitals – typically where the treatment is also used for other conditions.

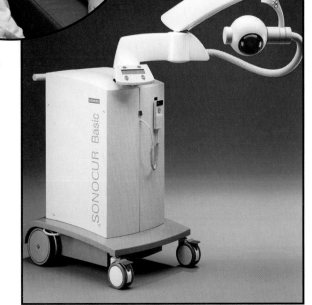

Sonocur, which heals tendon injuries with low-energy shock waves, is a painless, non-invasive alternative to surgery.

## Surgical solution
# A warm welcome for heat surgery

Inflamed or damaged tendons have become increasingly common, thanks to the active but ageing baby boom generation. And sometimes, there is just no escaping the need for surgery to take care of especially stubborn injuries. Now, a new kind of surgery available in the United States repairs tendons with a tiny 'wand' that's inserted through a small – 2.5cm (1in) – incision and heals the injury with mild heat. The whole procedure takes about 20 minutes, requires only mild sedation and gets patients back to their regular activities in a matter of days.

This is completely novel and a far cry from conventional tendon surgery. The 'open' procedure involves reaching the tendon through large incisions and scraping away diseased tissue with small spoon-like instruments.

After surgery, rehabilitation is lengthy and complications are common. Rugby players and footballers may feel that such a radical procedure is worth the trouble, but it's not the kind of thing the average victim of tennis elbow or jumper's knee would want to endure.

Almost all joint injuries are caused by overuse.

Endlessly repeated motions (such as tennis strokes) can damage tendons – the dense, fibrous attachments responsible for moving bones when the muscles generate energy. Usually, the best treatment is simply to wait for the tendon to heal itself, perhaps with the help of new noninvasive healing aids such as low-energy shock wave treatment or ultrasound-guided needle therapy.

But if the problem goes beyond painful inflammation (tendinitis) to more serious degradation of the tendon fibres, called tendinosis, it can hurt just to lift a coffee cup or walk up stairs, let alone play sports. Surgery may be needed, and that's where the new heat-based surgical method comes in.

**How it works** Dubbed Topaz by its manufacturer, ArthroCare Corporation, the new technology is a modification of existing 'ablation' methods that surgeons use when they need to burn through tissue. Because its high energy radiofrequency heat is so intense, ablation has never been an option for treating tendinitis or tendinosis.

But Topaz's controlled ablation uses a much gentler heat source that allows an orthopaedic surgeon to 'dissolve' damaged tendon tissue rather than burn it away. One therapeutic goal of the surgery is the removal of this scarred or damaged tissue, called debridement. But the heat treatment also hastens healing by promoting new blood vessel growth in the area.

**Availability** The Topaz technique became widely available in the USA in 2003 for tendon problems in the knee, shoulder, elbow, ankle and wrist. Topaz is usually recommended only for patients who haven't responded well to at least six months of other treatments and is less drastic than other surgery. But the treatment is not yet available in the UK.

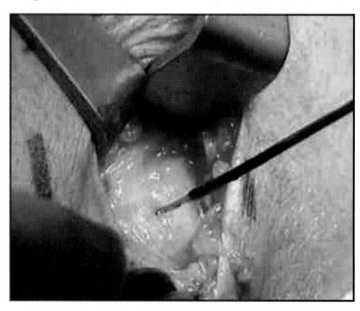

Surgery with Topaz uses a wand to dissolve damaged tendon tissue with gentle heat. It requires only a small incision, and patients recover within days.

## PATIENT PROFILE

### Life is no longer a pain in the elbow

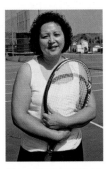

*The surgery known as Topaz allowed Silvia Dauphin to play tennis again – without pain.*

Silvia Dauphin got tennis elbow the ordinary way – by playing tennis. However, there was nothing at all ordinary about the way she finally freed herself from the consequent tendon pain that had been worsening since she was in her twenties.

At age 44, Silvia answered an advert in a San Diego newspaper and became a volunteer subject in the final testing phase of a new electrosurgery technique that heals tendons with heat. Several months after her surgery, Silvia was pain-free, and the new treatment, known as Topaz, had won US government approval.

Silvia found that advertisement at just the right time. She had gradually damaged the tendon in her right elbow as a young player, before much was known about safe grips and suitable racket weights. She had to give up tennis for most of her thirties, but she took it up again when she wanted to introduce her daughter to the sport. 'I love to play so much that I didn't really care about the pain,' Silvia says. 'I'd just suffer afterward and ice it down for hours.'

She had tried the usual tendinitis treatments – including high doses of anti-inflammatory drugs ('They just killed my stomach,' she says), pressure armbands, and a couple of cortisone shots ('They worked, but the pain came back in a few months'). Eventually, she learned that her tendon problem had advanced beyond the inflammatory stage (tendinitis) to more serious structural damage (tendinosis). Meanwhile, the pain got worse. 'It got to the point where I had to switch arms just to lift plates out of the cupboard,' she says. 'I figured I was going to live with this my whole life.'

Surgery was the only answer. What was it like to have a wand-like instrument aiming heat at the damaged tendon tissue through a small incision? Silvia can't tell you. 'They asked me to count backwards from 10, and I didn't make it to 6 before the anaesthetic took effect,' she says.

What she can tell you is that the procedure didn't take much more than 10 or 15 minutes. 'When I woke up, I looked at my right elbow and saw about an inch of sutures, but I didn't feel any pain,' she says. 'They gave me some Vioxx [an anti-inflammatory drug], but I only took the first one. I didn't need it.'

She was told to take it easy for six months, but she felt so good after four months that she began doing some light rallying on the tennis court. Later, the overhead shots and zinging serves returned to her game as well. 'I was amazed,' she says. 'I could do business as usual. I never feel my tendon at all now.'

As a result of the new procedure Silvia Dauphin traded in her pain for a little mark on her elbow. 'That scar?' she says. 'It's nothing.'

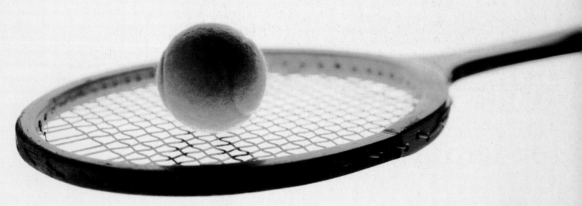

# REPRODUCTION AND SEXUALITY

## THE NEXT BIG MEDICAL STORY FROM CHINA MAY BE A NEW METHOD OF BIRTH CONTROL FOR MEN

Worldwide the race is on to find an effective new male contraceptive. Meanwhile, new birth-control techniques – including a vasectomy that involves a clip instead of a snip – have revolutionized sterilization for both sexes, and the Today Sponge offers a new alternative for women.

There is also news for couples who want a baby, from a natural extract that may boost male fertility and high-tech ways of weeding out 'weak' sperm to progesterone therapy to prevent premature births.

For women whose reproductive years are over, the bad news about hormone replacement therapy (HRT) continues. New research reveals that women receiving HRT therapies that combine oestrogen and progesterone double their risk of breast cancer. One bright spot: researchers are working harder to find new treatments for hot flushes, and a drug used to prevent epileptic seizures may help.

Finally, turn to page 220 for a look at the successors to Viagra.

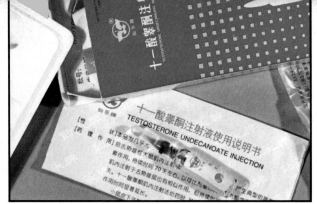

Men in China have been receiving injections of testosterone as part of a long-term study into an innovative form of contraception.

## Drug development
# Beyond the condom – a new era in male contraception

Women have had several reliable forms of birth control to choose from for more than 40 years. But men are still relying on a method that dates back to the ancient Egyptians – a device vulnerable to tearing and slippage.

That may be changing, as technology and science eventually catch up with biology. In early 2003, 1,000 men in China began to participate in a study of monthly testosterone injections as a birth control method. The World Health Organization (WHO) and the Chinese government are sponsoring the trial.

**How it works** When healthy young men are given supplements of testosterone, it shuts down production of testosterone in the testes, preventing them from making sperm, says Christine Wang, a professor at Harbor-UCLA Medical Center and Research Institute in California, and a member of the WHO committee overseeing male contraceptive research. Dr Wang comments that side effects are minimal and the infertility is temporary.

**Availability** Each participant will receive injections for two years, with the entire study expected to be completed some time in 2007. That may mean a birth control method for Chinese men, but scientists in the UK are concerned that the doses of testosterone required to suppress sperm production entirely are associated with side effects such as acne and weight gain. Current British research into male contraception is concentrated on hormonal implants and pills. There is

## TOP TRENDS

### TODAY SPONGE KILLS SPERM

A contraceptive sponge called Today is set to broaden the range of birth-control options open to women in Britain. The sponge – a small white foam cylinder impregnated with spermicide – is inserted into the vagina like a tampon.

Originally marketed in the USA more than a decade ago, the Today sponge fell victim to manufacturing problems, but production was recently revived by Allendale Pharmaceuticals, and the sponge became available in North America again in March 2003.

It will be the latest in a series of similar barrier devices, including Pharmatex and Protectaid, to be introduced in Europe since 1984. Also under development is Avert, a sponge with a much lower concentration of spermicide than its predecessors, lowering the risk of irritation.

Sponges containing spermicide became popular in the 1990s, but have since fallen out of fashion in Britain after gaining a reputation for unreliability.

### 'MORNING-AFTER' PILL GAINS WIDER ACCEPTANCE

The easy availability of Levonelle, the so-called 'morning-after' pill, which stirred up controversy among politicians and in the media appears to be gaining wider acceptance. In 2002, over 350,000 UK prescriptions for the drug were issued, with an extra 30,000 doses sold over the counter without a prescription.

If taken within 72 hours of unprotected sex, the pill – a high-dose of oral contraceptives – reduces the risk of pregnancy by 89 per cent. When the decision to make it available over the counter was announced in 2001, Conservative health spokesman Dr Liam Fox said he was 'alarmed and appalled' though the move was hailed as 'excellent' by Liberal Democrat MP Jenny Tong, a former family planning doctor.

The FPA (Family Planning Association) said: 'Emergency contraception has a vital role to play, either when contraception has failed or after unprotected intercourse.'

In the USA, since its approval in 1999, the pill has been used by an estimated 6 per cent of women and is being heralded as one reason for drops in abortion rates in some states. It has become available without a prescription in four states – New Mexico, California, Washington and Alaska – and can also now be obtained over the internet.

particular interest in an implant that is currently undergoing trials involving 120 men in Europe and the USA between the ages of 18 and 45. Developed by the Dutch company Organon, the implant uses etongestrel, a form of progesterone used to block sperm production, and could be effective for up to three years. Since it is delivered through tiny rods placed under the skin of the arm, it is impossible for men to forget to take it.

Men with the implant will need relatively low-dose testosterone injections every four to six weeks to maintain their sex drive. 'The results to date show completely reversible blockage of sperm production without major side effects,' says Dr Fred Wu, who is heading the study at Manchester Royal Infirmary. Organon hope to have the implant on the market before the end of 2005.

Why is it taking so long to develop a reliable male birth control method? The reasons are many.

- While a woman produces just one egg each month and is fertile for only a few days a month, a man produces up to 100 million sperm a day and is fertile continuously.
- Getting testosterone into the body is not easy. To date, there is no viable testosterone 'pill'. Instead, the hormone is available through less convenient patches, creams, injections and implants.
- Any male contraceptive would compete on the market with already profitable female contraceptives, limiting company incentives to develop such a product.
- Since men don't get pregnant and thus don't have quite as much incentive to prevent a pregnancy as women do, there is uncertainty about how much women could trust them to take a daily pill.

## Potential new male contraceptive identified by Oxford researchers

A drug used to treat a rare metabolic disorder known as Gaucher's disease shows unexpected potential as a male contraceptive – at least in mice.

The drug, known as NB-DNJ, works by disrupting the way the body produces fatty substances called glycosphingolipids. In people with Gaucher's, these substances accumulate in the spleen, liver, lungs, bone marrow and, in rare cases, the brain. They also play a critical role in sperm formation, as researchers from the Glycobiology Institute at Oxford University discovered while testing the drug in mice.

Specifically, NB-DNJ inhibits the action of tiny parts of the sperm called acrosomes, which help the

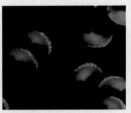 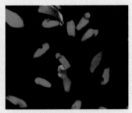

*Tiny acrosomes, essential for fertilization, are seen here on the sperm, marked in green.* *After treatment with the Gaucher's drug, these sperm have virtually no acrosomes.*

sperm to penetrate the egg's protective coating. It also interferes with the sperm's ability to make its way to the egg – its effect is like tying an anchor to an Olympic swimmer. The drug had no effect on the male sex hormone testosterone, which is necessary for

sex drive, or on the fertility of the female mice. When researchers stopped giving the drug to the male mice, the mice regained their fertility with no ill effects.

As the drug has been shown to be safe in Gaucher's patients (at doses ten times larger than those that may be required for contraception), the way is open for clinical testing, which was due to begin by the end of 2003. The findings were published in December 2002 by the US National Academy of Sciences.

### World-wide clinical trials for new drug

One of the first types of male contraception to be tested in large-scale studies could reach the market within a few years. The drug (which may be developed as an implant or injection) is a combination of testosterone and progestogen, the synthetic form of the female hormone progesterone. Progestogen not only halts egg production in women but also stops sperm production in men. Unfortunately, it significantly reduces testosterone production, too – which is why it has been combined with testosterone in the new drug.

Clinical trials will take place at hospitals and research centres around the world. They are the result of a partnership between two multinational pharmaceutical companies that have both worked for years to bring a male contraceptive to the market: NV Organon, a subsidiary of the Dutch company Akzo Nobel, and the German drug firm Schering AG.

Key discovery

# A different type of vasectomy – a clip rather than a snip

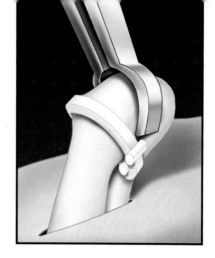

In the Vasclip procedure, a tiny clip is placed around the vas deferens, closing off the tube so that sperm can't pass through.

For all those men who have sworn never voluntarily to subject their reproductive parts to the surgeon's knife comes a new form of vasectomy that promises to be quicker, less painful – and snip-free. In fact, its creator thinks the procedure is so different from a traditional vasectomy that it began marketing the device that makes it possible – Vasclip, a tiny plastic clip about the size of a grain of rice – as an 'alternative to vasectomy' in the spring of 2003.

**How it works** In a traditional vasectomy, the vas deferens, the two tubes through which the fluid containing sperm flows on its way out of the testes, are cut or burnt (cauterized). With Vasclip, however, a clip is snapped around each of the vas deferens; the procedure resembles putting a clamp on a hose.

While a traditional vasectomy usually takes 15 to 20 minutes to carry out, the Vasclip procedure takes less than 10 minutes, says Dr David Kirby of St. Luke's Hospital in Duluth, Minnesota. 'When men are sitting there awake, they're apprehensive, and they get tense,' says Dr Kirby, who participated in clinical trials on Vasclip. 'This is much quicker. There is less tissue trauma and there is no cautery – so they don't see or smell the smoke – and since there's less dissection of the tissue, there's a much lower chance of bleeding.'

Clinical studies on 124 men found that the new procedure significantly reduced the incidence of complications, with less than 1 per cent of men who had Vasclip reporting any significant swelling, compared with up to 15 per cent of those who had the traditional vasectomy procedure. And none of the men who had the Vasclip procedure developed infections, compared with up to 6.9 per cent of those who had ordinary vasectomies.

In addition, since the Vasclip procedure causes less damage to the vas deferens, it may be easier to reverse. In the UK, about 32,000 men have vasectomies each year and around 3 per cent seek to have them reversed.

**Availability** The Vasclip company, which makes the device, introduced the procedure in the USA in 2003 and plans to export it to other countries throughout the world. It is due to be launched in Europe in early 2004.

Doctors use this device, which resembles a small stapler, to apply the Vasclip.

# ALSO in the NEWS  Fish oils equal intelligence

Fish oils could help to boost the intelligence of your unborn child. A study in the USA found that pregnant women who took 2 teaspoons of cod-liver oil daily, beginning in their 18th week of pregnancy and continuing until three months after delivery, had children who scored significantly higher on a standardized intelligence test at the age of 4 than children of mothers who took a placebo (in this case, corn oil). Cod-liver oil and other fish oils contain a class of essential fatty acids called omega-3s. The two most potent forms of omega-3s – eicosapentaenoic acid (EPA) and docosahexaenoic acid (DHA), needed for optimal brain development – are found in abundance in cold-water fish such as salmon, trout, mackerel and tuna.

## Key discovery
# Sterilization for women – no surgery required

A narrow telescope is inserted, through which a catheter, with the implant attached to its tip, is passed. The implant is placed in the fallopian tube. In the next three months, tissue grows over the implant, blocking the tube.

Essure is the first medical sterilization technique for women that does not involve surgery or an incision. It works by stimulating the formation of scar tissue to block the fallopian tubes and offers an alternative to the 43,000 women in the UK each year who undergo the well-established form of sterilization known as tubal ligation.

### PATIENT PROFILE

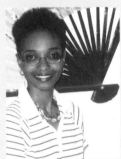

LaTia Mayer found an easy answer in Essure.

## The simplest sterilization

With a 7 year-old stepdaughter and a 7 year-old daughter of her own, LaTia Mayer had decided that her family was complete. She and her husband had no desire for more children. But LaTia's husband didn't want a vasectomy, and she wasn't keen on the idea of a tubal ligation. Then she heard a radio report about a clinical study involving Essure. Three months later, she decided to participate. Half an hour after she had entered the clinic, it was all over.

'It was great,' says LaTia, a 33 year-old receptionist. 'Quick, easy and painless.' By eleven o'clock that morning, she and her husband were back and sitting down to an early lunch. 'I'm just so glad this came along when it did,' she says. 'It was the best option.'

**How it works** Essure involves the insertion of a flexible titanium microinsert – a tiny metal implant – into each of a woman's fallopian tubes. The implants are inserted through the vagina using a hysteroscope, or narrow telescope, normally under local anaesthesia or intravenous sedation. The presence of the implants induces the formation of scar tissue that eventually blocks the fallopian tubes, preventing conception. A woman with Essure implants should use an additional form of contraception for three months after the procedure while the scar tissue forms. The procedure is also known as selective tubal occlusion.

Unlike tubal ligation and hysterectomy – the only other permanent sterilization techniques available for women – the procedure requires neither an incision nor general anesthesia. It is irreversible.

The total time taken for insertion of the implants is about half an hour, and women can usually return home 45 minutes after it has been completed and resume normal activities.

'The patient is on and off the table in 35 minutes,' says Dr David Levine, who directs the Women's Diagnostic Center at St. Luke's Hospital in St. Louis, Missouri. 'And 75 per cent of the patients we evaluated during the clinical trial didn't even need any pain relief after the procedure.'

Women who have had a previous tubal ligation that failed, and those with significant tubal disease from infection or uterine cavity scarring, are probably not good candidates for the Essure implants, says Dr Levine, a pioneer of the technique.

**Availability** Essure was introduced in the UK and Ireland in 2002 but is available in only a few areas. It has been mentioned as a possible replacement for laparoscopic tubal ligation (of which around 43,000 procedures are performed annually) and vasectomies (around 32,000 annually), but it will not become more widely available until its clinical effectiveness and cost-effectiveness have been evaluated.

# High-tech help
# Separating the boys from the girls

More than 500 birth defects, including haemophilia and X-linked mental retardation (the most common cause of inherited mental retardation), are linked to gender. In the UK and USA, such defects occur in 1 in every 1,000 live births.

Until fairly recently, would-be parents with a family history of such conditions had to choose between expensive in vitro fertilization, adoption and remaining childless; others decided simply to roll the dice and hope to avoid the one-in-four chance that they would have a child born with the sex-linked condition. Now, a technique called MicroSort, originally developed by US scientists to sort bull sperm, sorts male from female sperm, enabling couples to choose the sex of their babies before conception via artificial insemination.

In October 2002, research into the first 300 live MicroSort births was presented at the Society for Reproductive Medicine's national meeting in Seattle. Keith Blauer, medical director of MicroSort, which is based at the Genetics & IVF Institute in

Fairfax, Virginia, reported that the technique was 91 per cent successful for couples seeking girls and 73 per cent successful for those seeking boys. There was no evidence that the procedure damaged the sperm's DNA: babies that were conceived using MicroSort had the same rate of birth defects as those conceived without it.

**How it works** MicroSort relies on the fact that 'girl' sperm (those with an X chromosome) are much larger than 'boy' sperm (those carrying a Y chromosome) and contain about 2.8 per cent more DNA, explains Dr Blauer. In the procedure, a special dye is applied to sperm to highlight their DNA, then the sperm are sent through a machine called a flow cytometer, which uses a laser beam to make the DNA glow. The more DNA a sperm has, the brighter it glows and the more likely it is that it carries the X chromosome. The sperm are then sorted based on brightness, with the appropriate sperm collected for artificial insemination.

To ensure that the sample contains as much of the right sperm as possible, a small portion is evaluated using a DNA analysis called FISH (fluorescence in situ hybridization). This technique uses DNA probes that attach to either the X or Y chromosome in sperm and emit a red/pink colour for X-bearing sperm and green for Y-bearing sperm.

Parents who undergo MicroSort to avoid a sex-linked disorder have free access to the procedure, while those who simply want a child of a particular gender pay about £1500. This second option is not

## PATIENT PROFILE

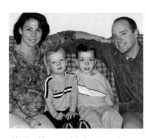

Kathy Krug, with her two boys and a girl on the way. The sex was chosen with MicroSort.

### It's a girl!

In February 2003, Kathy Krug of Virginia, USA, the mother of two sons, was thrilled to learn that she was expecting a girl. One of Kathy's sons has haemophilia, which is a bleeding disorder carried through the mother's genes and passed on to male babies only. For this pregnancy, Kathy and her husband, Cliff, chose artificial insemination using sperm selected by MicroSort.

They are very fortunate, says Kathy, because the technology exists and because it is available near them. She learnt about MicroSort via a friend who works at the Genetics & IVF Institute in the nearby town of Fairfax. Without the technique, she and her husband probably wouldn't have tried for more children, she says, even though they have always wanted a large family.

Her twin sister, Eileen, who also has a son with haemophilia, hasn't been so lucky. She has tried three times to get pregnant using MicroSort and artificial insemination with no success but hopes to break the pattern on her fourth attempt.

available in the UK, where sex selection is permitted for medical reasons only – not because one gender is preferred over the other.

All parents who have had the procedure in the USA are taking part in a government-approved trial, which will eventually include 750 participants. So far, says Dr Blauer, about 15 per cent of couples have used MicroSort to avoid genetic defects, and the rest used it for 'family balancing'.

Although the idea of choosing a child's gender is controversial, in 2001 the American Society of Reproductive Medicine endorsed the use of sorting techniques such as MicroSort for family balancing. The committee recommended the following in regard to the parents:

● They should be informed fully about the risks of failure.

● They should agree to accept fully children of the opposite sex if the gender selection fails.

● They should be counselled about having unrealistic expectations about the behaviour of children of a preferred gender.

● They should be offered an opportunity to participate in research to track and assess the safety, efficacy and demographics of preconception selection.

**Availability** In October 2002, MicroSort teamed up with the Huntington Reproductive Center of Southern California to provide a West Coast MicroSort office. Many clinics across the USA have cooperation agreements with the Genetics & IVF Institute and send frozen sperm to the institute for sorting, says Dr Blauer.

In Britain various measures are used for sex selection on medical grounds, such as screening of embryos, but these do not include preconception techniques.

# New test spotlights damaged sperm

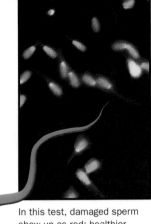

In this test, damaged sperm show up as red; healthier sperm appear green.

When a couple is infertile, many people assume that it is the woman who has a physical problem. But 30 to 40 per cent of all cases of infertility stem from a problem with the man's sperm. Even some men with what seem to be plenty of healthy, active sperm have trouble getting their partners pregnant – and, if they do succeed, miscarriage is often the result. Until recently, doctors had trouble establishing what was wrong with these men's sperm. But a new test can help.

The test, called sperm chromatin structure assay (SCSA), goes beyond simple sperm counts to look at the health of individual sperm and determine if there are any DNA abnormalities that would make conception and healthy pregnancy difficult or impossible.

**How it works** SCSA can identify a condition called sperm DNA fragmentation, explains Philip Werthman, a urologist and male infertility specialist in Los Angeles. Consider the double-helix design of DNA, resembling a twisted ladder. With DNA fragmentation, there are breaks in the rungs connecting the two sides of the ladder. This damage can prevent the sperm from fertilizing the egg. Even if the egg is fertilized, such sperm brings with it so much damaged DNA that the woman miscarries.

In the test, sperm cells are stained with a fluorescent dye and passed through a laser beam, which causes the dye to emit coloured light. Green sperm have very low levels of fragmented DNA, while red sperm have moderate to high levels. Although the egg can sometimes make some minor repairs to damaged sperm, sperm with moderate to high levels are too damaged for the egg to mend.

The test has reinforced the theory that men, like women, have a ticking reproductive clock. Using SCSA, researchers in Seattle discovered that the sperm of men older than 35 showed more DNA damage than that of younger men. For men with sperm damage that is not age-related, the good news is that, once the cause of the damage is identified – a virus, exposure to chemicals or toxins, heat, a varicose vein squeezing the testicle – the problem can often be corrected, and the sperm will return to normal.

**Availability** SCSA is awaiting approval in the USA by the Food and Drug Administration (FDA), which may be granted in 2004. Until then, the test is being used on an investigational basis. It is not yet available in the UK.

## Eggs may send out a 'siren call'

Ever since it was first discovered that there were such things as sperm and eggs, people have been trying to find out how one finds its way to the other. It turns out that

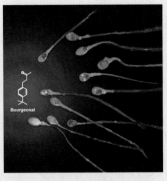

*It seems that an egg that is ready to be fertilized may emit a smell that attracts the sperm.*

sperm have a kind of 'nose' and, it is suggested, may be able to 'sniff out' the unique scent of an egg that is ready to be fertilized.

In a March 2003 issue of *Science* magazine, German and American scientists announced that they had found a protein on sperm, called hOR 17-4, that was similar to the olfactory proteins in the nose – that is, a protein designed to smell.

The idea that sperm can 'smell' is not new, but the scientists found out what the sperm respond to by searching for compounds that bind to hOR 17-4, also known as an odorant receptor. One of those compounds, called bourgeonal, made sperm swim faster and sent them swimming towards areas with high concentrations of the compound, suggesting that eggs may release bourgeonal as a sort of siren call. If that is the case, bourgeonal may one day be used to enhance fertility.

The scientists also identified a compound called undecanal that seems to block the effects of bourgeonal, suggesting a new avenue of research into contraceptives. The next step is to verify that the egg does indeed release bourgeonal or a similar compound. Those studies are now under way.

## Fertility from the forest

An extract from the bark of a pine tree that grows along the coast of south-west France may improve the health of sperm in men with fertility problems. The extract, called pycnogenol, is one of the most potent antioxidants known. Researchers in the American state of New Jersey gave 19 men with fertility problems 200mg of pycnogenol daily for three months. The patients' semen samples were examined at the beginning and end of the study. The researchers found that the antioxidant significantly improved the quality and function of sperm.

The likely reason is that pycnogenol protects sperm from the damage by oxidation that threatens all cells. The results of the study were published in the October 2002 issue of the *Journal of Reproductive Medicine*. Pycnogenol is available in the UK through specialist internet websites.

*The supplement comes from the bark of the tree.*

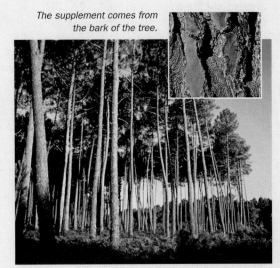

*Pycnogenol, which contains a mix of bioflavonoids (antioxidant compounds also found in fruits and vegetables), is extracted from pines growing on the coast of south-west France.*

## Rare syndrome that predisposes children to cancer may be linked to IVF

When specialists in the Netherlands noticed a higher than usual occurrence of a rare childhood cancer among children conceived using in vitro fertilization (IVF), they decided to investigate. The cancer, retinoblastoma, is a malignant tumour of the retina, the structure inside the eye that reflects light. Research revealed that the risk of retinoblastoma after IVF was 7.2 times higher than in children conceived naturally. The finding reflects a warning issued in 2003 by Cancer Research UK that a rare childhood illness is four times as common in babies born after IVF treatments. The condition, called Beckwith-Wiedmann syndrome, predisposes children to birth defects and a number of childhood cancers. It normally affects between two and five children in every 100,000.

## Drug development
# New hope despite breast cancer?

A medicine used to prevent and treat cancer may have some use as a fertility drug, according to a small study carried out at New York's Cornell University.

The anti-oestrogen drug tamoxifen, which is currently used in the treatment of breast cancer, was originally developed as a morning-after contraceptive, designed to prevent a fertilized egg from implanting in a woman's uterus if she had had unprotected sex. That initiative was a failure. The drug

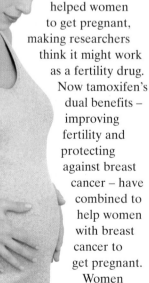

Tamoxifen, typically used to treat breast cancer, also increases egg production.

actually helped women to get pregnant, making researchers think it might work as a fertility drug. Now tamoxifen's dual benefits – improving fertility and protecting against breast cancer – have combined to help women with breast cancer to get pregnant. Women who have or have had the cancer may be left infertile by chemotherapy treatment. They cannot take traditional fertility drugs designed to increase their egg production because those drugs work by increasing the production of oestrogen, which can trigger the growth of breast cancer.

At the moment, women diagnosed with breast cancer who have in vitro fertilization (IVF) – either to freeze the resulting embryos before beginning cancer treatment or to help them become pregnant after treatment – rarely encounter success. Enter tamoxifen. Called a selective oestrogen-receptor modifier, tamoxifen belongs to a class of drugs that mimic the actions of oestrogen in the body but do not apparently have the same potentially harmful effects on breast tissue as natural oestrogen.

**How it works** 'Tamoxifen fools the brain to make it think that the ovaries are not working hard enough,' says Dr Kutluk H. Oktay of Cornell University, one of the main authors of the new study. 'As a result, the brain sends signals to the ovaries to make them work harder, which results in production of extra eggs. We wanted to hit two birds with one stone: while shielding the breast against oestrogen, which stimulates cancer cells, we can increase egg production.'

However, the research findings are dismissed by reviewers from Britain's NHS as being based on too small a sample to draw any strong conclusions about the effects of tamoxifen on the fertility of women with breast cancer. And Dr Oktay admits: 'Further research involving larger groups of patients would be necessary before the drug could be considered as a standard option for fertility treatment.'

The results were published in the January 2003 edition of the journal *Human Reproduction*.

## Key discovery

# Million Women study reveals latest HRT risk

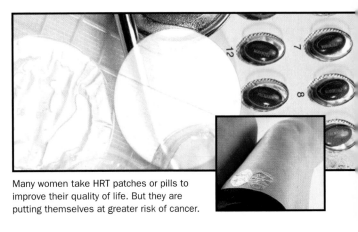

Many women take HRT patches or pills to improve their quality of life. But they are putting themselves at greater risk of cancer.

The biggest study ever conducted into the link between hormone replacement therapy (HRT) and breast cancer has concluded that women who are on a particular type of HRT are twice as likely to develop breast cancer as those who do not use it. The results, published in the medical journal *The Lancet* in August 2003, dealt another blow to the reputation of the drugs, which are used by an estimated 1.5 million women in the UK.

The Million Women study involved research into the medical histories of 1.1m British women between the ages of 50 and 64 who were free of cancer when they entered the national screening programme. It was funded by Cancer Research UK, the NHS Breast Screening Programme and the Medical Research Council.

Women who took combination oestrogen and progestogen therapies – about half of all those on HRT in the study – were found to be doubling their risk of developing breast cancer. Combination therapies are widely prescribed because oestrogen-only therapies are known to increase the incidence of cancer of the womb-lining.

But oestrogen-only therapies – taken by four out of ten HRT users in the study – increased breast cancer risk by only 30 per cent, posing a dilemma for women and their doctors.

The study also indicated for the first time that the increased breast cancer risk started after between one and two years of HRT use – challenging the belief that the increased risk developed only after long-term use. The risks grew larger the longer the HRT treatment continued.

The authors of the study calculate that during the past decade the use of HRT in the UK has resulted in an extra 20,000 cases of breast cancers in women between the ages of 50 and 64 – and that three-quarters of these cases are due to combination therapies. Rates of survival from breast cancer have improved considerably in recent years, and the researchers point out that it is too early to estimate

extra cancer deaths due to HRT. Valerie Beral, an author of the report who directs the Cancer Research UK epidemiology unit, said: 'Women need to weigh the increased risk of breast cancer by the addition of progestogen [to oestrogen] against the risk of uterine cancer. Comparing the risk is by no means simple, and women may well want to discuss options with their doctor.'

**RESEARCH ROUND-UP**

### Epilepsy drug to relieve hot flushes

Hormone replacement therapy (HRT) is one of only two treatments available in the UK for hot flushes, so – with the safety of HRT under review – researchers are seeking alternatives.

One promising candidate is gabapentin, a drug typically used to treat epilepsy, neuralgia and phantom limb pain. A study published in the US journal *Obstetrics and Gynecology* in February 2003 found that the drug significantly reduced the frequency and severity of hot flushes in menopausal women. Similar positive results occurred in a Mayo Clinic study of 24 women published in November 2002.

In the 2003 study, 59 menopausal women who had at least seven hot flushes a day were given either gabapentin or a placebo. The drug reduced hot flushes by more than half after 12 weeks of treatment, while the placebo cut them by about a third. (Hot flushes are notoriously sensitive to the placebo effect.) It should be noted that four patients in the gabapentin group withdrew from the study after experiencing dizziness, rash, heart palpitations and swelling.

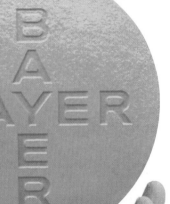

### Drug development
# Move over, Viagra

It is hard to believe that it has been five years since Viagra (sildenafil) became the butt of countless late-night television jokes and one of the biggest-ever moneymakers for drug manufacturer Pfizer.

In 2001, the year for which the most recent figures are available, more than 750,000 prescriptions for the impotence drug were written in the UK alone, at a cost to the NHS of £22 million. However, two medications are now offering Viagra some serious competition.

In February 2003, drug manufactuer Eli Lilly launched Cialis (tadalafil) in Europe, Australia and New Zealand, while GlaxoSmithKline and Bayer won European approval in March 2003 to sell their new impotence drug, Levitra (vardenafil). Analysts expected both drugs to receive US government approval by the end of 2003. They were already available from other countries via the internet some months earlier.

All three drugs are taken orally and all work by inhibiting an enzyme called PDE-5. That action relaxes smooth muscle cells in the penis, enabling more blood to flow in and out of the organ and helping to create an erection.

However, the manufacturers of the two newcomers highlight some significant differences between their products and the little blue pills. Cialis, for instance, is said to work for up to 24 hours after it has been taken, compared with Viagra and Levitra, which work for about 5 hours. While Viagra must be taken 60 minutes before intercourse, Cialis can be taken anywhere between 30 minutes and 12 hours in advance.

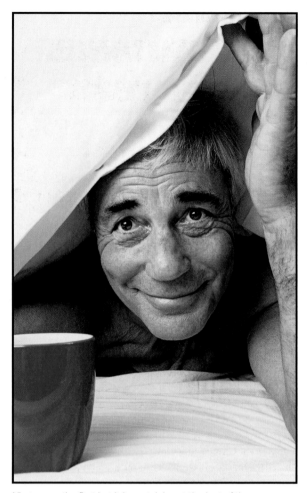

Viagra was the first but it is certainly not the last of the impotence drugs. Two new competitors are in the same drug class and target the same enzyme. More are likely to follow.

Cialis appears to be at a disadvantage when it comes to side effects, however, with participants in studies reporting headache, upset stomach, and back pain, compared with the facial flushing and headache seen in some men taking Levitra. Viagra is also known to cause flushing and headache, as well as altered or bluish vision.

The new drugs have a long way to go to beat Viagra, however. The *Wall Street Journal* calls it 'one of the drug industry's most successful products in recent years', with worldwide sales of $1.7 billion (£1 billion) in 2002. Doctors have written 120 million Viagra prescriptions since its introduction.

In Britain, all treatments for erectile dysfunction are available privately – and on the NHS provided that a patient meets defined medical criteria or is suffering severe distress as a result of impotence.

Drug development
# New warnings on HRT risks

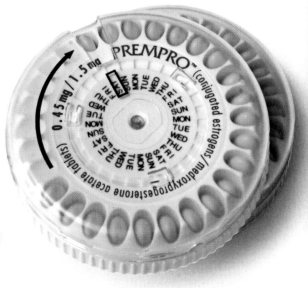

The UK's committee on safety of medicines has issued new warnings to prescribers about HRT products for use by postmenopausal women. It has also advised that patient information on all HRT products should be fully updated to reflect the results of the Million Woman study, published in August 2003 (see page 219).The study showed that women who took combination oestrogen and progestogen therapies were doubling their risk of developing breast cancer.

The US Food and Drugs Administration (FDA) has also issued a so-called 'black box' warning – the strongest step it can take to warn consumers of the potential risks from a medication, in response to the federally-funded Women's Health Initiative (WHI). In both the UK and USA, advice to prescribers has been updated to highlight the increased risk of heart disease, heart attacks, strokes and breast cancer linked to HRT, and to emphasize that oestrogen products are not approved for the prevention of heart disease.

Prescribers are also being advised to offer oestrogen products at the lowest dose and for the shortest possible duration when the benefits of alleviating severe menopausal symptoms outweigh the risks. And current HRT product information in the UK strongly encourages women to take part in the national mammography and cervical smear programmes, to be 'breast aware' and to report any unusual findings to their doctor without delay.

Until now in the USA, only Prempro, a combined oestrogen and progestogen product used by women in the WHI study carried the warning. But the FDA says that it should be assumed that all oestrogen-containing products pose similar risks unless proven otherwise. In the UK, there are 21 combined HRT products and 24 oestrogen-only preparations.

The warnings may not dissuade those who find HRT alleviates uncomfortable menopausal symptoms. However, health experts suggest that those who take it should periodically halt the treatment to see if menopausal symptoms, which reduce with age, actually return.

---

**RESEARCH ROUND-UP**

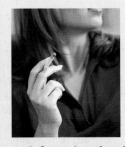

## Where there's smoke, there are hot flushes

Women who are looking for an alternative to HRT for relief from hot flushes should try stubbing out their cigarettes. A study published in February 2003 in the US journal *Obstetrics and Gynecology* found that smoking may lead to more severe or more frequent hot flushes during the menopause. In the study, current smokers were nearly twice as likely to experience moderate or severe hot flushes as women who had never smoked, and were more than twice as likely to suffer from daily hot flushes. The more the women smoked, it was shown, the more hot flushes they had.

The researchers also found a connection between obesity and hot flushes. Women with a body mass index (BMI) greater than 30, considered obese, were more likely to have frequent and severe hot flushes than women with a BMI under 25, considered a healthy weight. The BMI is a measurement that assesses weight in relation to height.

# ALSO in the NEWS

### Freezing shrinks fibroids

More than 60,000 hysterectomies take place in the UK each year, meaning that one in five of all women in the country will have a hysterectomy at some point in her life. The most common reason for a hysterectomy is fibroids – non-cancerous tumours on the inside or outside of the uterus. While the tumours can be symptomless, some women may have severe pain, bloating, pressure and bleeding.

Now, researchers in the US state of Utah have made a discovery that could do away with the need for so many operations. They found that using a device that freezes fibroids while they are still in the uterus can shrink the tumours, possibly making hysterectomy unnecessary. The device, called CryoGen Cryosurgical System, has already been approved by the US government for the treatment of abnormally heavy menstrual bleeding, which is another common reason for hysterectomy. However, the treatment is not yet available in Britain.

The procedure for fibroids, called laparoscopic cryomylysis, takes about 30 minutes and is performed in an outpatient facility. The doctor inserts a slender tube through a small incision in a woman's abdomen, then threads the probe through the tube into the tumour and releases a freezing gas.

In the study, whose results were presented at a meeting of the American College of Obstetrics

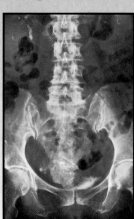

and Gynecology, 20 women with large fibroids underwent the procedure. All but one reported that their symptoms had disappeared or greatly improved in two weeks and doctors found their tumours had shrunk by an average of 57 per cent after six months.

# Smear tests set to reveal more

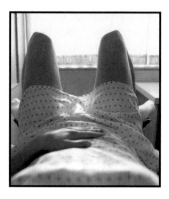

A visit to a family planning or sexual health clinic could become more revealing for women who have a certain kind of cervical smear test. Rather than simply learning whether a test has identified the presence of precancerous cells, the women will discover if they have been been infected with the virus that causes cervical cancer, called the human papillomavirus (HPV). Detection of the virus will determine whether the woman needs further tests and treatment.

The HPV test is a new partner to the cervical smear test available in the UK every three to five years to women between the ages of 20 and 64. As well as identifying HPV, the test can detect the viruses that cause chlamydia and gonorrhea.

Originally approved for use in women with abnormal smear test results, the HPV test became more generally available in the USA last year.

**How it works** As in the traditional smear, doctors take one sample of cervical and upper vaginal cells, but when they send it to the laboratory they ask for the new test to be carried out along with the old. The analysis can identify HPV, which is known to cause up to 90 per cent of cervical cancers.

The US Centers for Disease Control and Prevention estimates that between 50 and 75 per cent of sexually active adults will harbour the virus at some point. While most infected women get rid of it with no problem, some develop a persistent, symptomless infection that can eventually lead to precancerous changes in cervical cells. There is no treatment for HPV, but testing for the virus lets doctors know whether to keep a close watch for signs of cancer. If cancer does develop, the earlier it is found the better the chance of a full recovery.

If a woman tests positive for HPV, she is given another smear every 6 to 12 months. Women whose

## FALL IN CANCER DEATHS
# NHS INTRODUCES MORE TARGETED SMEAR PROGRAMME

In a bid to provide effective screening for the age group at highest risk of cervical cancer, the NHS is to roll out a more targeted smear programme over the next five years.

Until now under the NHS Cervical Screening Programme, all women aged 20 to 64 have been invited to have a cervical smear test every three to five years. Following new proposals from Cancer Research UK, all women aged 25 to 49 will be offered the test every three years; those aged 50 to 64 will be offered it every five years.

While it is acknowledged that cervical screening is not perfect, it can prevent 80 to 90 per cent of cancer cases in women who attend for regular smears. The incidence of cervical cancer in England and Wales fell by 42 per cent between 1988 and 1997 and cervical screening is now believed to save approximately 1,300 lives per year.

However, the optimal frequency of screening has been a subject of debate since the scheme was introduced.

The NHS move follows the publication in 2003 of new findings by Cancer Research UK, using data supplied by the NHS Cancer Screening Programmes.

'We are always looking for ways in which we can improve the quality of the programme and offer greater protection for women, while protecting them from over-screening,' said Julietta Patnick, the programmes' director.

The new recommendations, which reflect that the frequency of cervical screening should change according to a woman's age, are the following:

● Women under 25 years should not be screened.
● Women aged 25 to 49 should be screened every three years.
● Women aged 50 to 64 years should be screened every five years.
● Women over 65 should only be screened if they have not been screened since the age of 50.

tests are negative and who have normal smears – meaning no precancerous abnormalities were detected – do not need either test again for three years, according to American Cancer Society (ACS) guidelines. Those women have less than a 0.2 per cent risk of developing cervical cancer, while the risk for women with an abnormal smear test and a positive HPV test is 6 per cent or higher.

The likelihood that HPV will lead to precancerous cell changes is greatest in women over 30. In the UK about 3,200 women are diagnosed with cervical cancer each year; there were 927 deaths from cervical cancer in 2002.

**Availability** A pilot study is underway in the UK to evaluate the case for limited HPV testing. In the USA, the test is available to women over 30.

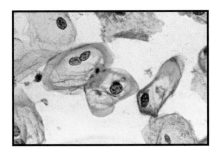

Most cases of cervical cancer are caused by the human papillomavirus, the same virus that causes genital warts.

RESEARCH ROUND-UP

## More accurate smear test adopted

After years of debate over the benefits of a more expensive method of analysing cervical smears, known as liquid based cytology (LBC), the NHS has finally decided in its favour.

The test will replace the conventional smear test which is analysed on a slide in a laboratory. For the LBC test, the cell sample is suspended in liquid and a spot of thin cells is extracted for analysis, thereby removing blood, vaginal secretions and other extraneous matter from the sample and potentially making it easier to read.

Its introduction in England, says the NHS, will:
● Reduce the number of 'inadequate' tests and hence the number of women who have to be recalled for testing.
● Reduce pressure on a skilled workforce. They will have fewer inadequate smears to look at and clearer samples to report.
● Reduce levels of anxiety...due to the quicker reporting time and a reduction in the number of women whose tests have to be taken again.

Progress in prevention

# A new solution to old problem of prematurity

Premature birth is the major cause of death in normal babies, and about 1 in 10 mothers in the UK go into premature labour. In the USA, more than 476,000 babies annually – 1 in 8 – are born too early, a 27 per cent increase on the number of premature births 20 years ago. This is the biggest problem in obstetrics, says Paul Meis, professor of obstetrics and gynaecology at Wake Forest Baptist University in North Carolina. The increase has occurred despite improvements in prenatal care and diagnosis.

While doctors have ideas about the reasons for the increase, such as the use of in vitro fertilization (IVF) techniques that result in more multiple births (often associated with prematurity), they don't know how to prevent it. But the results of a large study suggest that weekly injections of a synthetic form of the hormone progesterone may hold the key.

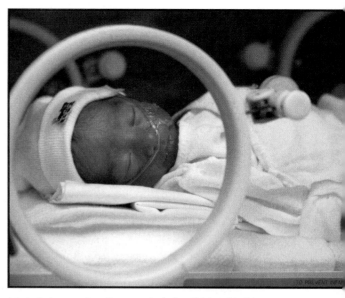

A baby born more than three weeks before its due date is considered premature. Premature babies are deprived of vital development time and may leave the uterus with organs that cannot sustain life.

## RESEARCH ROUND-UP

### Bed rest makes no difference

For decades, doctors prescribed bed rest for pregnant women at risk of delivering their babies prematurely. In fact, many women spend at least a week of their pregnancies in bed. There's just one problem: it doesn't work.

A report published in the December 2002 issue of the American journal *Obstetrics and Gynecology* finds no evidence that bed rest helps to prevent premature births. In fact, of the four trials conducted on the use of bed rest in women who were pregnant with twins, two found no benefit and two showed bed rest actually increased the chance of premature birth. The study's author, Robert L. Goldenberg, professor of obstetrics at the University of Alabama, also found no benefit from drinking plenty of fluids, using home uterine monitors, or sedation – other methods commonly prescribed to prevent premature labour.

**How it works** Progesterone plays an important role in prolonging pregnancy by relaxing the uterine muscle so that it does not start to contract, exerting anti-inflammatory effects that suppress the immune system (and prevent it from 'attacking' the foetus as a foreign object), and preventing the formation of what are called gap junctions – spaces between individual cells in the uterus that begin the cascade of events that results in labour.

In the 1960s and 1970s, some small-scale trials were carried out on the use of progesterone to prevent premature delivery, but no major studies were ever completed. 'We wanted to revisit this old treatment that seemed to have fallen out of favour,' says Dr Meis, who belongs to a research network consisting of 19 clinics operating under the auspices of the US National Institutes of Health.

The research units enrolled 459 pregnant women who had already experienced at least one premature delivery (one-third of the women had had more than one). Beginning in their 17th week of pregnancy, about two-thirds of the women received injections of a form of progesterone known as 17-alpha-hydroxyprogesterone caproate, or 17P, and the rest received a placebo.

The difference between the two groups was so significant – the rate of premature births among those who got 17P was reduced by more than one-third – that the trial was halted early so that the women in the placebo group could receive the drug. Another study that is currently in progress will test the efficacy of the drug used in combination with omega-3 fatty acids, or fish oils, deficiencies of which have been associated with premature births.

Combining the two, says Dr Meis, might reduce the rate of premature labour even further. He presented the results of the progesterone study at the annual meeting of the Society for Maternal–Fetal Medicine in February 2003.

Research into a mechanism that may influence the activity of progesterone at the time of labour is also under way at London's Imperial College.

**Availability** Although 17P has not yet been approved for use in the prevention of premature labour, doctors in the US are nevertheless free to prescribe it, notes Dr Meis, who says he is willing to administer it to patients who have already had one premature delivery and are at risk of having another: 'I think clinicians need to make their own decision as to whether or not to use it. I certainly would not say that it is the standard of care at the present time; I can only advocate its use for women with a previous preterm birth.' Likewise, some doctors in others countries have started to give progesterone in high-risk pregnancies.

# ALSO in the NEWS

## Coffee is given a break

New research appears to show that as long as a pregnant woman drinks no more than three cups of coffee a day, she is probably not increasing her risk of having a premature, very small or stillborn baby. For years, researchers have debated the issue, with some studies linking even moderate coffee consumption to low-birthweight babies or miscarriage, and others showing little effect.

In a study published in the *American Journal of Epidemiology*, researchers at Yale University evaluated 2,291 pregnant women who delivered single babies between 1996 and 2000. They tested urine samples for levels of caffeine, cotinine and creatinine (all found in coffee) and repeated the tests at intervals to track the women's coffee consumption.

When the researchers compared the results with the babies' health, they found that coffee intake did not increase the risk of low birth weight or pre-term delivery and had no effect on foetal growth. But there does seem to be a limit.

A Danish study published earlier in the *British Medical Journal* found that pregnant women who drank four to seven cups of coffee a day had an 80 per cent increased risk of stillbirth compared with women who didn't drink any, and those who drank eight or more cups had a 300 per cent increased risk.

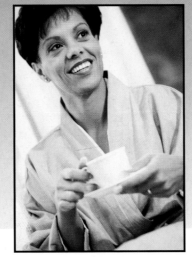

## More pregnancies for older women

At 50, many women are facing the menopause. But a few – particularly in the USA – are looking at a very different phenomenon: new motherhood, thanks to assisted reproductive techniques such as donor eggs and in vitro fertilization. And according to a study published in the *Journal of the American Medical Association*, for healthy women, there is no clear medical reason not to.

The study looked at 77 women between the ages of 50 to 63, all of whom were postmenopausal and used donated eggs. It found that the women's rates of pregnancy, multiple gestation (twins, triplets, etc.) and miscarriage were similar to those of younger women who received donated eggs. The older women, however, were reported to have a higher risk of pre-eclampsia (a serious condition of pregnancy involving high blood pressure and fluid retention) and gestational diabetes, and most of their babies were delivered by caesarean section.

The numbers of women over 50 who give birth in the USA is small but growing. According to the Center for Disease Control and Prevention, there were 239 births in the USA to women aged 50 to 54 in 2000, up from 174 in 1999. There is no comparable UK figure for women over 50 but, in ten years, births to women over 40 (16,300 in 2001) have risen by 50 per cent.

# RESPIRATORY

## FORMER US PRESIDENT JIMMY CARTER PROBABLY NEVER MET A PEANUT HE DIDN'T LIKE

But thousands of other people who are allergic to peanuts would rather chance an encounter with just about anything else. Soon they may have less to worry about, thanks to an injection of a revolutionary new allergy drug that could turn accidental ingestion of peanuts into a minor threat instead of a deadly crisis.

Talking of health threats, if you're a long-time smoker aged 50 or over, there's now a quiz you can take to find out your risk of developing lung cancer in the next 10 years if you keep smoking, and if you stop now. For people who have emphysema – usually smokers and ex-smokers – the results of a long-term US study on lung volume reduction surgery are finally out. Find out which emphysema patients are most likely to benefit from the procedure.

Also in this chapter, how eating fish in the first year may protect young children from asthma and allergic rhinitis, proof of the link between thunderstorms and asthma attacks and a good reason to avoid indoor hot tubs.

**Drug development**

# Tough nut – can new drug crack peanut allergy?

Advertisers, caterers and anyone giving a children's party these days has to be wary of peanuts in food. Life-threatening allergies are on the rise and no-one quite knows why – though numerous theories abound. A survey on the Isle of Wight showed that sensitivity to peanuts tripled among pre-school children between 1993 and 1999, If applied to the rest of the UK, this would mean that more than one in 70 children is now allergic to peanuts

Unlike an allergy to, say, milk, pet hair or pollen, a peanut allergy can be very serious. In the UK, the severe allergic reaction that some people experience after eating peanuts is responsible for at least 10 deaths a year. The only way to prevent this reaction, known as anaphylaxis, is to avoid peanuts – which is surprisingly difficult these days as everything from gravy to snacks and sweets seems to contain some kind of peanut product.

That's why news of an experimental drug for peanut allergies drew such excitement from US researchers, doctors and patients in 2003. The drug, currently dubbed TNX-901, prevented reactions in allergic patients when they ingested capsules of ground peanuts. If future studies bear out the positive results, the drug could revolutionize the treatment not only of peanut allergies but of all allergies, says Dr Hugh A. Sampson, director of the Jaffe Food Allergy Institute at Mount Sinai School of Medicine in New York. Dr Sampson was the lead researcher for a study on the drug published in the *New England Journal of Medicine* in March 2003.

**How it works** Administered by injection, the drug is what's known as a monoclonal antibody, that is a laboratory-engineered, custom-designed antibody. (Antibodies are proteins that identify and neutralize invaders, such as viruses, that the body perceives as threats.) It's nearly identical to the human antibody immunoglobulin E (IgE), which plays a starring role in allergies.

Normally present at very low levels in the body, IgE is found in larger quantities in people who have allergies. If you are allergy-prone, the first time that you're exposed to an allergen, your body begins to make large amounts of corresponding IgE anti-bodies. The antibodies then attach to the surfaces

### Baby lotions linked to peanut allergy

There are numerous theories as to why peanut allergies might be on the rise – from the idea that more women eat peanuts while pregnant to the increasing popularity of soy formulas for infants; some experts suspect that soy is a peanut allergy trigger. Now, a study from Great Britain has found that using lotions and creams that contain peanut oil can sensitize children to peanut protein, eventually resulting in peanut allergies.

There are plenty of products that do not use peanut oil, so it is probably best to read through the list of ingredients and choose one of these. The study was published in a March 2003 issue of the *New England Journal of Medicine*.

### Another excuse not to vacuum

High-end vacuum cleaners with high-efficiency particulate arrest (HEPA) filters are supposed to provide cleaner environs for people with allergies. But do they? Researchers from a hospital in Manchester tested five HEPA vacuum cleaners, along with some older, non-HEPA models, in homes with cats. Then they measured the amount of dander – scurf from the pets' coats – in the air.

Rather than clearing the air, both types of vacuums significantly increased the amount of inhaled dander. The HEPA vacuums worked better, however, in a testing chamber. It appears that vacuuming in the home increases airborne dander by pulling it from clothes, skin and other surfaces.

of cells known as mast cells, which in turn spit out chemicals, such as histamine, that are responsible for the wheezing, sneezing, runny eyes, and the itching that is associated with allergies. By binding to receptors, or 'locks', on the mast cells meant for IgE, TNX-901 prevents the real IgE from locking on. 'Basically, you've got a lot of mast cells sitting around with very little IgE,' says Dr Sampson. 'They're like guns with no triggers.'

In the study, Dr Sampson and his colleagues gave 84 patients with a history of peanut allergies a small, medium or large dose of the drug once every four weeks for four months. Two to four weeks after the final dose, the patients took a capsule containing ground peanuts. Although some participants experienced a reaction, it was quite mild. It took the equivalent of 9 peanuts to trigger a reaction instead of the half peanut it took without the drug, and five people ate the equivalent of 24 peanuts with no reaction.

That, concludes Dr Sampson, should translate into protection against most unintended consumption of peanuts. Even better: the drug should work against all allergies, all of which result from the same IgE/mast cell process. The only drawback, he says, is that people will need to continue injections every two to four weeks, possibly for the rest of their lives.

**Availability** Despite its promise, the new drug is still several years away from going to market. Phase III clinical trials in the USA became stalled in mid-2003 because the three companies that were involved in developing the drug were arguing over the rights to develop it.

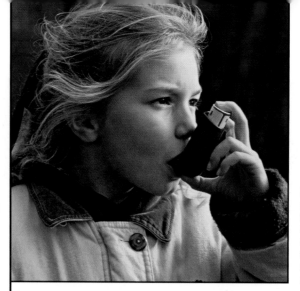

If your child has asthma even though there's no history of asthma or allergies in your family, a surprising underlying problem may be to blame.

**Key discovery**

# Acid reflux may lurk behind asthma in children

If your child has asthma that's difficult to control, another underlying condition may be to blame. Treat that condition and your child's need for asthma medication may be drastically reduced, according to the results of a recent study.

The condition is acid reflux, also known as gastro-oesophageal reflux disease (GORD), in which highly acidic stomach fluid backs up (refluxes) into the oesophagus, the long tube that connects the mouth to the stomach. Before you assume that your child doesn't have it, consider this: previous research indicates that at least half of all children who have asthma also have GORD. Asthma attacks can be triggered when a small amount of the fluid that makes its way to the oesophagus is inhaled into the lungs, or when the irritated oesophagus makes the person cough as a reflex.

In a small study reported in the April 2003 issue of the US journal *Chest*, 27 children with both asthma and evidence of GORD either took medications to treat the reflux (drugs called proton-pump inhibitors) for one year or underwent a common surgical procedure to fix it. As a result, the children's overall need for asthma medications was reduced by more than 50 per cent, and their use of inhaled corticosteroids dropped by 89 percent, says Dr Vikram Khoshoo Ph.D., lead study author and a paediatric gastroenterologist at West Jefferson Medical Center, New Orleans.

If your child has asthma as well as heartburn or a sensation of stomach acid rising into the throat, ask the doctor whether reflux could be playing a role, Dr Khoshoo suggests – especially if your family has no history of asthma or allergies, or if the asthma is becoming increasingly hard to treat.

# ALSO in the NEWS

## That potential 'kiss of death'

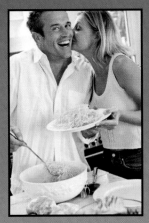

Do you have any kind of food allergy? Before you pucker up for that goodnight kiss, you'd better be sure what your darling had for dinner. An article published in the February 2003 issue of the *Mayo Clinic Proceedings* describes the case of a 20-year-old woman who went into anaphylactic shock just after kissing her boyfriend. She wasn't allergic to the young man but to the shrimp he'd eaten an hour before. 'To my knowledge, this is the first report of a life-threatening reaction to shellfish transmitted by passionate kissing,' wrote Dr David P. Steensma the Mayo Clinic doctor who treated her. So now, at least for the highly allergic, lovebirds dreaming of where a kiss might lead have another outcome (albeit unlikely) to envision – death. An ironic side note: both the young woman and her boyfriend worked at a seafood restaurant when the incident occurred. After treating her with epinephrine, doctors prescribed another remedy: quit the job.

## Can fish diet beat childhood asthma?

It has been suggested that consumption of fish and polyunsaturated fatty acids could have a protective effect against inflammation in the airways and the development of asthma and other allergic diseases.

To test this theory, researchers from the Norwegian Public Institute of Health conducted a study of 2,531 Norwegian children, charting their health from birth over a period of four years.

Within that group, 47.6 per cent had eaten fish during their first 12 months. The researchers found that the incidence of both asthma and allergic rhinitis was lower among the fish-eating infants.

'Fish consumption in the first year of life may reduce the risk of developing asthma and allergic rhinitis in childhood,' they concluded in a study published in the *Journal of Asthma* in June 2003.

## Heeding call for asthma monitoring

Mobile phones may one day replace plastic peak flow meters as the best way to monitor lung status in people with asthma. More than 5.1 million people in the UK have asthma and about half have to regularly check their lung capacities by blowing hard into a peak flow meter and tracking the results so that their doctors know if their medications should be changed. But it's hard to get people – especially children – to do it. Now a company based in Oxford has designed software that enables mobile phones to capture data from a small electronic flow meter, about the size of an asthma inhaler, that attaches to the phone. The phone reminds owners to use the flow meter twice daily, then it sends the results to a computer for analysis. If the computer detects signs of a problem, it emails the patient's doctor, who then contacts the patient. The company, E-San, was conducting trials in mid-2003.

## Thunderstorms spark asthma attacks

When there's a thunderstorm in the forecast, casualty departments expect a rush of patients with asthma attacks – a phenomenon charted in a new study. Researchers at the University of Ottawa Health Research Institute in Canada examined four years of records from a children's hospital, comparing asthma attacks with weather patterns, airborne allergens and pollution. They found that asthma-related hospital visits jumped 15 per cent during thunderstorms and suspect the increase is related to fungal spores, which almost double in number during thunderstorms. Their findings were published in the March 2003 issue of the US journal *Chest*.

Researchers at Southampton General Hospital in December 2002 compared asthma sufferers who presented with acute symptoms after a thunderstorm, with a control group of asthma sufferers. After they had examined airway inflammation in both groups, they too concluded that some asthmas can probably be sparked by a storm-induced grass pollen deluge.

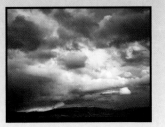

Alternative answers

# New doubts cast on echinacea

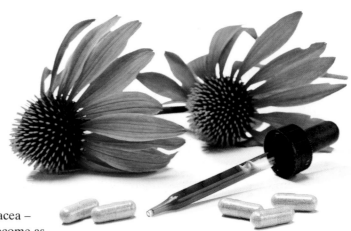

For many people, the herbal remedy echinacea – taken in capsules, teas, or tinctures – has become as much a part of the cold-and-flu arsenal as bed-rest and a hot lemon drink. But no one seems to know for sure whether it actually *works*. That's because, like many herbs, echinacea hasn't been as rigorously analysed as a pharmaceutical drug might be.

Now a careful scientific clinical trial (double-blind, placebo-controlled) on echinacea has found that it worked no better than a placebo (dummy pill) in improving cold symptoms. The results were published in the December 2002 issue of *Annals of Internal Medicine.*

Researchers at the University of Wisconsin at Madison recruited 148 students with colds. Half received capsules containing powdered echinacea; the other half received placebos. Both groups began taking the capsules soon after their cold symptoms began (in most cases, within 36 hours).

The students took four capsules six times the first day, then three times daily thereafter until their colds went away. Each day, they completed a questionnaire about their symptoms. Researchers then compared the duration and severity of 15 separate cold symptoms (dry cough, sore throat, runny nose, and so on) on each day of the study.

The result? Echinacea capsules apparently had no effect. In each of the student groups colds lasted an average of about six days.

That doesn't mean the herb is worthless, however, says lead researcher Dr Bruce P. Barrett, assistant professor of family medicine at the university. 'I'm not convinced that our trial is the final word,' he said, because so many other trials have suggested that echinacea *does* have benefits.

Part of the problem may also be that there is no standard echinacea product – a point highlighted in an article in the British magazine *Doctor* in 2001. The chemical composition of preparations currently on the market in the UK and elsewhere can differ greatly as some contain the roots, some the flowers, some the whole plant. To add to the confusion, different species and different methods of extraction are used by different manufacturers.

The article concludes: 'Although some positive evidence exists, an evidence-based approach cannot support recommending echinacea for prevention and treatment of the common cold,' and adds: 'If a patient wants to try echinacea, it must be a personal choice and any risk must be taken by the individual.'

---

**RESEARCH ROUND-UP**

### Nose spray takes the sting out of flu jab

US patients who go to their GPs for a dose of the annual flu vaccine may soon be getting it from a nasal spray rather than a needle. FluMist, the first nasal spray flu vaccine available in the USA, was approved by the Federal Drug Administration in June 2003. Children, who also receive the vaccine in the States, will undoubtedly welcome the new product.

'They leave the office happy,' says Dr Robert Belshe director of the Center for Vaccine Development at Saint Louis University and lead researcher on studies that tested the vaccine.

It is not yet approved for the under-fives, because a safety study found that children in that age range may be more likely to have wheezing after the treatment. Nor is it approved for adults aged 50 and older, because safety and effectiveness haven't been proven for that group. And because it is the first flu vaccine to use live viruses rather than inactivated ones, it's not intended for people with weakened immune systems. However, more research is planned. The spray vaccine will protect people from the same strains of flu virus each year as the injected type, Dr Belshe says.

## Surgical solution

# Less lung means a better life – for some

To identify someone with the lung-destroying disease emphysema, just look for the characteristic barrel-shaped chest. This physical oddity occurs as oxygen-starved lungs grow larger and take up more space in the chest cavity, causing the diaphragm to flatten and making it even harder for the lungs to move air in and out. Most emphysema patients go on to develop chronic obstructive pulmonary disease (COPD), which in the UK is responsible for 6 per cent of all deaths in men and 4 per cent in women. As much as 9 per cent of all sickness absences in the UK are attributed to emphysema and associated NHS costs have been estimated at more than £800 million.

In recent years, lung volume reduction surgery (LVRS), in which 20 to 30 per cent of the lung is removed has been considered of potential benefit to some patients. While not a cure, it seems to improve breathing by creating more room in the chest.

But in the past several UK trials have failed to establish a significant difference in survival rates between emphysema patients who had undertaken LVRS and those relying on conventional medical treatment. A trial currently underway, however, seems more positive about the procedure.

In its commissioning policy for the trial, the West Midlands Development and Evaluation Service says that LVRS 'appears to be effective and is likely to be cost-effective'. Due to be completed this year, the trial involves 40 patients at the Heartlands Hospital in Birmingham, the Papworth Hospital in Cambridge and the Royal Hallamshire Hospital in Sheffield.

In the USA a landmark study, published in a May 2003 issue of the *New England Journal of Medicine* and paid for by Medicare (the government insurance programme for the elderly) and other government agencies, suggests that for about 10 per cent of people with emphysema, the surgery can both extend life and improve quality of life.
**How they found out** The study, begun in 1996, enrolled 1,218 people with severe emphysema at 17 sites across the United States. Half received surgery

and half received conventional drug treatment. All were followed for about three years. The researchers studied patient survival, exercise capacity (as measured by a bicycle stress test), lung function, quality of life, shortness of breath, and illness and hospitalization rates.

After one year, the exercise capacity of 15 per cent of patients who had the surgery increased significantly, compared with 3 per cent in the drug treatment group. They also had higher scores on questionnaires designed to measure their quality of life. After two years, however, the scores for quality of life and exercise capacity returned to their pre-surgery starting point.

But a small group of patients, whose disease was limited to the upper lobes of the lungs and who were able to do little exercise prior to surgery, not only lived longer than those in other groups but also had increased lung function.

The results may help to define who might benefit from LVRS. But lung reduction surgery is just one therapy among many that can help emphysema, says Dr Barry Make, senior professor at the National Jewish Medical and Research Center in Denver, and one of the study researchers.

Given that in the USA an estimated 3 million people – most of them over 65 – suffer from emphysema, drug companies have also targeted the disease, and a plethora of new treatments is expected in the near future.

### Lung reduction surgery

In minimally invasive lung reduction surgery, a tiny video camera and surgical instruments are inserted through three to five incisions. The camera allows the surgeon to guide the instruments. Lung volume is usually reduced by 30 to 40 per cent.

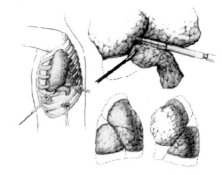

*Source: University of Pittsburgh Medical Center*

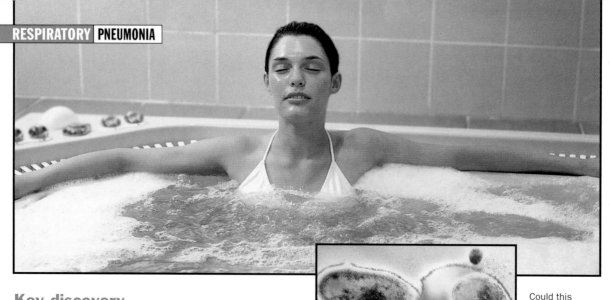

Could this lung-irritating bacterium – be lurking in your hot tub? For US tub owners with indoor tubs, the answer is 'yes'.

## Key discovery

# Bubble, bubble, hot tub trouble

Hot tub bubbles may soak away stress, but could also make you sick, say US doctors at the Mayo Clinic in Rochester, Minnesota. They reported two cases of 'hot tub lung disease' in the November 2002 issue of *Mayo Clinic Proceedings*.

The disease, a form of lung inflammation, is caused by *Mycobacterium avium* complex (MAC). It thrives in the warm, moist environment of a spa, as chlorine loses much of its disinfectant properties at temperatures higher than 29°C (84°F), says study author Otis B. Rickman D.O., a pulmonary critical care fellow at the Mayo Clinic. MAC is carried on the bubbles in hot tubs, which are the perfect size to be inhaled into the lungs, he says.

Hot tub lung disease – earlier reported at the American Thoracic Society's conference in 2000 – appears to be related to a hypersensitivity to MAC – almost like an allergy. The more patients use their indoor hot tubs, the more likely they are to develop the condition. Symptoms include fever and short-ness of breath, with X-rays showing shadows on the lung that can be confused with pneumonia.

**Clear the air** Dr Rickman is not aware of any outbreaks in outdoor tubs, probably because of the cleansing effects of sunlight on water and better ventilation outdoors.

No MAC cases have been reported in the UK. However, an Irishman died from legionnaires' disease in May 2003 after inhaling the vapour from a hot tub at a house he had merely gone to view.

# ALSO in the NEWS

## Better treatment for bronchiolitis?

Most children have had a bout of bronchiolitis, an acute viral infection of the lower respiratory tract with wheezing, runny nose, cough, fever and irritability. For years, US doctors have treated the infection with drugs such as corticosteroids and adrenalin. British GPs, however, take a more conservative approach and tend to suggest fluids and paracetamol for the fever, unless a child is very distressed and requires admission to hospital.

After evaluating 83 studies on the use of drugs for treating bronchiolitis, the US Agency for Healthcare Research and Quality (AHRQ) endorses the British approach, concluding that the drugs don't work and corticosteroids have potentially serious side effects. Researchers also found that a carefully conducted medical history and physical examination is as effective for diagnosing the disease as more expensive lab tests and chest X-rays. However, it was reported that palivizumab (Synagis), a new antiviral drug, helps to prevent the infection in children with a lung condition called bronchopulmonary dysplasia and children under six months who were born prematurely.

# New quiz can measure smokers' lung cancer risk

It is common knowledge that smoking increases your risk for lung cancer. But how much smoking? How much increased risk? Until recently, doctors had no idea. Now they do. Using data from a large study conducted with 18,172 former smokers, US researchers from Memorial Sloan-Kettering Cancer Center in New York City and the Fred Hutchinson Cancer Research Center in Seattle came up with a formula that accurately predicts a person's risk of developing lung cancer. The formula is based on age, sex, smoking history and any exposure to asbestos. The results were published in a March 2003 issue of the *Journal of the National Cancer Institute.*

The researchers calculated that a 51 year-old woman (one of the study subjects) who smoked a pack a day for 28 years and stopped smoking nine years earlier had less than a 1 per cent risk of developing lung cancer in the next 10 years, assuming she didn't start smoking again. Any female of a similar age who had never smoked would have a 0.07 per cent risk.

Another study subject, a 68 year-old man who currently smoked and had smoked two packs a day for 50 years, was estimated to have 15 to 20 times the risk of someone like the female ex-smoker, with an 11 per cent risk of lung cancer if he quit smoking immediately and a 15 per cent risk if he continued to smoke at his current level.

Lead researcher Dr Peter Bach, of Memorial Sloan-Kettering, sees two main ways in which this information can be used by the public and by researchers. First, it will provide a better screening tool for clinical trials designed to test ways to prevent lung cancer in smokers.

'Researchers want to select study participants who are at very high risk of getting the disease,' says Dr Bach. Until now, they have had no way of identifying who those people were, 'so everyone was really flying blind.' In the past, for instance, no one knew if it mattered if the person had smoked for 20 years or for 30 years. 'Now we're able to show that it matters,' he says.

The quiz will also be useful for helping people and their doctors decide if they should undergo a screening test called spiral CT, which can identify some lung cancers at a very early stage, as it will enable doctors to identify those with the highest risk of lung cancer – the best candidates for the test.

Designed for people who are 50 to 75 years old and have smoked for 25 to 55 years, the lung cancer prediction quiz is available online at: http://jncicancerspectrum.oupjournals.org/cgi/content/full/jnci;95/6/470/DC1.

In the UK, a spokesman for Action on Smoking and Health (ASH) said the test could be very useful because: 'Risk is a difficult concept to communicate. People understand that smoking is harmful but many smokers fail to take on board that the risks apply to them.

' If this test is successful at communicating personal risk, it could be very valuable.'

## What's your risk?

Here are sample quiz results, showing the lung cancer risk for five people with different smoking histories.

| PERSONAL PROFILE | LUNG CANCER RISK PERCENTILE | | | | |
| | 5th | 25th | 50th | 75th | 95th |
| --- | --- | --- | --- | --- | --- |
| Age | 51 | 54 | 58 | 56 | 88 |
| Average number of cigarettes smoked per day | 20 | 20 | 25 | 40 | 40 |
| Years smoked | 28 | 35 | 40 | 44 | 50 |
| Years since quitting | 9 | 0 | 3 | 0 | 0 |
| Asbestos exposure | NO | NO | NO | NO | NO |
| 10 year risk if no further smoking (%) | 0.08 | 1.50 | 4.10 | 5.60 | 10.80 |
| 10 year risk if continued smoking | NA | 2.80 | NA | 8.40 | 14.90 |

*Source: Journal of the National Cancer Institute.*

# SKIN, HAIR AND NAILS

## WHEN IS A ROLL OF DUCT TAPE MORE THAN A ROLL OF A DUCT TAPE?

When it's a remedy for warts. A US study at an army medical centre in Washington found that giving warts the sticky treatment usually gets rid of them within a month.

Once you have dealt with your wart, how about tackling that acne? New research has shown that laser light therapy can offer a quick, painless, and lasting solution to the condition that distresses so many teenagers. If you're an older adult battling the face-reddening disorder rosacea, a new gel derived from wheat can stop you from seeing red when you look in the mirror.

Finally, an injectable drug represents a brand-new, gentler treatment approach to the maddening skin condition known as psoriasis.

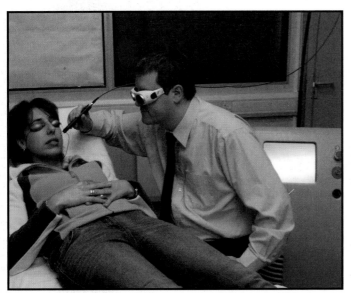

Laser cure for teenage curse: N-Lite uses a laser light beam to kill *P. acnes*, the bacterium that causes acne, without harming the skin.

## High-tech help
# Laser treatment clears up acne

Acne affects about 90 per cent of teenagers in the UK and as many as one in 20 adults. While the creams, ointments and oral antibiotics currently available help some people, many find them ineffective and the drugs are not without their side effects. The success of the acne 'wonder drug' Isotretinoin (Roaccutane), for example, has been clouded by claims that it can lead to depresssion and even, in some cases, suicide.

But a new treatment has recently been developed that dermatologists hope may herald the beginning of a new era in acne control. The N-Lite laser, pioneered at the University of Wales, Swansea, produced a 50 per cent improvement among those taking part in NHS trials in January 2003 and it completely cleared the acne in 10 people. Researchers at the London Hammersmith Hospital tested the drug on 41 volunteers who had all failed to respond to conventional acne treatments. They were given a five-minute session with N-Lite and monitored for three months. Results showed that 81 per cent saw a significant improvement and, in 58 per cent of tests, acne was reduced by 50 per cent. Consultant dermatologist Dr Tony Chu, who ran the trials, said, 'This really is the first major advance in acne treatment in 30 years.'

**How it works** Acne is caused by bacteria. When tiny sebaceous glands near the skin's surface start overproducing an oily substance called sebum, skin pores become blocked,

## TOP TRENDS
### BOTOX FANS PARTY ON

Ever since the spring of 2002, when the US Food and Drug Administration (FDA) approved facial injections of botulinum toxin type A to smooth out crow's feet and wrinkles, sales of the drug have soared in the USA, and Botox parties have become all the rage. Although not licensed for cosmetic use in the UK, Botox can be used by doctors but they must accept personal responsibility for any ill-effects.

Botox is injected into the skin and it works by temporarily paralysing the muscles. The results are evident three to seven days after treatment and they last for three or four months. The FDA have warned, however, that more than 4 in 10 people suffer side effects, such as drooping eyelids, although most are minor and temporary. Dr Peter Misra from the National Hospital of Neurology and Neurosurgery also cautions: 'In this atmosphere of "Botox parties" – where champagne-sipping socialites are infected with botulinum toxin – it is easy to forget that it is a potent neurotoxin and that its very long-term effects are still unknown.'

Meanwhile, potential uses for Botox are growing. An article in the *Archives of Dermatology* in January 2003 reported that injecting Botox into armpits reduces body odour. Other research points to potential benefits for chronic back pain, migraines and urinary incontinence.

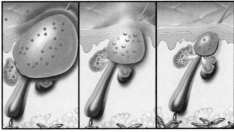

**BEFORE**  **DURING**  **AFTER**

ClearLight, a light therapy approved in late 2002 in the United States and available at private clinics in the UK, can reduce acne by about 70 per cent. A band of high-intensity light triggers the proliferation of natural substances that attack and destroy the acne bacteria. Full-face treatments take about 15 minutes.

and the bacteria multiply in the accumulated sebum. Laser light attacks the acne bacteria and also boosts the skin's natural healing process. Treatment is painless, with no reported side effects and a single treatment, costing £300, lasts for three months.

**Availability** N-Lite is currently used to treat psoriasis in the UK although some private clinics are using it in the treatment of acne. But Dr Chu admits that more tests are needed. In the USA another light therapy treatment called ClearLight was approved in late 2002 by the Food and Drugs Administration. This treatment, available at some private dermatology clinics in the UK, uses high-intensity blue (rather than skin-damaging ultraviolet) light to kill bacteria. An NHS trial at the Royal Gwent Hospital in 2001 showed that eight 10-minute sessions could banish 70 per cent of spots.

# ALSO in the NEWS

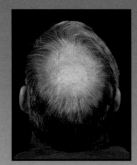

### A 'cultured' cure for baldness?

When researchers in Israel tested a new technique for healing wounds a few years ago, they discovered that it also appeared to aid hair regrowth in people who had sustained head injuries. Now, the same researchers are convinced that a rub-on gel made from cell culture medium – the substance in which skin cells are grown in the laboratory – will provide a better hair-growing treatment than other formulas. Study results published in February 2003 in the *Dermatology Online Journal* boost their theory.

The researchers tested a cell culture medium supplemented with three hormones (insulin, thyroxin, and growth hormone) on half of a group of 48 balding men, who applied the gel daily. After six months, their average hair count had increased by 17.1 per cent. The rate of hair loss also slowed, and existing hair grew faster. The authors of the study believe that the cell culture medium works by delivering nutrients (including amino acids) to the hair follicles.

# LIGHT THERAPIES TACKLE
# SCARS AND STRETCH MARKS

Acne scars and stretch marks are skin flaws that we have to live with – or do we? If you're determined to get rid of them, light therapy may help.

Both N-Lite and Smoothbeam – a very similar treatment approved by the US Food and Drug Administration in late 2000 – use lasers to penetrate the skin and stimulate new growth of collagen (the fibrous protein that builds healthy new skin) in the scarred area. Clinical trials of N-Lite have shown an average reduction in acne scar depth by nearly 50 per cent with a single treatment. Some private clinics in the UK offer N-Lite treatment for acne scarring.

Another light-emitting device, ReLume, takes a different tack. A lot of long-term acne scarring and the majority of stretch marks that are at least two years old are examples of what dermatologists call hypopigmented skin – areas that appear lighter against natural skin colour because of decreased pigmentation. By aiming controlled doses of ultraviolet-B (UVB) light at the scarred area, ReLume stimulates production of melanin, the substance responsible for skin colour. After the treatment, the area more closely resembles the colour and texture of the surrounding skin.

The results are often visible after the first few weeks of twice-weekly treatments. The full regimen typically lasts seven weeks. The effects aren't permanent, though, so monthly sessions are necessary. ReLume is currently being marketed in the UK and is likely to be available at private dermatology clinics soon.

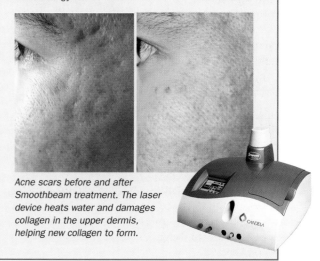

*Acne scars before and after Smoothbeam treatment. The laser device heats water and damages collagen in the upper dermis, helping new collagen to form.*

## Drug development

# Smart new psoriasis jab aims only for troublemakers

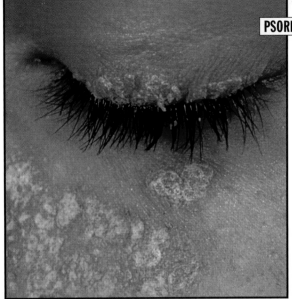

Psoriasis is an itchy, burning skin condition marked by red, scaly patches, which affects around one in 50 people in the UK. Although there are various ointments, ultraviolet light therapies and drugs available that may help to relieve the condition, these are not always completely effective and some can suppress the immune system.

But now those with moderate to severe psoriasis may find relief in a new injectable psoriasis drug called alefacept (Amevive), which hit the US market in February 2003. Known as a 'biologic' drug, alefacept is the vanguard of a whole new treatment approach for psoriasis. It was created by Biogen, a biotechnology company in Massachusetts, who work with proteins from living cells instead of the synthetic chemicals used by pharmaceutical companies. Since biologics are more at home in the body, they're better able than traditional drugs to target the problem cells and leave the rest of the body alone.

That difference translates into two huge advantages for people with psoriasis. For one thing, alefacept is safer, since its immune-suppressing action is much more narrowly focused than that of existing drugs, which sometimes affect the entire immune system. What's most exciting, though, is how well its finely tuned action works.

In the studies leading up to its approval by the Food and Drug Administration, between 40 and 56 per cent of the volunteers who received alefacept instead of a placebo saw their psoriasis symptoms cut by half within two to three months. Those who stayed on the medication longer, completing two 12-week courses of weekly injections instead of just one, did even better, with 75 per cent of them experiencing at least a 50 per cent improvement in symptoms. What's more, the benefits lasted seven months or longer after the last shot of the second course.

**How it works** Psoriasis, like rheumatoid arthritis, is caused by a misguided immune system attack. In this case, specialized white blood cells called T cells become overactive. They travel to the skin and cause its cells to reproduce at 10 times the normal rate, causing itching, scaling, and other symptoms. Alefacept's mission is to keep the T cells in line and 'punish' any that do step out of line. Like a schoolteacher who knows that some kids are more likely to misbehave in the presence of certain others, alefacept works by blocking receptors on T cells to prevent contact with other 'activating' cells that would start the skin-damaging process. At the same time, it helps other special cells identify and eliminate already overactivated T cells.

**Availability** Alefacept is recommended for people with moderate to severe psoriasis, not for those with mild cases. Because alefacept is a protein, it would be digested and rendered useless if taken orally, so 12 weekly injections into a vein or muscle are required. Further research is needed, however, into the long-term effects of using this drug.

Studies have also been conducted on alefacept in the UK but the Committee for Proprietary Medicinal Products has demanded further research into the drug before European approval is granted. Therefore it is likely to be a few years still until alefacept is available in the UK.

But this is just the beginning of the revolution. A number of new biologics are performing well in clinical testing, and ongoing studies being carried out on the rheumatoid arthritis drug infliximab (Remicade) have revealed that this drug may also provide effective treatment of moderate to severe cases of psoriasis.

## Drug development
# An antidote for the red flush

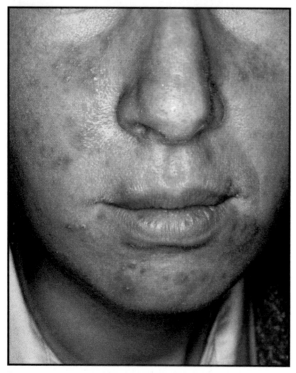

Rosacea occurs most often in fair-skinned people aged 30 to 50. The skin becomes red and may develop acne-like pimples.

Those suffering from the face-reddening skin condition known as rosacea have a new ally in their struggle to keep their skin clear. A gel known as azelaic acid (Finacea), a natural substance derived from wheat, was approved in March 2003 by the US Food and Drug Administration as a rosacea treatment. Water-based and free of fragrance and alcohol, it works at least as well as (and perhaps better than) metronidazole, the existing topical medication.

About one per cent of people in the UK suffer from this skin condition. The disorder usually begins as occasional blushing and flushing, and for the lucky ones, it stays that way. But the redness tends to become more persistent over time. Worse still, papules and pustules (pimply facial protrusions) often appear. In its most serious form, rosacea can cause a bulbous red nose, a condition known as rhinophyma.

**How it works** Dermatologists aren't sure how azelaic acid reduces rosacea symptoms – although this is hardly surprising since they're not sure what causes the condition in the first place. The problem could be inflammatory (the result of an over-blown immune response), infectious (caused by multiplying microorganisms), hormonal (the flushing episodes mimic those of menopausal women, who are at increased risk for rosacea), and/or vascular (that is, caused by a blood flow problem; people with rosacea are two to three times more likely to have migraine headaches, which are vascular in nature). Its antibacterial properties, along with its anti-inflammatory action, may also help it fight rosacea.

Results from a study presented to the American Academy of Dermatology in March 2003 confirmed that twice-daily applications will get the red out. In the UK, azelaic acid is currently used in a slightly different formulation as an acne treatment (under the brand name Skinoren). Approval for Finacea in the UK is expected in 2004 and the product has already been launched in Germany and Finland.

# ALSO in the NEWS

## A well-rounded answer to the painful problem of ingrown toenails

Ingrown toenails are painful and unfortunately very common. A bad cut, the wrong shoes, or a crushing mishap can embed one or both sides of the nail in the soft skin, where it will keep growing if it's not treated. However, help is at hand in the form of a new over-the-counter sodium sulphide gel, which was approved in October 2002 by the US Food and Drug Administration (FDA).

The treatment comes complete with an application ring that you slip over your toe, positioning the small gel-dispensing opening right where the nail is ingrown. A specially formed bandage strip holds the ring in place. The nail-softening action of the gel relieves pain and causes the nail to lift out in about a week. Following the FDA ruling, drug manufacturer Schering-Plough was expected to put a sodium sulphide ingrown toenail medication (complete with a ring applicator) on the US market sometime in 2003. Sufferers will hope that an application for a European or UK licence will follow.

## Alternative answers
# A sticky new cure for warts

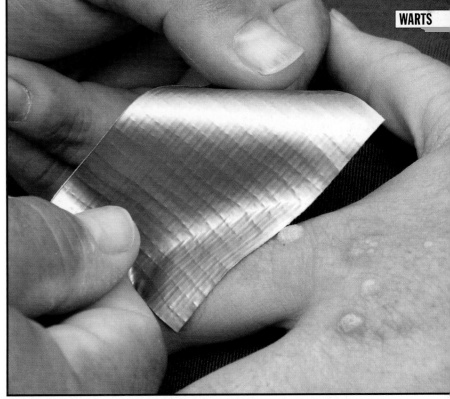

It's not just a garage staple anymore: new research has revealed that duct tape wrapped around warts seems to stimulate the body to fight the infection underneath.

Duct tape, also known as gaffer tape, is the favourite aid of electricians, plumbers and handymen because of its amazing versatility – it can be used for just about anything, from neatly bundling cables together to patching a hole in an old leather sofa. But now it appears duct tape has a medical use as well – for curing warts.

Don't laugh. A serious study led by investigators at an army medical centre found that sticking duct tape on the unsightly growths will usually get rid of them within a month or two. In fact, based on the research, duct tape looks like the treatment of choice for warts – faster, surer, safer, cheaper, and easier than traditional methods.

Although it may seem unlikely, the whimsical, nonthreatening nature of using a piece of sticky silver tape as a medical treatment is a strong point in duct tape's favour. Many wart sufferers are children under 16, who find it difficult to stick to a course of treatment. And who can blame them? Cryotherapy, the most common method of wart removal, requires repeated applications of liquid nitrogen to freeze the warts. The treatment, which can cause an uncomfortable burning sensation, is an intimidating experience for many kids. By comparison, using the tape patches can be lots of fun for children – which is why the researchers think they will be more likely to follow through the duct tape treatment.

Most important, though, is that duct tape may actually work better than cryotherapy. The researchers gathered 51 young people (ages 3 to 22) with warts in Tacoma, Washington. While 25 of them underwent cryotherapy every two to three weeks, the rest were sent home with free duct tape and instructions for using it. After two months, the duct-tape team had scored a clear victory. According to results published in the October 2002 issue of *Archives of Pediatrics & Adolescent Medicine*, the warts completely disappeared in 23 of the 26 subjects who used tape, most of them within a month. Only 15 of the 25 who received cryotherapy saw their warts vanish.

**How it works** To use duct tape as they did in the study, cut a piece that will just cover the wart. Stick it on and leave it there for six days. When you take the tape off, soak the area in water for a few minutes, then use an emery board or pumice stone to file away whatever dead skin has accumulated. Leave the wart uncovered overnight and apply a new patch in the morning. Repeat the procedure until you're wart-free.

What is it about duct tape that cures warts? Researchers suspect that the secret lies in covering the skin. Those hard, bumpy growths that we call warts are actually symptoms of a common viral infection, and it's likely that the skin irritation caused by the tape rallies your immune system to fight off the virus once and for all. No more infection, no more warts.

Before treating a child's warts, consult a paediatrician. And if a wart doesn't clear up within two months, try a different therapy.

# URINARY TRACT

## A WRINKLE CURE MAY BE THE ANSWER TO EMBARRASSING LEAKS

Doctors have started injecting the wrinkle cure Botox into the muscles around the urethra to treat incontinence. If an overactive bladder is your problem, a new skin patch may soon be able to help; already available in the USA, it has all the benefits of oral drugs without the dry mouth and constipation. That means fewer frantic dashes to the bathroom. And, speaking of the bathroom, men who are suffering from urinary problems brought on by an enlarged prostate may now find relief from the impotence drug Viagra.

For the thousands of people who suffer from kidney disease and are hoping to avoid complete kidney failure, there is tantalizing new evidence that the cholesterol-lowering drugs known as statins can slow down the progress of the disease. Finally, find out what you should be eating and drinking to stave off dreaded urinary tract infections.

**Drug development**

# Botox can help bladder control

Botox (botulinum toxin type A) – renowned for its ability to banish facial wrinkles – is being hailed as a possible treatment for urinary incontinence.

A purified protein derived from the bacterium *Clostridium botulinum*, administered by a few tiny injections, Botox blocks the nerve impulses that trigger muscle contractions. It was first used in the early 1980s to treat muscle disorders such as eye ticks. In cosmetic applications, it paralyses the muscles of the face that are used in frowning and raising the eyebrows. When these muscles relax, the fine lines and wrinkles smooth out.

In March 2003, scientists in Taiwan published the results of a successful test of Botox for the bladder. The study involved just 20 subjects, but each had serious incontinence problems brought on by an underactive muscle in the bladder wall. This muscle, called the detrusor muscle, is meant to contract to expel urine when the time is right. The researchers used Botox to paralyse another muscle group in the urinary tract (the sphincter muscles in and around the urethra). The aim was to equalize the pressure along the urinary tract and thereby re-establish normal excretion of urine. The strategy worked. There was marked improvement in bladder control in 18 of the patients within two weeks. Some were even able to remove catheters inserted to control urine flow. The study complemented research by the University of Pittsburgh a year earlier that explored the use of Botox for incontinent patients with overactive detrusor muscles. The symptoms caused by either an overactive or underactive detrusor are often the same – leakage, an urgent need to urinate and frequent visits to the bathroom at night. The Pittsburgh researchers injected Botox into the overactive detrusor muscle rather than the urethral sphincters.

Botox is not yet licensed for this treatment in the UK, but specialists are using it to treat incontinence and say that it remains effective for 9-12 months.

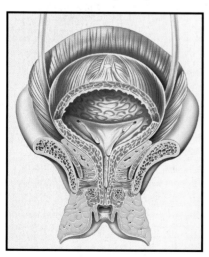

By paralysing the sphincter muscles around the urethra (the tube through which urine exits the body), Botox improves bladder control in people with serious incontinence.

**RESEARCH ROUND-UP**

## HRT may lead to leaks

As well as running an increased risk of breast cancer (see page 219), women who are taking hormone replacement therapy (HRT) now have something else to consider – bladder control. Research results released in April 2003 show that older women who take the hormones oestrogen and progestogen to offset the effects of menopause have at least double the normal risk of developing urinary incontinence.

The findings were based on information gathered over a four-year period from 1,208 women whose average age was 66. The longer the women took hormones, the higher their likelihood of developing bladder problems.

The study's authors do not know why HRT negatively affects bladder control, but a feature the women had in common may point to an explanation: all of them, whether they were on HRT or not, had a history of cardiovascular disease. Oestrogen was once thought to be a preventive treatment for urinary incontinence; it is now regarded as a possible cause.

## Drug development
# A patch calms an overactive bladder – with no side effects

If you put eight British people in a room, one of them, statistically speaking, will have an overactive bladder. For the other seven to understand what that unfortunate person is going through, they would have to remember what it was like to be travelling in the back seat of a car at the age of four desperate to urinate. Or they would need to recall early childhood episodes when they failed to make it to the bathroom in time – and then they would have to imagine the frustration and embarrassment of feeling like that virtually all the time.

Fortunately, a drug called oxybutynin has been available for some 25 years to counteract the various symptoms that come under the heading of 'overactive bladder'. Those symptoms include a persistent urge to urinate, interrupted sleep from frequent nocturnal bathroom visits and, for many, the involuntary release of urine (incontinence).

Taken orally, oxybutynin is very effective at reducing urgency, frequency and incontinence, but its users usually pay a price in side effects – most notably, a dry mouth and constipation. One way or another, they experience discomfort.

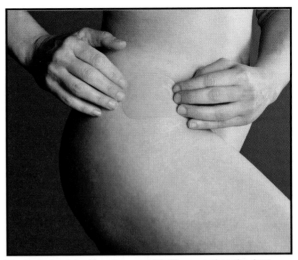

The Oxytrol patch offers the same bladder control as the drug oxybutynin, and works at less than half the dose of the oral drug.

But incontinence sufferers worldwide received good news in February 2003 when the US Food and Drug Administration (FDA) approved a new oxybutynin-releasing skin patch called Oxytrol that calms overactive bladders with no observable side effects. Simply by applying the small, thin, clear patch to their abdomen, hip or buttock, people with overactive bladders – in the USA, an estimated 33 million people – can get relief for up to four days. A study released after approval had been granted showed that the new patch may also clear the way for higher and more effective doses of the drug.

**How it works** Transdermal systems, or skin patches, work by releasing a steady, controlled dose of medication through the skin and directly into the bloodstream. The method has several distinct advantages over drugs taken orally. One advantage is that patients don't need to swallow a medicine. Instead, they simply apply the adhesive patch and forget about it for four days – you can even shower or swim with the patch on – while a steady supply of oxybutynin calms the nerves responsible for urgency-producing bladder contractions.

Another advantage of the oxybutynin patch is that the medication does not have to work its way through your digestive system. Because the liver and gastrointestinal tract are not required to process the oxybutynin, the digestive by-products that cause a dry mouth and constipation are never produced, so there are no troublesome side effects.

**Availability** Oxytrol is available at pharmacies in the USA on prescription only. The patch is not yet available in the UK.

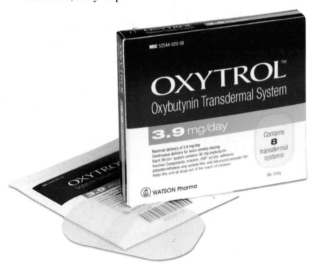

**Drug development**

# Anti-cholesterol drugs may slow the progress of kidney disease

If you have been diagnosed with kidney disease, your overriding aim is to stop the condition from reaching the ominously named 'end stage', when it becomes kidney failure. At that point, the kidneys can no longer eliminate waste from the bloodstream in the form of the urine. The only thing that can keep you alive is regular dialysis, a procedure that takes several hours to filter your blood through a machine. Early detection, dietary restrictions and medications to lower blood pressure and eliminate excess fluid from your body are still the most effective ways to prevent the progression of kidney disease.

But what if there were a class of powerful and readily available drugs that could do more to stop kidney disease from worsening? According to new research, such drugs already exist, and they are called statins. Statins have been one of the great pharmaceutical success stories, helping millions of people worldwide to reduce their risk of heart disease by controlling their cholesterol levels. Results of a study published in the *American Journal of Kidney Disease* in March 2003 suggest that they can also help people with kidney disease.

After a year of giving daily doses of the statin drug Lipitor (atorvastatin) to half of 56 volunteers with kidney disease, researchers from the University of Southern California made two encouraging discoveries. The patients who took Lipitor were excreting a lot less protein in their urine than they had before taking the drug, while the others (who continued to receive standard care without statins) saw little or no change. Because too much protein in the urine is a marker for kidney disease, this is considered a good indication that the Lipitor was helping the kidneys.

The other promising result had to do with a natural waste product called creatinine. Levels of creatinine in the blood rise as kidney function weakens. A standard kidney disease test measures creatinine 'clearance' through the urine – that is, the more creatinine expelled, the less accumulates in the blood. Over the course of the study, creatinine clearance dropped significantly in the patients who did not take Lipitor, while those who did kept about the same clearance levels as when they started.

**How it works** While the results suggest that Lipitor (and probably other statins) can slow down the progress of kidney disease, it is still a mystery how the process works. The study's authors do not believe that the drugs' ability to inhibit liver enzymes involved in the production of cholesterol is a factor.

**Availability** Statins will not be adopted as an treatment for early-stage kidney disease based on this relatively small study and the even smaller studies and animal experiments that preceded it. But the findings clear the way for a larger study to confirm the results.

Key discovery

# Its relaxing effect seems to endow Viagra with twin powers

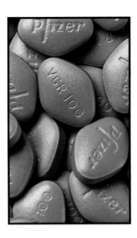

Since its introduction in 1999, Viagra (sildenafil) has helped many men to overcome erectile dysfunction, revitalizing the sex lives of countless couples. Now, British researchers have discovered that those blue pills can solve another common problem.

For older men, urinary difficulties, often caused by an enlarged prostate gland, can turn the simple act of urinating into a frustrating and sometimes painful challenge. And many men with urinary problems also experience erectile dysfunction. It seems that Viagra may alleviate both conditions.

British urologists asked 100 men who complained of erectile dysfunction to fill out questionnaires about their sexual and urinary problems. Researchers used the questionnaires to measure the severity of the subjects' symptoms, then the men were each given a three-month supply of Viagra. After three months of observation and many questionnaires,

the connection between Viagra use and better urinary function was clear. Before the men had begun using Viagra, there was no correlation between the scores for the severity of erectile dysfunction and those for the severity of urinary discomfort, but as the study progressed a link became apparent. Consistently, as the first score improved, so did the second. The researchers could determine that it was the Viagra use itself – not the resulting improvement in the men's ability to achieve erections – that was clearing up the urinary symptoms. And the worse the urinary symptoms at the start of the study, the better the improvement in erectile dysfunction at the end of the three months.

**How it works** In an article published in the December 2002 issue of the *British Journal of Urology*, the authors proposed an explanation for Viagra's twin powers. The drug produces erections not by directly stiffening the penis but by relaxing key genital tissue so that blood can flow into it more easily. While Viagra is present in that part of the body, it may improve urine flow as effectively by relaxing similar tissue lining the urethra.

**Availability** Viagra has been on the market and widely prescribed for several years. The researchers do not recommend that men with urinary symptoms but no erectile problems start using it. They do suggest, however, that taking Viagra makes perfect sense for men who have both.

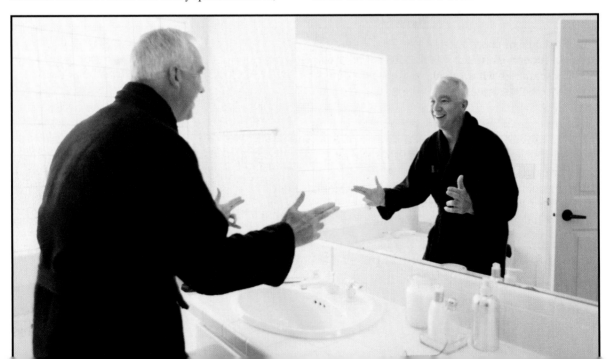

Alternative answers

# Say 'cheese!' – plus yoghurt and fruit juice

Many women who have recurrent bladder infections take advantage of the well-known benefits of cranberry juice. Now new research indicates that regular consumption of any kind of fresh juice, along with a steady diet of cheese and yoghurt, offers protection from urinary tract infections, of which bladder infections (cystitis) are the most common.

Researchers in Finland compared the eating and drinking habits of 139 women with bladder infections with those of 185 women in the same age range who were free of infection. Those who ate fermented milk products – yoghurt and cheese – at least three times a week were more than 75 per cent less likely to have had recent infections, and regular fruit-juice drinkers were more than 33 per cent less likely to have had them. Any berry juice (not just cranberry) that is freshly squeezed or made from a concentrate with no added sugar seems to have the same beneficial effect. (A wide range of juices can now be found at supermarkets and healthfood stores.)

The researchers, whose results were published in the March 2003 issue of the *American Journal of Clinical Nutrition*, suspect that the 'friendly' bacteria in yogurt and cheese make it harder for infection-causing bacteria (usually *E. coli*) to find their way from the rectum up the urethra, the tube that carries urine out of the bladder.

The preventive power of fruit juice may be attributable to concentrated forms of natural chemicals that evolved in plants to protect the plants themselves from infections.

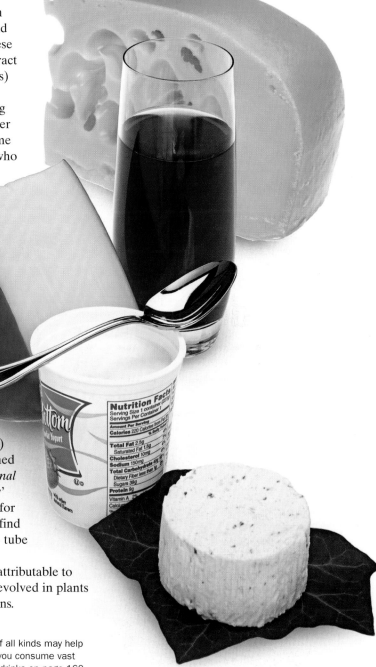

Beyond cranberry juice: yoghurt, cheese and fruit juices of all kinds may help protect against infections of the urinary tract. But before you consume vast quantities of fruit juice, read about a disadvantage of the drinks on page 160.

# Index

**253**

# Credits